ROUTLED(

MW01707812

Volume 12

SYMPTOM-FOCUSED PSYCHIATRIC DRUG THERAPY FOR MANAGED CARE

SYMPTOM-FOCUSED PSYCHIATRIC DRUG THERAPY FOR MANAGED CARE

S. JOSEPH

Routledge
Taylor & Francis Group
LONDON AND NEW YORK

First published in 1997 by The Haworth Medical Press, Inc.

This edition first published in 2019
by Routledge
2 Park Square, Milton Park, Abingdon, Oxon OX14 4RN

and by Routledge
711 Third Avenue, New York, NY 10017

Routledge is an imprint of the Taylor & Francis Group, an informa business

British Library Cataloguing in Publication Data
A catalogue record for this book is available from the British Library

ISBN: 978-1-138-60492-6 (Set)
ISBN: 978-0-429-43807-3 (Set) (ebk)
ISBN: 978-1-138-32444-2 (Volume 12) (hbk)
ISBN: 978-1-138-32458-9 (Volume 12) (pbk)
ISBN: 978-0-429-45085-3 (Volume 12) (ebk)

Publisher's Note
The publisher has gone to great lengths to ensure the quality of this reprint but points out that some imperfections in the original copies may be apparent.

Disclaimer
The publisher has made every effort to trace copyright holders and would welcome correspondence from those they have been unable to trace.

S. Joseph, MD, PhD, MPH

Symptom-Focused Psychiatric Drug Therapy for Managed Care

Pre-publication REVIEW

"This book, written by a gifted and active clinical psychiatrist with expertise in psychopharmacology, provides busy, medically oriented psychiatrists with an up-to-date view of how to use the whole array of psychotropic medications. Dr. Joseph uses his considerable clinical wisdom in psychopharmacology to impart a philosophy of care relevant to the current practice of psychiatry in managed care settings. This is a thoughtful and comprehensive overview of practical clinical psychopharmacology for the busy clinician."

Andrew Brotman, MD
Clinical Professor of Psychiatry,
Harvard Medical School;
Chief of Psychiatry,
Deaconess Hospital,
Boston, Massachusetts

Symptom-Focused Psychiatric Drug Therapy for Managed Care

S. Joseph, MD, PhD, MPH

HMP

The Haworth Medical Press
An Imprint of The Haworth Press, Inc.
New York • London

Published by

The Haworth Medical Press, an imprint of The Haworth Press, Inc., 10 Alice Street, Binghamton, NY 13904-1580

DISCLAIMER
Medicine is an ever-changing science. As new research and clinical experience broaden our knowledge, changes in treatment and drug therapy are required. While many suggestions for drug usages are made herein, the book is intended for educational purposes only, and the author, editor, and publisher do not accept liability in the event of negative consequences incurred as a result of information presented in this book. We do not claim that this information is necessarily accurate by the rigid, scientific standard applied for medical proof, and therefore make no warranty, expressed or implied, with respect to the material herein contained. Therefore the patient is urged to consult his or her own physician prior to following a course of treatment. The physician is urged to check the product information sheet included in the package of each drug he or she plans to administer to be certain the protocol followed is not in conflict with the manufacturer's inserts. When a discrepancy arises between these inserts and information in this book, the physician is encouraged to use his or her best professional judgement.

Cover design by Donna M. Brooks.

Library of Congress Cataloging-in-Publication Data

Joseph, S. (Sonny)
Symptom-focused psychiatric drug therapy for managed care / Sonny Joseph.
p. cm.
Includes bibliographical references and index.
ISBN 0-7890-0194-2 (alk. paper)
1. Mental illness–Chemotherapy. 2. Psychopharmacology. 3. Psychotropic drugs. I. Title.
[DNLM: 1. Psychotropic Drugs–therapeutic use. 2. Mental Disorders–drug therapy. 3. Managed Care Programs. QV 77.2 J83s 1997]
RC483.3.J67 1996
616.89'18–dc20
DNLM/DLC
for Library of Congress

96-26946
CIP

To my beloved parents, my first teachers, for their encouragement and support of my educational endeavors, which at one point seemed endless, and to all the tèachers who continued to encourage and support me. Also to my wife Mary, and our children, Susan, Lisa, and Annie.

Note: The author has attempted to ensure that the drug doses are consistent with standards of modern psychiatric practice. However, psychiatry being a complex science, the individual physician's judgment, based on professional knowledge of the individual patient, determines the dosages and course of treatment for a particular patient. Clinical practice patterns are evolving processes based on new research, clinical experience, and availability of new drugs. The reader should review the latest package insert provided by the manufacturer of the medications mentioned in the book.

CONTENTS

ABOUT THE AUTHOR

S. Joseph, MD, PhD, MPH, is a board-certified psychiatrist and licensed clinical psychologist in Orlando, Florida. He is also certified in Geriatric Psychiatry and Addiction Psychiatry and possesses professional training in clinical hypnosis. He received his Master's degree in Public Health from Harvard University and completed his psychiatric specialization at Thomas Jefferson University Hospital in Philadelphia. Dr. Joseph's educational background spans the North American continent. He completed his medical training at the Universidad de Cuidad Juarez in Mexico, his PhD in clinical psychology at the University of Ottawa in Canada, his clinical clerkship in psychiatry at Massachusetts General Hospital, and part of his public health training at the Massachusetts Institute of Technology. Based on his vast experience as a practitioner of psychiatry and psychology, he believes that medication and psychotherapy are equally important for the optimal psychiatric treatment outcome. His success in managing challenging cases validates this belief. Dr. Joseph is a member of the American Medical Association, the American Psychiatric Association, and the American Psychological Association.

Foreword

Dr. Joseph, a gifted practicing psychiatrist, expert psychopharmacologist, and clinical psychologist, has written a book on the practical, most up-to-date therapeutic approaches on medication treatment for psychiatric ills. Like a cookbook with recipes on "How to Cook," this is a book with recipes on "How to Treat." This book is a gold mine of information! Its treatment regimens will be the gold standard for the treatment of psychiatric disorders. It is a clearly written and easy-to-understand book that allows beginners, more experienced psychiatrists, psychiatric residents, family physicians, and medical students to access information on prescribing medicines for simple and complex psychiatric conditions. For other mental health professionals, this is a book to help you and your patients understand the medications they are taking as an adjunct to therapy.

What is especially interesting and unique is the chapter dealing with special patients such as celebrities, friends, and other doctors. And what really captures interest in that chapter are answers to *patients' questions*, including:

- Do I have a chemical imbalance?
- Can I be tested for a chemical imbalance?
- I don't have depression, I have anxiety. Why are you giving me an antidepressant?
- Why do I need to take a medication when my depression is understandable?
- Does depression run in the family? Will my children get it?
- What is the best medicine for depression? I want the best medicine there is.

The book describes the intelligent use of multiple medication combinations to achieve *rapid symptom resolution* safely and efficiently, a necessity in this managed-care environment. The book closes with 100 psychopharmacological cases that outline the specific medication regimens used for specific illnesses and the rationale for their use.

This book helps you enter the inner sanctum of psychiatry, and lets you exit with the knowledge and expertise of a gilt-edged, sage expert in the field.

E. Michael Gutman, MD
Fellow, American Psychiatric Association;
Past President, Florida Psychiatric Society;
Diplomate, American Board of Forsenic Psychiatry

Preface

This book describes highly practical pharmacological techniques in the uses of simple as well as complex combinations of medications to treat the more common psychiatric disorders among adults. Diagnostic principles and treatment strategies and their nuances are explained in a straightforward and practical manner, along with descriptions of the clinical decision-making process. One hundred clinical cases presented in Part II illustrate the application of the diagnostic and treatment concepts described in Part I. Discussion of diagnostic and treatment principles emphasizes outpatient management techniques to minimize or avoid inpatient psychiatric hospitalization. Clinical ideas, insights, and techniques are discussed throughout the book.

Most texts currently available do not describe practical medication combinations and specific dosing guidelines. This is the specific goal of this text. The emphasis is on a highly practical clinical approach; theoretical considerations and neurochemistry are not dealt with here. The limited discussion of diagnosis is for the purpose of emphasizing practical decision making and for treatment selection. Systematic presentation of diagnoses is available in many fine textbooks as well as in the major diagnostic reference source, the *Diagnostic and Statistical Manual of Mental Disorders*, Fourth Edition. The most commonly encountered diagnoses and specific treatment guidelines are described here. Most of the diagnostic and treatment concepts, especially those of symptom-focused treatment and combination psychopharmacotherapy, are derived from years of busy and extremely successful office and hospital practice experience. This book helps clinicians understand patients' problems from a psychopharmacological perspective that is practical and effective. Varied clinical presentations are reduced to treatable symptoms with specific medication and dosage recommendations so that even physicians who are not experienced with a medication or combination of medications will feel more comfortable in using these interventions.

In Part II, 100 cases are presented from the author's case files. The cases were not chosen at random but specifically chosen to illustrate various diagnostic and treatment issues including the following:

– Rational use of multiple drugs and specific dosing strategies
– Complex diagnostic decision making encountered in actual practice
– Symptom-focused treatment

– Outpatient treatment of severe disorders
– Treatment along the spectrum of simple to complex
– Side effects and their management
– Treatment failures
– Suicide risk
– Successful practice guidelines

Patient identity is disguised to ensure confidentiality. Clinical history, treatment course, medication doses, and treatment outcome are real. Cases were selected to illustrate different principles, but occasional overlap may be present.

The first paragraph of each case briefly describes the presenting complaints and symptoms, along with past psychiatric history, family psychiatric history, and medical history, if relevant. Personal and social history is largely omitted except in several cases where it was thought to have some bearing on diagnosis. This is followed by "Current Diagnosis," which lists one or more diagnoses or symptoms that are the focus of treatment. *DSM-IV* diagnoses are used for the most part, but keep in mind that there are occasions in actual practice when it is not immediately possible to arrive at a formal diagnosis. Unofficial diagnostic terms are therefore occasionally listed to identify clinical problems that need medication treatment. "Current Treatment" lists the patient's most recent medications and dosages.

The second paragraph summarizes the treatment course. Each case concludes with a paragraph titled "Comments," which discusses salient diagnostic and treatment issues or topics that are directly or indirectly related to key issues raised by the case. Most of the comments have a practical clinical focus. On rare occasions, concepts of a controversial or philosophical nature are presented.

The cases should give a "hands-on" feeling to physicians who are interested in learning balanced use of various psychotropic medication combinations. Cases are arbitrarily grouped into three classes:

Simple Cases:	Cases 1-32
Moderately Complex Cases:	Cases 33-66
Complex Cases:	Cases 67-100

The cases may also be classified in the following manner. Most simple cases can be diagnosed and managed by a primary care physician. The majority of the moderately complex cases require the expertise of a psychiatrist for accurate diagnosis and proper management although a primary care physician interested and experienced in psychopharmacologic treatment could manage some of these cases. Virtually all of the complex cases require the expertise of a psychiatrist proficient in psychopharmacology. A variety of diagnoses and medication combinations are presented, from the simple to the most complex. A few of the most highly complex cases presented have proved challenging even to some of the most experienced psychiatrists.

Practical diagnostic and treatment concepts are discussed at a fairly advanced level, assuming some familiarity with psychiatric diagnosis and psychotropic medications on the part of the reader. This book is written primarily for psychiatrists, psychiatric residents, and other physicians; however, various mental health professionals such as clinical psychologists, clinical social workers, psychotherapists, counselors, and psychiatric nurses should find the book educational and instructive. Medical students are likely to find the discussion too clinically advanced for their level of comprehension, although someone considering psychiatric specialization may find it interesting, motivating, and informative. Beginning and experienced clinicians should find the book useful in their daily clinical practice. This book is directed toward the busy practicing clinician, not to the researcher. While the clarity of the material makes it easily accessible, there is the concern that an insufficiently trained person could assume a similar simplicity in diagnosis and treatment of mental illnesses. This book is not intended as a "cook book" for nonphysicians; it is the author's opinion that such use could be dangerous.

Please note that clinical impressions, opinions, and evaluations of medications are primarily based on the author's clinical practice experience and on information gathered from professional sources listed under "Bibliography," and might represent clinical art and wisdom rather than scientifically tested and validated facts. There is no intent that this text should reflect a compilation of published research. For example, the ranking of medications as "best for milder" or "for more severe conditions" is based on clinical judgment and experience. These are examples of choices I would make, given a particular scenario, in order to achieve a positive response as rapidly as possible. There is no medication that is universally good or bad. However, it is a common clinical observation that a particular medication may be generally superior for treating a specific symptom and yet may be inferior in treating another symptom. Similarly, a medication that gave excellent results in one individual may not be tolerated by another individual for the same indication despite a controlled trial showing that the medication is superior to others. Nevertheless, general evaluative statements based on cumulative clinical practice experience are presented for the clinician. The reference list contains the sources that were consulted to compile factual information included in this book.

I am grateful to Anne Carney, MD, for her conscientious review of the manuscript and for the numerous constructive suggestions made; to Pearlene Gardberg, PsyD, for her review of early drafts and for useful comments; to Nancy Janisz, MS, for assisting with the preparation of the manuscript; and to Mary Randall, BSN, RNC, for her technical editorial assistance. I am also grateful to Ruth Gelfand, my office manager, for her efficient management of the practice, which enabled me to devote my attention and efforts to clinical matters and the writing of this book.

S. Joseph
Orlando, Florida

Acknowledgments

I would like to individually thank Bill Cohen, publisher, and all the editors and the production staff at The Haworth Press, including Bill Palmer, Patricia M. Brown, Sandy Jones Sickels, Margaret Tatich, Becky Miller-Baum, Peg Marr, Susan Trzeciak Gibson, Lisa J. Franko, Dawn Krisko, Paula Patton, and Donna M. Brooks. I would also like to thank Dr. Michael Gutman and Dr. Steven Sharfstein for their reviews of the book.

Introduction

When a patient elaborates on his or her presenting problem, the psychologically/psychodynamically oriented clinician conceptualizes the clinical material in terms of conflicts, defenses, patterns, symbolic meanings, and motives; however, a physician with a pharmacological orientation translates the same clinical material into symptoms, and neurotransmitter dynamics.

A physician specializing in psychiatry must have a working knowledge of about 70 primary psychotropic medications and some familiarity with medications prescribed by other physicians, since patients are frequently on nonpsychiatric medications. The psychiatrist should also be able to manage the side effects of the primary psychiatric medications using other medications, which makes psychopharmacological treatment more medically complex than is initially apparent. Many of the psychotropic medications are rather complicated, with problematic multisystem side effects. Examples are clozapine, lithium, valproic acid, carbamazepine, tricyclic antidepressants (TCAs), monoamine oxidase inhibitors (MAOIs), and antipsychotics. Compared to the number of medications typically associated with some of the medical specialties, the number of primary medications with which a psychiatrist has to be thoroughly familiar is significantly greater.

Frequently, for optimal treatment of a psychiatric patient, combinations of psychotropic medications have to be used; hence, a thorough knowledge of a wide variety of medications and medication combinations is required.

Effective psychotherapists reduce the numerous and varied complaints, behaviors, thoughts, and symptoms into a few fundamental conflicts, patterns, or defenses, usually within their particular theoretical framework. Such an approach gives the therapist the ability to better understand the patient and to design an effective intervention without being confused by seemingly disparate symptoms and behaviors described by the patient. Therapy will usually lack direction, purpose, and progress in the absence of understanding the patient's problems in terms of a few fundamental concepts. Similarly, when prescribing a medication, the physician must reduce the patient's behaviors to fundamental symptoms or etiologies that can then be treated. For example, eating disorders, paraphilias, and somatoform disorders frequently have an obsessive-compulsive basis, yet the behaviors and symptoms are so diverse that unless such a reductionistic approach is taken, the physician is likely to be overwhelmed with what would seem like incongruous clinical material.

Obviously, one must be careful not to become oversimplistic; several distinctive symptom complexes that are optimally responsive to different classes of psychotropic medications can coexist. Some behaviors may be understood as antisocial or malingering, for which no effective psychopharmacological intervention is currently available, enabling the physician to so advise the patient and the referral source. If what appears to be an obsessive-compulsive behavior is understood as a manifestation of underlying psychosis, then the choice of medication is an antipsychotic rather than an antiobsessional drug. Suffice it to say that effective psychopharmacological intervention requires a psychopharmacological understanding of the patient's history, complaints, and symptoms, just as effective psychotherapy depends on a psychosocial understanding of the patient's history, presenting symptoms, and complaints. Symptoms vary in severity, and so there is considerable variation in the dose of medication. In general, mild symptoms require only low doses, and severe symptoms require high doses (as illustrated in Figure 1). This general observation is based on clinical experience. For instance, mild psychotic symptoms respond well to a low dose of an antipsychotic while severe psychosis requires a relatively high dose for an adequate response.

It is important for the prescribing physician to know the meaning and exact morphology of symptoms. For example, insomnia could be due to caffeine intake, depression, or psychosis. Besides discovering the etiology, the prescribing physician also has to know the type of insomnia: initial, middle, or terminal. The choice of medication is different for the various etiologies of insomnia, as well as for the three general types of insomnia (as will be discussed later in the text). Similarly, an obsessive-compulsive symptom could be a manifestation of obsessive-compulsive disorder or prodromal phase of schizophrenia.

Considerable clinical judgment is involved in modern clinical psychiatric practice. The recent introduction of selective serotonin reuptake inhibitors (SSRIs), venlafaxine and nefazodone, and new antipsychotics such as clozapine, risperidone, and olanzapine are making psychiatric practice ever more effective, exciting, and challenging. Patient management involves much more than diagnosing patients and prescribing medication. A

FIGURE 1. The Linear Relationship Between the Severity of Symptoms and Medication Dose

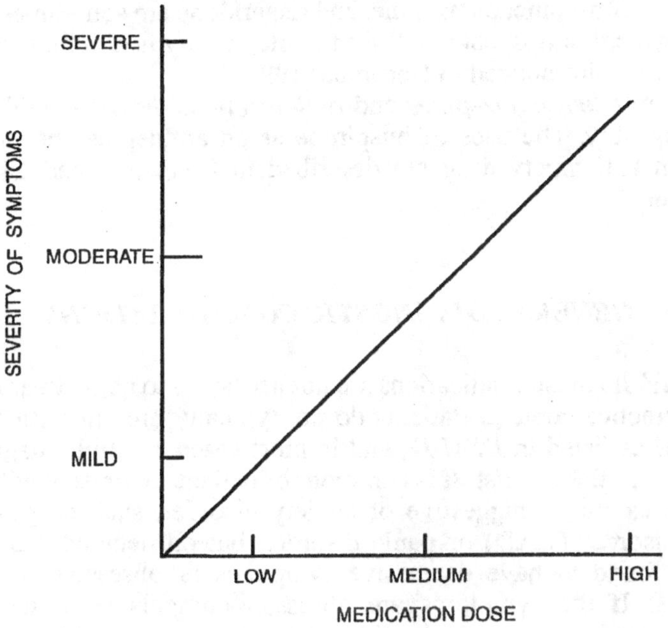

clinician has to form and maintain rapport, medicate appropriately, anticipate resistance and overcome it, diagnose and manage side effects, and motivate the patient to complete the treatment. Psychotherapy, in addition, is universally helpful and should be encouraged by the clinician even if the primary etiology is thought to be biological in nature.

The term *tricyclic antidepressant* (TCA) is loosely used to include both tricyclic (imipramine, desipramine, amitriptyline, nortriptyline, doxepin, clomipramine, trimipramine, and protriptyline) and tetracyclic (maprotiline and amoxapine) groups of drugs. Selective serotonin reuptake inhibitors (SSRIs) include fluoxetine, sertraline, paroxetine, and fluvoxamine, as well as venlafaxine, which is truly an inhibitor of serotonin and norepinephrine reuptake. Nefazodone has multiple actions in the synapse as outlined in Chapter 4. The term *monoamine oxidase inhibitor* (MAOI) is used to include phenelzine and tranylcypromine. The manufacturing of isocarboxazid (Marplan) was discontinued by Roche Laboratories several years ago.

"Traditional" antipsychotics include all currently available antipsychotics except olanzapine, risperidone, and clozapine. They include all phenothiazines, haloperidol, thiothixene, chlorprothixene, loxapine, and molindone. Clozapine, olanzapine, and risperidone are sometimes referred to as "atypical antipsychotics." Sertindole, an atypical antipsychotic, is expected to be introduced in December 1996.

The words *benzodiazepines* and *antianxiety medications* will be used interchangeably. The uses of buspirone as an antidepressant augmentor and as an antianxiety drug are described in Chapter 2 and Chapter 8, respectively.

GENERAL DIAGNOSTIC CONSIDERATIONS

DSM-IV diagnostic indications are not necessary to begin treatment in a clinical practice context. Patients do not typically present with clear-cut symptoms as listed in *DSM-IV*, and in most cases, multiple diagnoses of varying severities coexist. It is common for patients to present with symptoms, for example, suggestive of anxiety disorder, such as generalized anxiety disorder (GAD) or panic disorder, but on detailed examination they are found to have depressive symptoms or obsessive-compulsive symptoms. If the symptoms are obsessive-compulsive in nature, the choice of medication could be limited to clomipramine or serotonergic medications, which could also address both depression and anxiety. It should be noted that obsessive-compulsive disorder primarily is an anxiety disorder in which anxiety is bound to specific obsessions and compulsions. Similarly, it is common for patients with psychosis to present with anxiety and depressive symptoms, and they might even deny any psychotic symptoms on direct interview. Paranoid patients typically will not reveal any of their psychotic symptoms, but will simply report the secondary depression and anxiety. Hence, the psychiatrist must be extremely perceptive and should have the ability to identify subtle symptoms; he or she should have a low threshold for suspecting the presence of more serious underlying problems in patients presenting with anxiety and depression, the common presenting complaints.

The symptoms of anxiety and depression in psychiatry are like "fever" and "pain" in general medicine. It is important for the primary care physician and the mental health professional to explore the presence of underlying problems such as psychosis, manic tendencies, obsessive-compulsive tendencies, and personality disorder in patients complaining of anxiety and/or depression. For example, a psychotic patient with paranoia and hostility can present with depressive symptoms. If this patient is started only on an antidepressant, there is the real risk of the patient becoming even more paranoid. Similarly, it is important to recognize a history of mania, the presence of which deserves careful supervision of an antidepressant treatment and probable prophylactic coverage with an antimanic medication.

Underlying mild psychosis is frequently missed by primary care physicians and even by psychiatrists unless a thorough history and collateral information are obtained. Florid psychosis or severe mania, which are easy to diagnose, do not usually present in the office; therefore, a high level of vigilance is required in an office setting to be able to make the proper primary as well as secondary diagnoses.

Psychiatric diagnosis is a clinical diagnosis, not a laboratory-based diagnosis, at least presently and in the foreseeable future. (The routine ordering or use of dexamethasone suppression test [DST] and thyrotropin-releasing hormone stimulation test [TRHST] for diagnosing depression, psychological tests, and neurophysiological studies should be discouraged.) Of the tests and procedures that are available, psychological tests are the most useful in a clinical setting and only in select cases. Other procedures such as hypnosis and sodium amytal interview are neither reliable nor necessary for diagnostic purposes, and have no significant therapeutic value except perhaps with dissociative disorders.

THE ART OF PSYCHIATRY

Effective psychiatric treatment requires tact; therapeutic alliance; reassurance; perseverance; creative medication strategies; ability to predict, identify, and resolve resistance; persuasion; and a host of other skills subsumed under the general term "art." The author believes that psychiatric management and sustained clinical improvement, to some extent, are dependent on the art of the individual clinician. The more complicated the case and the treatment, the more art is necessary for a successful and lasting outcome. In an individual-practice setting, the attending psychiatrist is personally and directly involved with the patient throughout the treatment course, whereas in a research institution, intermediaries such as research assistants, residents, medical students, technicians–as well as the rigors of the research design–unwittingly interfere with the art of psychiatry. These considerations are important not only in complicated cases but also in less complicated cases, such as simple depression or anxiety disorders. Let me illustrate this idea using a simplified hypothetical case.

Treatment Approach A

A psychiatrist has his or her assistant conduct a thorough evaluation, including psychological testing and various lab studies, including thyroid function tests, dexamethasone suppression test, topographical brain mapping, and a CAT scan. The psychiatrist reviews the voluminous data and makes the correct diagnosis of major depression and obsessive-compulsive disorder, prescribes an SSRI, and asks the patient to return to the office in two weeks. The patient notices partial improvement in symptoms but stops taking the medication after one week because of nausea, fails to keep his or her next appointment, and seeks treatment by another psychiatrist.

Treatment Approach B

Another psychiatrist directly interviews the patient, arrives at the same diagnosis of major depression and obsessive-compulsive disorder, based on the clinical interview, and prescribes the same SSRI as the psychiatrist in Treatment Approach A. However, this psychiatrist explains the diagnosis and reassures the patient by maintaining eye contact during the interview and explaining the common side effects. The patient continues to take the medication despite the initial nausea, which subsides after about eight to ten days, and reports significant improvement in symptoms when seen for the follow-up office visit two weeks later.

In Treatment Approach A, a technically correct diagnosis and proper treatment were identified, but the treatment failed. In Treatment Approach B, the therapeutic alliance automatically formed because of the psychiatrist's personal attention and interest improved the medication compliance. Although the case and the outcomes described above are hypothetical, the phenomenon illustrated by the case is real.

It is a common observation that in the absence of therapeutic alliance, patients find reasons to rationalize their noncompliance, which leads to treatment failure. This is more applicable in a complex specialty such as psychiatry. Thus, one could have the most brilliant psychiatrist correctly diagnose a patient and suggest the best treatment, only to have the treatment fail. Even in the practice of biological psychiatry, bedside manner and therapeutic alliance are extremely important. These concepts are more relevant when managing complicated psychiatric disorders such as bipolar disorder, schizoaffective disorder, or borderline personality disorder. In a controlled-study context, it is often difficult to incorporate the informal and intangible therapeutic processes that can enhance compliance. Moreover, considerable reassurance, persuasion, and determined trials on various adjunctive medications are frequently necessary for eventual success of complicated treatments that use mood stabilizers or clozapine, for example. While large, controlled, double-blind studies are extremely important and valuable in discovering trends, superior outcomes can often be expected with an individual approach that incorporates the artful practice of psychiatry involving clinical judgment, intuition, and individualized treatment, which are essential for a successful clinical practice. Superior technical knowledge and skills are not sufficient for effective psychiatric practice, as opposed to another field of medicine such as radiology or surgery. The relationship with the patient is the foundation on which technical knowledge finds usefulness in the field of psychiatry.

MANAGED CARE AND PSYCHIATRIC PRACTICE–GENERAL CONCEPTS

The application of the concept of managed care has always been present in one form or another in clinical medicine. The patient's finances, insurance, informed consent requirements, and the physician's duty to manage the patient efficiently and economically have, in the past, served the managed care functions in an informal sense. It is unfortunate that clinicians (physicians included) as well as numerous for-profit treatment centers have abused the generous limits of insurance companies in the past by overutilization of services. Years of this abuse resulted in the need for closer scrutiny and tighter limits on the medical treatment process. In the field of psychiatry, which is the familiar specialty to me, there has been considerable overutilization of services, particularly in the area of psychiatric hospitalization. One major culprit responsible for the overutilization is the profit pressures that naturally emerge when services are provided strictly as a business (for profit), as occurred with the proliferation of for-profit institutions in the 1980s. Psychiatrists, being human, were not immune to the temptation induced by such liberal limits. For-profit psychiatric institutions, and to some extent not-for-profit institutions as well, had to have the cooperation of psychiatrists to further the for-profit operations. There is no doubt that institutions and individual psychiatrists became rich in the process. The resulting formalized managed care became a virtual necessity, not only to restrict overutilization, which is a desirable goal, but also to shift the profit to insurance companies.

Hospitals and insurance companies are business entities that operate for the ultimate goal of earning the maximum profit. Some physicians also operate with the singular motive of profit. A strong profit motive tends to lead to overutilization. It is sufficient to say that managed care was inevitable in the face of overutilization.

What is wrong with insurance companies wanting to retain some of the profits? Fundamentally, businesses exist for profit. The higher the profit, the better. Ideally, the best business is the business that provides the least goods or services while earning the maximum profit. Like most things in life, the ideal rarely exists in the pure form. The point is: the provision of services or goods is a necessary evil that must be curtailed as much as legally and ethically possible in order to further the business interests. When health care was permitted to evolve into a business, it should not have been surprising that the full spectrum of business practices would come into play. A high percentage of physicians do not approach their medical fields as businessmen. It has to do with why most physicians chose medicine as their career. If you ask an individual why he or she wanted to become a doctor, the usual replies are, "I wanted to help people," "I wanted to cure illnesses," or "I liked the idea of helping people get well." Few will say that the primary goal of choosing medicine as a career was to make money. In fact, to highlight profit as a motive is considered offensive, although I suspect that this may be changing. On the other hand, if you ask a health insurance company president or executive why he or she chose the health insurance field, the answer is likely to be something like "It is a good business," "It is a growing field," or "There are lots of opportunities," meaning there is an opportunity to make money. It is important to understand the basic attitudinal difference between direct health care providers, including doctors, nurses, and other health care professionals, and the third-party payers, whose legitimate business goal must be to pay the least so that the business is maximally profitable. In a business environment, this attitude is not only desirable, but also necessary.

Although most physicians enter the medical profession primarily because of its service appeal, there are many opportunities for temptation and greed to prevail, and the profit motive can sometimes become primary. Physicians must always remain responsive to the patient's needs and look after the patient's medical interests. If they do not vigorously pursue this goal, others will step in to fill the need, just as social service agencies or prosecuting attorneys have come to the aid of children neglected or exploited by parents. Underutilization can result in suboptimal patient care with great potential for harm to the patient, as well as poorly quantifiable additional expenses such as costs associated with patients presenting with advanced disease, contracting diseases due to lack of preventive care, suboptimal quality of life, lack of productivity, and burden to society and family. Overutilization of services can escalate the cost of health care to the extent that many people would not be able to afford it. Needless to say, both are to be avoided. The ideal goal of managed care is to foster appropriate and needed medical services by "managing" or controlling overutilization.

Driven by pure business motives, numerous insurance companies–HMOs and PPOs included–could be irresistibly tempted to increase profits by refusing to authorize needed services. The stigma of mental illness, the impaired cognitive abilities, lack of motivation, and the diminished functional capacity present among many patients suffering from emotional disorders make them less likely, compared to nonpsychiatric patients, to take initiative for asserting their right to receive appropriate treatment, or to complain about or appeal denial of needed services. Opportunistic politicians and shrewd third-party payers are well aware of this, making the mental health field a wide-open area for exploitation by cutting funding for mental health services (in the case of a politician), denying needed services, placing excessive procedural requirements so that the emotionally disordered patients have difficulty following or severely limiting access to care, with considerable impunity. Employer-driven benefit programs, including health benefits, are understandably driven primarily by the ultimate motive of profit. Employee welfare is one of many intangible factors that, in the long term, could benefit the employer by making the employee maximally functional so the employee will be capable of and motivated for working for the employer. However, employee benefits programs cost money for the employer. When employee turnover rate is high, as is true with many low- and medium-paying jobs, there is less incentive for the employer to provide benefits to employees with no prospects for any return on the money expended. Therefore, it is unrealistic to expect that most employers will consistently be motivated to provide any more benefits than what are the absolute minimum required by law or industry ethics. We cannot expect the employer to assume a parental or protective role toward the employees. Neither can we expect a truly caring and patient advocacy role from the insurance company because both businesses and insurance companies function essentially for generating profit. Therefore, it is up to clinicians, patients' families, and social service agencies to advocate for patient health benefits and provision of adequate services despite the risk of being unfairly perceived as self-serving. If the physician is not ultimately a patient advocate, then who will be?

At the same time, the insurance relationship is between the patient and the insurance company, not between the physician and the insurance company. Even in cases in which a physician is directly employed in a clinical capacity by an insurance company, the physician is paid to care for the patient. Savvy insurance companies recognize that physicians are prone to appropriate the maximum resources for their patients, and so have been known to provide incentives to the physician to *not* provide every needed service to the patient. A capitation-based arrangement is an example of one such incentive. In effect, the physician is acting like an insurance company in such an arrangement. This is a conflictual role at best, and at its worst is quite dangerous.

Managed care strives to deliver appropriate and needed medical services in the most efficient and economical manner–an admirable goal with which few would take issue. In fact, physicians should always have this goal regardless of whether or not care is managed by a third party. The diagnostic and treatment techniques described in this text are consistent with this managed care goal. The treatment techniques afford the physician a means to treat the patient in the most efficient and economical manner, without overutilization. Perhaps this point needs repeated emphasis: economical does not necessarily mean least expensive. It means the treatment that enables the patients to function at their highest potential with a minimum of side effects or complications. Some of the most commonly used medications are the least expensive, while others are very costly. For example, among benzodiazepines, the author prefers lorazepam because of its versatility (by mouth [po], intramuscular [IM], and intravenous [IV] use, and lack of active metabolites) and low cost (due to generic form). However, among antipsychotics, olanzapine and risperidone are preferred, despite their expense, because of their favorable side-effect profiles, including low tardive dyskinesia risk. Among antidepressants, the serotonergic antidepressants are generally preferred to tricyclics. Refer to Table 1 for a list of prices of various commonly used psychotropic medications.

Some insurance companies manage the expense by generating a drug formulary that is limited to inexpensive drugs. In relevant cases, the physician should inform the patient of the availability of other more desirable drug options that are not in the formulary and let the patient make the decision whether or not to choose the medication from the formulary (which may not incur any out-of-pocket expense for the patient) or to go out of the formulary, thereby incurring additional out-of-pocket expenses. Remember, the fundamental concept is that the insurance contract is between the patient and the insurance company, not between the physician and the insurance company. Applying this principle to this context reveals that the drug formulary is an arm of the insurance company. Hence, if the

TABLE 1. Prices of Various Psychotropic Medications

Drug Name	Dose		Number of Pills per Month	Approximate Price in U.S. $ as of 8/95
fluoxetine (Prozac)	10 mg	HS	30	60
fluoxetine (Prozac)	20 mg	BID	60	105
sertraline (Zoloft)	100 mg	AM	30	60
paroxetine (Paxil)	30 mg	AM	30	58
venlafaxine (Effexor)	100 mg	BID	60	58
fluvoxamine (Luvox)	100 mg	BID	60	105
nefazodone (Serzone)	200 mg	BID	60	48
mirtazapine (Remeron)	30 mg	HS	30	60
clomipramine (Anafranil)	50 mg	TID	90	96
clomipramine (Anafranil)	75 mg	BID	60	85
bupropion (Wellbutrin)	100 mg	TID	90	73
bupropion SR (Wellbutrin SR)	150 mg	BID	60	79
bupropion SR (Wellbutrin SR)	100 mg	QID	120	153
imipramine (Tofranil)	50 mg	TID	90	12
divalproex sodium (Depakote sprinkle)	125 mg	TID	180	55
divalproex sodium (Depakote)	250 mg	TID	90	55
divalproex sodium (Depakote)	500 mg	BID	60	65
carbamazepine (Tegretol)	200 mg	BID	60	12
gabapentin (Neurontin)	400 mg	TID	90	100
lamotrigine (Lamictal)	100 mg	BID	60	105
lithium (Eskalith CR)	450 mg	BID	60	26
lithium (Lithobid)	300 mg	TID	90	26
lithium carbonate	300 mg	TID	90	10
doxepin (Sinequan)	10 mg	HS	30	7
amitriptyline (Elavil)	10 mg	HS	30	5
risperidone (Risperdal)	1 mg	HS	30	60
risperidone (Risperdal)	2 mg	HS	30	95
risperidone (Risperdal)	3 mg	HS	30	119
risperidone (Risperdal)	4 mg	HS	30	158
olanzapine (Zyprexa)	5 mg	HS	30	150
olanzapine (Zyprexa)	7.5 mg	HS	30	150
olanzapine (Zyprexa)	10 mg	HS	30	220
haloperidol (Haldol)	5 mg	HS	30	8
clozapine (clorazil)	25 mg		30	44
clozapine (clorazil)	100 mg		30	103
zolpidem (Ambien)	10 mg		30	50
estazolam (Prosom)	2 mg		30	50
lorazepam (Ativan)	1 mg		30	50
temazepam (Restoril)	15 mg		30	7
naltrexone (Revia, Trexan)	50 mg		30	148
selegiline (Eldepryl)	5 mg	BID	60	130

Note: The dosages of all antidepressants (except doxepin 10 mg, amitriptyline 10 mg, and fluoxetine 10 mg) are at the medium dosage range and are fairly comparable. For example, fluoxetine 40 mg (two 20 mg capsules) is fairly comparable to sertraline 100 mg one tablet per day. Such an estimation is necessary for meaningful cost comparison.

patient's choices are limited due to restrictions imposed by the insurance company, that is an issue between the patient and the insurance company. Having informed the patient of the availability of drugs that are more desirable outside the formulary, the physician should, of course, offer to choose the best medication among the formulary drugs for the individual patient.

The approach taken in this text is efficient, effective, and economical diagnosis and management of the psychiatric patient. This approach necessitates outpatient treatment whenever possible, rapid treatment strategies, and a careful, balanced, and rational combination of medications for comprehensive and aggressive management when more than one medication is indicated. My approach does not endorse using the cheapest medication unless it is the most effective medication. However, it does recommend choosing the most effective medication for the particular patient.

As illustrated in this text and the clinical cases, nearly all psychiatric medications currently available have been found effective for one or more patients. There is no *one* medication that is good for everybody or bad for everybody. Medication tolerance and effectiveness are highly individual matters. Patients with identical diagnoses can have different symptom profiles and may need different medications or combinations of medications. On the other hand, patients with different diagnoses can respond well to the same medication. These issues are described in the text along with clinical examples.

Managed care is

- efficient diagnosis and treatment,
- effective treatment (to the greatest extent possible),
- cost-effective treatment,
- avoidance of overutilization, and
- emphasis on primary and secondary prevention.

Managed care is not

- underutilization (suboptimal treatment),
- stalling or avoidance strategies (even if legally valid),
- prescribing the cheapest medications rather than the most effective medications (unless the most effective medication happens to be the cheapest),
- management using underqualified staff, or
- undertreatment.

Responsible managed care organizations do not deliberately engage in the practices noted in the latter list. However, since managed care is an evolving area, it remains a fertile field for unscrupulous companies to make a quick profit–especially when new managed care companies are being formed almost every week.

The diagnostic and treatment techniques and the 100 clinical cases described in this book are consistent with the author's understanding of what managed care is and should be, as listed above. Essentially, it is smart medicine. The concept of managed care brings into better focus the need for efficient and economical diagnosis and treatment. The numerous clinical case studies reinforce the success of using this methodology with regard to these foci of managed care systems.

RATIONAL POLYPHARMACY: THE MEDICAL MODEL AND EVOLUTION IN PSYCHIATRIC DRUG THERAPY

Polypharmacy carries the negative connotation of involving too many drugs, conflicting drugs, and a lack of physician care and attention to the complete drug list because multiple specialists are together prescribing a mishmash of medications with toxic potential. More precisely, however, the word polypharmacy in its pristine form means "multiple drugs." While the negative connotation indicates too many, the more correct definition, as adhered to in this text, should have a positive connotation of only as many drugs as necessary, each for a specific target symptom, each evaluated individually for efficacy and side effects and adjusted optimally, with the elimination of each one that is no longer necessary. The phrase *rational polypharmacy* might be semantically more relevant in this context.

Polypharmacy is the rule in most medical specialties. Generally, the ideal management objective is to employ the least number of medications needed to achieve optimal improvement. In some cases, one medication may effectively address multiple symptoms, whereas in other cases, multiple medications are necessary for optimal symptom control. In the former case, a patient with three or four distinct and disparate symptoms can be treated with one medication, whereas in the latter case, a person with three or four different symptoms may need three or four medications from different classes, depending on the specific symptoms. In rare instances, multiple medications may be necessary for the optimal control of one symptom. The following simplified hypothetical examples will illustrate this point.

1. A healthy 30-year-old patient presents with depressed mood, obsessive rumination of the fear of dying of cancer, mild compulsive cleaning behavior, anxiety attacks, and anger outbursts. In this example, there are four different target symptoms:

1. Depressed mood
2. Obsessive-compulsive features
3. Anxiety
4. Anger

All of the above symptoms might effectively be treated with one medication, for instance with one of the serotonergic antidepressants* such as fluoxetine, sertraline, paroxetine, venlafaxine, mirtazapine, and fluvoxamine, or with clomipramine, or with one of the tricyclic antidepressants (TCAs) or monoaxmine oxidase inhibitors (MAOIs). The author prefers a first trial on serotonergic antidepressants (SSRIs), then clomipramine, then TCAs, and lastly MAOIs, primarily because of the benign side effect profile of SSRIs. The ideal goal is to treat the symptoms using one medication. This is quite possible if the symptoms are as listed above. However, such economy is not always possible, as will be seen in the next hypothetical case example.

2. A healthy 30-year-old patient presents with symptoms such as depressed mood, frequent nightmares causing sleep disruption, paranoid ideation, and significant mood swings. The four different target symptoms are listed below:

1. Depressed mood
2. Nightmares
3. Paranoid ideation
4. Mood swings

This patient also has four different symptom foci. However, adequate resolution of these four symptoms could require the use of medications from four different classes as follows:

---

*The term "serotonergic antidepressants" is used loosely in this context to include all of the new generation antidepressants such as fluoxetine, sertraline, paroxetine, venlafaxine, fluvoxamine, and mirtazapine. Venlafaxine and mirtazapine have both serotonergic and noradrenergic effects.

Symptom	Medication Options
Depression	antidepressant, preferably an SSRI
Nightmares	benzodiazepine at bedtime, or low dose of a TCA at bedtime
Paranoia	low dose of an antipsychotic
Clinically-significant mood swings	mood stabilizer

3. A healthy 30-year-old patient presents with hostility. The only target symptom is hostility. This patient could require medications from different classes for the best outcome.

Symptom	Medications
Hostility	SSRI and antipsychotics at low doses (risperidone and olanzapine preferred due to favorable side effect profile)

The key concept is global improvement via symptom control, through treatment with effective medication for each symptom identified. The patients' complaints are translated into individual symptoms (no matter how many there might be), which are then targeted for treatment; progress is then followed in an organized and disciplined manner. Drugs that are not effective are eliminated, and drugs that become unnecessary over time are reduced or discontinued. Conversely, a symptom that improves partially may respond to increasing drug doses or addition of other medications as dictated by the clinical problem.

Unfortunately, when dealing with psychiatric problems, many excellent physicians do not think in the same clinically precise manner that they would employ if they were treating a nonpsychiatric illness. Again, a medical example illustrates this idea: a 42-year-old patient presents with symptoms of clear rhinorrhea, dyspnea upon exertion, postprandial bloating, premenstrual cramps, low backache, productive cough, and heartburn. Exam findings are those of a blood pressure of 175/102 and are otherwise consistent with benign etiologies for all of the above complaints. Additional history is a five-year history of borderline hypertension, a family history of essential hypertension, and a cyclic history of seasonal allergies, frequently with reactive airways. The diagnoses then are seasonal allergies with rhinorrhea, allergic asthma, probable lactose intolerance, essential hypertension, premenstrual syndrome, lumbar strain, bronchitis, and gastritis/reflux esophagitis. The primary care physician will have no hesitation in considering several medications from different classes:

Symptom/Diagnosis	Medication
Rhinorrhea	antihistamines, decongestants
Asthma	bronchodilators, steroids
Essential hypertension	diuretics, beta-blockers (both undesirable with asthma), calcium channel blockers, ACE inhibitors, alpha-2 agonists, peripheral vasodilators, etc. (and physical measures)
Lactose intolerance	lactase
Premenstrual cramps	nonsteroidal anti-inflammatory, oral contraceptive, aspirin, acetaminophen
Lumbar strain	nonsteroidal anti-inflammatory
Bronchitis	antibiotics
Gastritis/reflux esophagitis	H2 blockers, omeprazole, antacids

While this comparison between medical and psychiatric approaches has its limits (psychiatrists do not generally search for occult diseases as rigorously as medical practitioners look for cancers, for example), it does reinforce the point that when it comes to nonpsychiatric problems, physicians have no difficulty organizing the symptoms and prescribing a medication for each specific target symptom. Returning to the hypothetical case, this patient could be prescribed eight different medications for eight different problems. Fewer than eight medications could be considered suboptimal treatment. Some combinations of medications might be contraindicated, or in another circumstance one medication will serve for two or more symptoms. It is not at all uncommon to see a medical patient taking three, four, ten, or even more medications from different pharmacologic classes. As in psychiatry, this entire list of medications is not permanent, with medication for acute symptoms being eliminated as soon as the patient's condition allows, and with antihypertensives more likely to be a lifelong necessity. Physicians tend to think clearly, logically, and specifically when dealing with nonpsychiatric symptoms. The time has come in psychiatry for psychiatric specialists as well as primary care physicians to apply this same clinical precision on a more general scale (i.e., to use it in the management of psychiatric problems). Polypharmacy may be necessary for the optimal treatment of many psychiatric patients–particularly in recent years, when more and more new psychiatric medications with specific indications and effects have become available and when psychiatry is attempting to strengthen its identity primarily as a medical specialty. Some years ago, when there were only three or four classes of psychiatric medications available (each with many common side effects), and when medication effects were less specific, concurrent use of more than one class of medication was likely to lead to adverse effects. Examples are TCAs and traditional antipsychotics. Improved specificity of the main effects of the newer medications in the context of symptom-focused drug therapy enables precise titration of multiple medications to efficiently and expeditiously treat various symptoms or clusters of symptoms. An analogous scenario existed in the specialty of medical oncology many years ago, when most of the available cytotoxic drugs had broad spectrum effects and less specificity, which made it unnecessary and even dangerous to use more than one cytotoxic drug at a time. Cancer chemotherapy has now evolved to the point that combination drug treatment is the norm primarily due to the development of newer drugs that have more specific and limited actions during particular stages of the cell cycle and on targeted cell lines, thereby giving more control to the treating oncologist and resulting in more effective response with less unwanted effects. Although in symptom-focused psychiatric drug therapy, multiple medications are employed to treat fairly heterogenous symptoms, combination chemotherapy as a concept is still appropriate for modern psychiatric practice. Since "chemotherapy" has an oncologic connotation, the phrase "rational polypharmacy" might be more suitable for describing the use of multiple medications to treat psychiatric disorders by deliberately focusing on their constituent symptoms.

Even in psychotherapy, multiple therapeutic techniques ranging from supportive and cognitive-behavioral to psychodynamic are employed by a skilled therapist within a single session. Frequently these techniques are integrated to such an extent that for the experienced therapist, the multimodal interventions would come to mind spontaneously and naturally. Multiple pharmacological interventions can also be similarly orchestrated by the physician to provide optimal benefit to the patient.

A simplified hypothetical case will illustrate the application of the concept of rational polypharmacy in psychiatry. An individual presents to the office with depression characterized by depressed mood, insomnia, and loss of appetite. The patient also complains of heartburn.

Before 1990, a reasonable first-line medication choice for this patient would be one of the tertiary amine TCAs. For the sake of discussion, let me choose doxepin, which has antidepressant, sedating, appetite-stimulating, and H2-blocking properties–ideal target effects for this patient. However, the physician cannot increase the antidepressant effect by increasing the dose without also increasing the sedating effects. Moreover, other typical TCA side effects such as anticholinergic and cardiovascular effects could further limit the dosage escalation. In a sense, doxepin comes as a "package" with a broad spectrum of actions in the synapse. The physician cannot independently increase or decrease specific receptor antagonist or agonist actions to achieve a desired pharmacological outcome, whereas adjusting the total dose proportionally affects the whole spectrum of main effects and side effects. Now let me suggest several modern medication options that enable the physician to independently vary the doses of medications to achieve an optimal balance of desired main effects for a particular patient while minimizing the side effects.

In order to illustrate the concept of symptom-focused approach for teaching purposes, the following treatment options are presented, again using the same simplified hypothetical case. The term SSRI is used in a generic sense in this context to include all of the new generation antidepressants that have selective and specific actions on the synapse (such as SSRIs, venlafaxine, mirtazapine, bupropion, and nefazodone).

Option #1

Target Symptoms	Medication Options
Depressed mood	Any of the SSRIs
Insomnia	Low dose of a sedating TCA
Anorexia	Low dose of a TCA
Dyspepsia	Doxepin or amitriptyline which have H2 blocking properties

In option #1, insomnia, anorexia, and dyspepsia can all be improved with the use of a low dose of a TCA such as doxepin 10 to 25 mg HS, amitriptyline 10 to 25 mg HS, or trimipramine 25 to 50 mg HS. The dose of the SSRI and the TCA can be independently adjusted to obtain optimal effects.

Option #2

Target Symptoms	Medication Options
Depressed mood	Any of the SSRIs
Insomnia	Any of the hypnotics
Anorexia	Low dose of a secondary amine TCA
Dyspepsia	H2 receptor antagonist or antacids

In option #2, the physician has even better control of the pharmacological effects because each of the four medication doses can be precisely titrated to provide the optimal pharmacological action a particular patient needs.

Option #3

Target Symptoms	Medication Options
Depressed mood	Any of the SSRIs
Insomnia	Any of the hypnotics
(Anorexia)	No treatment
Dyspepsia	H2 receptor antagonist or antacids

In option #3, anorexia, which is a symptom of depression, is exploited by deliberately not treating it to achieve a desirable goal (for obese patients).

Option #4

Target Symptoms	Medication Options
Depressed mood	Any of the sedating TCAs
Insomnia	Any of the sedating TCAs
Anorexia	Any of the sedating TCAs
Dyspepsia	Any of the sedating TCAs

In option #4, the choice of a TCA such as doxepin at the full therapeutic dosage range (e.g., doxepin 100 to 250 mg daily) might still be ideal for an occasional patient.

Option #5

Target Symptoms	Medication Options
Depressed mood	Any of the stimulating antidepressants (bupropion or stimulating SSRIs)
Insomnia	Low-dose sedating TCAs or hypnotics
Anorexia	Low-dose sedating TCAs
Dyspepsia	Low-dose sedating TCAs, H2 blockers, or antacids

Numerous variations of medication options and dosages are possible depending on the particular characteristics of the target symptoms and the relative "weights" assigned to each of the symptoms. For example, antidepressants differ in their energizing and anxiolytic properties, making some of them more or less effective for different types of depression. Hypnotic medication choice is dependent on the specific type of insomnia: initial, middle, or terminal insomnia. Again, the dosage of the hypnotic can also vary based on the severity of insomnia. Anorexia may be left untreated in the case of an obese patient. If anorexia needs to be treated, any one of the TCAs may be chosen, with the particular side effect profile of the TCA influencing the choice. On the other hand, anorexia might improve spontaneously when depression responds to the antidepressant treatment, and therefore may not need targeted treatment. Dyspepsia can be treated using H2 receptor antagonists, antacids, or by modifying diet, depending on the severity. As is obvious by now, even for a simplified case as presented here, there is a multitude of treatment variations to suit individual needs. The treatment options and variations are countless for a complicated problem such as schizoaffective disorder, bipolar disorder, or borderline personality disorder. Numerous medication combinations and subtle variations are discussed throughout this text and in the case studies. The need for mastery of complicated medication interventions involving combination drug treatment and the need to secure compliance and cooperation from patients who are often ambivalent towards psychiatric treatment, makes psychiatry an enormously complicated, challenging, and exciting field.

Virtually all exacerbations and emotional "breakdowns" are precipitated by one or more psychosocial stressors. It is also important to be aware of the fact that emotional disorders can precipitate psychosocial disequilibrium. Therefore, whether or not psychosocial stressors precipitate or are precipitated by emotional disorders, psychotherapy is frequently necessary along with pharmacotherapy for optimal outcome. The fact that an emotional breakdown can be entirely attributable to psychosocial stressors does not imply that psychopharmacological interventions are unnecessary. Alluding again to a medical example, although poor hygiene may have precipitated an infection, once the infection becomes symptomatic, treatment consisting of good hygiene practices alone is not sufficient. Pharmacologic treatment using antipyretics and anibiotics is necessary along with good hygiene. Similarly, once the patient becomes psychiatrically symptomatic, the most efficient and effective treatment involves both medications and psychotherapy. A psychosocial and psychodynamic explanation is found or should be sought for abnormal mental phenomena so that the patient's illness is understood from a biopsychosocial perspective. The advantage of this comprehensive approach is that optimal interventions from all relevant modalities can be provided to the patient, maximizing the chances of a complete recovery.

Modern psychiatric practice will soon demand of the contemporary psychiatrist a sophisticated and integrated psychopharmacological approach grounded in fundamental psychodynamically based clinical skills. A symptom-focused approach and balanced, intelligent, and rational polypharmacy as outlined in this text should aid the practicing physician to evolve into an even more effective and efficient clinician and to maximally utilize the full range of psychotropic medication options available, both old and new. Inevitable and desirable evolution in psychiatric drug therapy has made it possible to practice rational polypharmacy, which every modern psychiatrist must learn in order to provide patients with the best care possible in an era of psychopharmacological revolution.

PART I: DIAGNOSTIC AND TREATMENT CONCEPTS

Chapter 1

Depression: Practical Diagnostic and Management Guidelines

DEPRESSION: GENERAL CONSIDERATIONS

Depressive symptoms, if interfering with one's functioning, should be treated regardless of the cause. Treatment requires evaluation of the symptoms in terms of their characteristics, severity, duration, and etiology. Depression and other psychiatric syndromes can be related to a number of factors.

Case in point, most medical conditions can cause depression. Certain medical conditions such as hypothyroidism, cerebrovascular accident, and Parkinson's disease frequently lead to depression. Other medical conditions such as chronic pain and diabetes can lead to increased frustration and stress, thereby precipitating depression. If the medical condition that is etiologically related to depression can be diagnosed and treated, depression is usually resolved. For example, thyroid supplements can reinstate euthyroid status and if hypothyroidism caused the depression, there should be resolution of depression with thyroid replacement. However, if a cerebrovascular accident causes depression, the treatment of depression must be symptomatic, using an antidepressant, since the cerebrovascular accident cannot be reversed.

There are many medical conditions that in varying degrees cause depression, or worsen depression. In many cases, treatment of the underlying medical problem may not lead to complete regression of the depressive symptoms. In some instances, medical treatment may cause the depression. Examples are cancer chemotherapy, some antihypertensives, and steroid treatment. In these latter cases, symptomatic treatment using antidepressants is usually necessary for optimal outcome.

In most cases, the chances are slim that an undiagnosed medical condition presents with depression, without other physical symptoms, signs, or complaints. For example, a brain tumor can present with depression; however, such a tumor frequently is accompanied by neurological symptoms or signs as well. The probability that a brain tumor will present with depression as the only symptom is remote except with frontal lobe tumors in rare cases. Nevertheless, there are probably cases reported where depression was the presenting symptom of a brain tumor. Does this necessitate obtaining a CT scan or MRI of the brain of every patient who presents with depression? The answer is an unequivocal no. However, physicians should be vigilant as to the existence of possible medical etiologies for various psychiatric symptoms by obtaining a thorough history, physical examination if indicated by the history, and laboratory studies, if needed, dictated by findings, if any, in the medical history, physical examination (if already done), and psychiatric symptoms. Endocrine, neurological, infectious, cardiovascular, rheumatological, gastrointestinal, reproductive, hematological, pulmonary and renal disorders, and nutritional deficiencies can cause or exacerbate depression. Hence underlying medical conditions, if amenable, should be treated for optimal psychiatric outcome. As mentioned earlier, in some cases diagnosis and treatment of the medical condition will correct the problem, but in most cases concomitant treatment of depression is necessary. Very frequently it is impossible to confirm whether or not a particular medical disorder is primary in causing depression. Any medical illness is a stress that can psychologically precipitate depression. Conversely, endogenous and reactive depression can stress the organ systems, causing physical symptoms, although the etiology is difficult to confirm and the precise mechanism is poorly understood.

It should be emphasized that as in other medical specialties, physical examination and laboratory studies should be guided by medical history. For example, if a patient complains of dizziness, vital signs including orthostatic blood pressure should be obtained. However, if a patient is seen in the office for depression with no medical complaints, a physical examination is usually not necessary. In a healthy patient with no medical complaints, the yield from routine physical examination and laboratory studies as they relate to the patient's presenting psychiatric complaints is very low in an office practice context. However, the psychiatrist should not hesitate to conduct a focused physical examination and laboratory investigation if the patient's history indicates the need because psychiatrists, by virtue of their primary medical training and qualification as physicians, are expected to continue to exercise basic medical judgment.

However, a thyroid profile is commonly obtained as part of the initial evaluation of patients with depression and anxiety. Even when thyroid abnormalities are discovered, treatment of the thyroid abnormality is frequently not sufficient to completely ameliorate the patients' presenting psychiatric complaints and symptoms. Psychiatric intervention is eventually needed in most of these cases for optimal resolution of their psychiatric problems. However, identification and correction of the thyroid abnormality paves the way for improved response to psychiatric intervention. Therefore, routine thyroid screening using the widely available and fairly inexpensive thyroid stimulating hormone (TSH) level is justified, particularly in females and in the elderly, in whom thyroid abnormalities tend to be relatively more common.

In some of the psychiatric inpatient and outpatient programs, a wide variety of laboratory studies including EEG and brain CT/MRI scans are obtained as part of the routine admission workup, regardless of the presenting complaints and without regard to the cost involved. Some psychiatrists obtain computerized topographic mapping of the EEG, dexamethasone suppression test, etc., fairly routinely. These tests are costly, represent overutilization in most cases, and do not provide essential and valid clinical information in most cases.

This is not to imply that laboratory studies are not to be obtained. There are valid reasons to obtain laboratory studies in many circumstances:

- Medical history and physical exam may point to the need for specific tests.
- Various baseline laboratory studies are useful and necessary prior to starting different medications such as carbamazepine (Tegretol), valproic acid (Depakene, Depakote), lithium, disulfiram (Antabuse), etc. Mandatory baseline laboratory tests are required prior to clozapine (Clozaril) administration.
- Periodic blood level monitoring and other laboratory tests are necessary for proper patient management involving various medications as listed above, including clozapine, which requires a weekly WBC.
- The elderly and the medically ill tend to have occult physical problems which may dictate the need for a greater reliance on a variety of laboratory screening tests.

The appropriate function of a physician is to use discretion based on clinical judgment and the clinical needs of individual patients. If indeterminate testing involving a large battery of tests is conducted routinely without relevant clinical justification and without regard to individual needs, clinical judgment is supplanted, paving the way for inaccurate or invalid conclusions. A medical technician could very well supervise such a task. Laboratory testing or procedures without clinical indication suggest inappropriate utilization of services, invariably driving up the cost of mental health care. For the most part, patients admitted to medical wards are tested on a more focused basis, whereas for some reason, patients admitted to most psychiatric units are tested indiscriminately. This is true even for patients who are repeatedly admitted and whose diagnosis is not in question. This observation is based on the author's experience of working in various inpatient psychiatric units in several major cities in the United States.

In addition to medical etiology, another important and common causative agent of depression is prescription medications, including antianxiety medication and antihypertensives. In many instances, substitution of medications is not possible, requiring treatment of depression using antidepressants. Most systemic medications listed in the *Physicians' Desk Reference (PDR)* can cause depression and anxiety; hence, it is not always practical to avoid medications for which depression and anxiety are listed in the *PDR* as side effects.

It is a commonly held belief that propranolol (Inderal) causes depression. In the several cases the author can recall where a patient on a beta-blocker presented with depression, switching the patient to ACE inhibitors or calcium channel blockers did not resolve depression, and the eventual resolution necessitated antidepressant treatment.

Compared to prescription drugs, alcohol and street drugs are more important and more common precipitants of depression and anxiety. Since they are not medically needed, they are entirely avoidable. Abstention from their use could relieve some or all symptoms of depression. Many patients "self-treat" their psychiatric symptoms by abusing alcohol and illicit drugs. Primary psychiatric problems frequently found among alcohol and drug abusers are depression, anxiety, cyclothymia, hypomania, attention deficit disorders, various phobias, and chronic pain. However, if a primary psychiatric disorder, which the author's experience suggests is present in most substance abusers, is not diagnosed and treated, the temptation and the drive to again "self-treat" with alcohol and illicit drugs will eventually resurface. Alcoholics and substance abusers should be strongly suspected of having an underlying treatable psychiatric disorder unless proven otherwise. Substance dependence is best seen as a symptom, not as a disease. This is why substance abuse treatment must not be limited to detoxification and rehabilitation treatment. A diligent search should be made to uncover probable underlying psychiatric disorders, so that appropriate psychiatric treatment can be initiated.

There is a tendency for polarized thinking among mental health professionals relating to psychiatric versus substance abuse disorders. At times, such thinking takes on concrete and fanatical proportions. For example, it is unfortunately common among substance abuse professionals to directly or subtly discourage patients from using prescription psychiatric medications. Usually this takes the form of devaluing the medication by labeling it "mind-altering," or a "chemical," or telling the patients that they are just substituting one drug for another. Over the years, I have seen many patients who have experienced relapses of their underlying psychiatric illnesses as a result of discontinuing psychotropic medications, as well as patients who have experienced relapses of their substance abuse, which could have been prevented by supporting the patients' pharmacological treatment of primary or secondary psychiatric disorders. Since the substance abuse and mental health fields attract a heterogeneous group of professionals, such unfounded attitudes and ignorance are unfortunately likely to continue. Mental health and substance abuse problems are related problems requiring comprehensive solutions, an important component of which is medication treatment of treatable underlying psychiatric problems.

My perspective has been that of seeing substance abuse as a symptom that requires both symptomatic treatment and, equally important, careful search for and treatment of the underlying psychiatric problems. In some cases, a specific diagnosable problem eludes the search, whereas in other cases, treatment is not available or is not accepted by the patient. Yet the psychiatrist has the responsibility to search for or identify the underlying problem, and to offer treatment, if available. Primary or secondary depression is very common among substance abusers, and merits aggressive treatment, in addition to abstention.

Depression can present in many diagnostic forms such as major depressive disorder, dysthymic disorder, adjustment disorder with depressed mood, schizoaffective disorder (depressed), bipolar disorder (depressed), etc. The future editions of *DSM* will probably have other titles and other categories of depression. For example, depressive personality disorder, minor depressive disorder, recurrent brief depressive disorder, mixed anxiety-depressive disorder, premenstrual dysphoric disorder, and post psychotic depressive disorder of schizophrenia are included in *DSM-IV* as diagnoses for further study for possible inclusion in *DSM-V*. All of these proposed diagnoses have predominant depressive symptoms. As mentioned throughout this book, from a practical clinical standpoint what matters most are the symptoms, not the specific diagnostic term. The main classes of depression according to *DSM-IV* are listed below, along with reproductions of diagnostic criteria sets.

Diagnostic Classifications of Depressive Disorders

There are four major classes of depression:

- Major depressive disorder (commonly known as major depression)
- Dysthymic disorder (also known as dysthymia)
- Depressive disorder not otherwise specified
- Adjustment disorder with depressed mood

MAJOR DEPRESSIVE EPISODE

Major depressive disorder is characterized by one or more major depressive episodes. According to *DSM-IV*, criteria for a major depressive episode are as follows:*

A. Five (or more) of the following symptoms have been present during the same two-week period and represent a change from previous functioning; at least one of the symptoms is either (1) depressed mood or (2) loss of interest or pleasure.

1. *Depressed mood most of the day, nearly every day, as indicated by either subjective report (e.g., feels sad and empty) or observation made by others (e.g., appears tearful). Note: In children and adolescents, can be irritable mood.*
2. *Markedly diminished interest or pleasure in all, or almost all, activities most of the day, nearly every day (as indicated by either subjective account or observation made by others)*
3. *Significant weight loss when not dieting or weight gain (e.g., a change of more than 5 percent of body weight in a month), or decrease or increase in appetite nearly every day. Note: In children, consider failure to make expected weight gains.*
4. *Insomnia or hypersomnia nearly every day.*
5. *Psychomotor agitation or retardation nearly every day (observable by others, not merely subjective feelings of restlessness or being slowed down).*
6. *Fatigue or loss of energy nearly every day.*

---

*Italicized text is reprinted with permission from the *Diagnostic and Statistical Manual of Mental Disorders*, Fourth Edition. Copyright 1994 American Psychiatric Association.

7. *Feelings of worthlessness or excessive or inappropriate guilt (which may be delusional) nearly every day (not merely self-reproach or guilt about being sick).*
8. *Diminished ability to think or concentrate, or indecisiveness, nearly every day, (either by subjective account or as observed by others).*
9. *Recurrent thoughts of death (not just fear of dying), recurrent suicidal ideation without a specific plan, or a suicide attempt or a specific plan for committing suicide.*

B. The symptoms do not meet criteria for a mixed episode.

C. The symptoms cause clinically significant distress or impairment in social, occupational, or other important areas of functioning.

D. The symptoms are not due to the direct physiological effects of a substance (e.g., drug of abuse, a medication) or a general medical condition (e.g., hypothyroidism).

E. The symptoms are not better accounted for by bereavement, i.e., after the loss of a loved one, the symptoms persist for more than two months or are characterized by marked functional impairment, morbid preoccupation with worthlessness, suicidal ideation, psychotic symptoms, or psychomotor retardation.

MAJOR DEPRESSIVE DISORDER

If more than one major depressive episode occurs, the major depressive disorder is classified as recurrent. The diagnostic criteria for major depressive disorder according to *DSM-IV* is as follows:*

Major Depressive Disorder, Single Episode

A. Presence of a single major depressive episode.

B. The major depressive episode is not better accounted for by schizoaffective disorder and is not superimposed on schizophrenia, schizophreniform disorder, delusional disorder, or psychotic disorder not otherwise specified.

C. There has never been a manic episode, a mixed episode, or a hypomanic episode. Note: This exclusion does not apply if all of the manic-like,

---

*Italicized text is reprinted with permission from the *Diagnostic and Statistical Manual of Mental Disorders*, Fourth Edition. Copyright 1994 American Psychiatric Association.

mixed-like, or hypomanic-like episodes are substance or treatment induced or are due to the direct physiological effects of a general medical condition.

Specify (for current or most recent episode):

- *Severity/psychosis/remission specifiers*
- *Chronic*
- *With catatonic features*
- *With melancholic features*
- *With atypical features*
- *With postpartum onset*

Major Depressive Disorder, Recurrent

A. Presence of two or more major depressive episodes. Note: To be considered separate episodes, there must be an interval of at least two consecutive months in which criteria are not met for a major depressive episode.

B. The major depressive episodes are not better accounted for by schizoaffective disorder and are not superimposed on schizophrenia, schizophreniform disorder, delusional disorder, or psychotic disorder not otherwise specified.

C. There has never been a manic episode, a mixed episode, or a hypomanic episode. Note: This exclusion does not apply if all of the manic-like, mixed-like, or hypomanic-like episodes are substance or treatment induced or are due to the direct physiological effects of a general medical condition.

Specify (for current or most recent episode):

- *Severity/psychosis/remission specifiers*
- *Chronic*
- *With catatonic features*
- *With melancholic features*
- *With atypical features*
- *With postpartum onset*

Specify:

- *Longitudinal course specifiers (with and without interepisode recovery)*
- *With seasonal pattern*

SEVERITY/PSYCHOSIS/REMISSION SPECIFIERS FOR MAJOR DEPRESSIVE EPISODE

The are several subcategories of major depression, based on severity level, presence or absence of psychotic symptoms, and degree of remission. The specific *DSM-IV* criteria for each of these specifiers are listed below:*

- ***Mild:*** *Few, if any symptoms in excess of those required to make the diagnosis and symptoms result in only minor impairment in occupational functioning or in usual social activities or relationships with others.*
- ***Moderate:*** *Symptoms or functional impairment between "mild" and "severe."*
- ***Severe without Psychotic Features:*** *Almost continual supervision required to prevent physical harm to self or others.*
- ***Severe with Psychotic Features:*** *Delusions or hallucinations. If possible, specify whether the psychotic features are mood-congruent or mood-incongruent:*
    - ***Mood-Congruent Psychotic Features:*** *Delusions or hallucinations whose content is entirely consistent with the typical depressive themes of personal inadequacy, guilt, disease, death, nihilism, or deserved punishment.*
    - ***Mood-Incongruent Psychotic Features:*** *Delusions or hallucinations whose content does not involve typical depressive themes of personal inadequacy, guilt, disease, death, nihilism, or deserved punishment. Included are such symptoms as persecutory delusions (not directly related to depressive themes), thought insertion, thought broadcasting, and delusions of control.*
- ***In Partial Remission:*** *Symptoms of a major depressive episode are present but full criteria are not met, or there is a period without any significant symptoms of a major depressive episode lasting less than two months following the end of the major depressive episode. (If the major depressive episode was superimposed on dysthymic disorder, the diagnosis of dysthymic disorder alone is given once the full criteria for a major depressive episode are no longer met).*

---

*Italicized text is reprinted with permission from the *Diagnostic and Statistical Manual of Mental Disorders*, Fourth Edition. Copyright 1994 American Psychiatric Association.

- ***In Full Remission:*** *During the past two months, no significant signs or symptoms of the disturbance were present.*
- ***Unspecified***

DYSTHYMIC DISORDER

The *DSM-IV* diagnostic criteria for dysthymic disorder are the following:*

A. Depressed mood for most of the day, for more days than not, as indicated either by subjective account or observation by others, for at least two years. Note: In children and adolescents, mood can be irritable and duration must be at least one year.

B. Presence, while depressed, of two (or more) of the following:

1. *Poor appetite or overeating*
2. *Insomnia or hypersomnia*
3. *Low energy or fatigue*
4. *Low self-esteem*
5. *Poor concentration or difficulty making decisions*
6. *Feelings of hopelessness*

C. During the two-year period (one year for children or adolescents) of the disturbance, the person has never been without the symptoms in criteria A and B for more than two months at a time.

D. No major depressive episode has been present during the first two years of the disturbance (one year for children and adolescents)–i.e., the disturbance is not better accounted for by chronic Major Depressive Disorder, or major depressive disorder, or in partial remission.

Note: There may have been a previous major depressive episode provided there was a full remission (no significant signs or symptoms for two months) before development of the dysthymic disorder. In addition, after the initial two years (one year in children or adolescents) of dysthymic disorder, there may be superimposed episodes of major depressive disorder, in which case both diagnoses may be given when the criteria are met for a major depressive episode.

---

*Italicized text is reprinted with permission from the *Diagnostic and Statistical Manual of Mental Disorders*, Fourth Edition. Copyright 1994 American Psychiatric Association.

E. There has never been a manic episode, a mixed episode, or a hypomanic episode, and criteria have never been met for cyclothymic disorder.

F. The disturbance does not occur exclusively during the course of a chronic psychotic disorder, such as schizophrenia or delusional disorder.

G. The symptoms are not due to the direct physiological effects of a substance (e.g., a drug of abuse, a medication) or a general medical condition (e.g., hypothyroidism).

H. The symptoms cause clinically significant distress or impairment in social, occupational, or other important areas of functioning.

Specify if:

- ***Early Onset:*** *if onset is before age 21 years*
- ***Late Onset:*** *if onset is age 21 years or older*

Specify if (for most recent two years of dysthymic disorder):

- ***With Atypical Features***

ADJUSTMENT DISORDER WITH DEPRESSED MOOD

Adjustment disorder with depressed mood presents with symptoms such as depressed mood, tearfulness, anhedonia, and feelings of hopelessness. For classification as an adjustment disorder, the symptoms must develop within three months of onset of an identifiable psychosocial stressor. The symptoms should cause either marked distress or significant impairment in social or occupational functioning. The symptoms typically resolve within six months of the termination of the stressor unless the stressor is chronic or the consequences are enduring. If symptoms resolve within six months, the episode is considered *acute* and if symptoms last six months or longer, the adjustment disorder is described as *chronic*. The treatment strategy is similar to that for depression.

ADJUSTMENT DISORDER WITH MIXED ANXIETY AND DEPRESSED MOOD

This diagnosis is used when symptoms of anxiety and depression are present in a person who meets other criteria for adjustment disorder. In general, for classification as an adjustment disorder, the symptoms must develop within three months of onset of an identifiable psychosocial stressor. The symptoms should cause either marked distress or significant impairment in social or occupational functioning. The symptoms typically resolve within six months of the termination of the stressor unless the stressor is chronic, or the consequences are enduring. If symptoms resolve within six months the episode is considered *acute*, and if symptoms last six months or longer, the adjustment disorder is considered *chronic*. The treatment of adjustment disorder with mixed anxiety and depressed mood is similar to that of depression and anxiety discussed in detail in this book.

DEPRESSIVE DISORDER, NOT OTHERWISE SPECIFIED

This category includes disorders with depressive symptoms that do not meet the full criteria for the various depressive disorders described above. Specific examples of depressive disorder, NOS, as given in *DSM-IV*, are reproduced below:*

1. Premenstrual dysphoric disorder: in most menstrual cycles during the past year, symptoms (e.g., markedly depressed mood, marked anxiety, marked affective lability, decreased interest in activities) regularly occurred during the last week of the luteal phase (and remitted within a few days of the onset of menses). These symptoms must be severe enough to markedly interfere with work, school, or usual activities and be entirely absent for at least one week postmenses.

2. Minor depressive disorder: episodes of at least two weeks of depressive symptoms but with fewer than the five items required for major depressive disorder.

3. Recurrent brief depressive disorder: depressive episodes lasting from two days up to two weeks, occurring at least once a month for 12 months (not associated with the menstrual cycle).

4. Postpsychotic depressive disorder of schizophrenia: a major depressive episode that occurs during the residual phase of schizophrenia.

5. A major depressive episode superimposed on delusional disorder, psychotic disorder not otherwise specified, or the active phase of schizophrenia.

6. Situations in which the clinician has concluded that a depressive disorder is present, but is unable to determine whether it is primary, due to a general medical condition, or substance induced.

---

*Italicized text is reprinted with permission from the *Diagnostic and Statistical Manual of Mental Disorders*, Fourth Edition. Copyright 1994 American Psychiatric Association.

If depressive symptoms are present, treatment is usually needed. Treatment can take many forms depending on the following factors:

- Etiology of symptoms
- Severity of symptoms
- Nature of symptoms
- Variety of symptoms
- Duration of symptoms
- Concurrent conditions

ETIOLOGY OF SYMPTOMS

Etiology of symptoms can be multiple, including medical disorders, hormonal effects, pain conditions, postpartum status, and drug effects (including alcohol and illicit drugs), or the symptoms might be of an unknown cause. Whenever possible the causative disorder or condition should be corrected. Two examples are depression related to hypothyroidism and chronic use of sedatives. However, in most cases, an identifiable or correctable etiological factor cannot be found; hence antidepressant treatment is initiated. Postpartum depression, bipolar depression, and endogenous depression are examples. In some cases, the etiological factor, even if identified, is not amenable to correction. In these circumstances, antidepressant treatment is indicated to overcome depression. Depression associated with steroid or cytotoxic medications, for which substitution may be neither available nor desirable, is one such example. If chronic pain is judged to be the etiological factor in precipitating depression, referral is usually made to a pain management program. If depressive symptoms are significant, antidepressant treatment can be initiated while concurrently attempting to correct the etiological factor. Thus, a careful search for treatable or correctable etiology is important in the evaluation of all patients. This process should be guided by patient history and the clinician's judgment, rather than by a standard battery of expensive tests for every patient.

SEVERITY OF SYMPTOMS

In general, mild to moderate depressive symptoms can be treated on an outpatient basis. Even severe symptoms can be treated on an outpatient basis unless the patient is suicidal, homicidal, or has other out-of-control behavioral or medical conditions that complicate the clinical picture. The presence of suicidal ideation does not necessarily require that the patient be hospitalized. In severe depressions, suicidal ideation is common. A thorough evaluation of suicidality will reveal information that will help the physician make an appropriate treatment recommendation. If the physician's clinical assessment suggests that the patient is of imminent risk to self or others due to mental illness, and if the determination is that inpatient hospitalization is necessary, and if the patient refuses inpatient treatment, the physician should initiate procedures for involuntary commitment. If the patient assures the physician that he or she will not act on suicidal and homicidal ideation, a clinical judgment must be made as to whether or not the patient can be relied upon. Significant others may be available to stay with the patient, thus providing an element of security. If this is the case, they should be directed to contact the physician regarding any concerns or changes in the patient's condition.

In most situations in which the patient states that he or she will not follow through on a suicidal or homicidal act, the statements should be accepted at face value unless there is reason to believe otherwise. The physician cannot be a detective or an investigator or a police officer, hence the common practice is to make decisions based on available clinical information while adhering to patients' rights laws. A physician cannot prevent a determined patient from attempting suicide or homicide. Ultimately the responsibility for the patient's actions rests with the individual patient.

Also deserving consideration for inpatient treatment are complicating medical conditions such as severe anorexia and weight loss, as well as out-of-control behavior problems such as dependence on alcohol or drugs. In the author's experience, most severe symptoms can be treated on an outpatient basis if the patient is cooperative, even in the presence of suicidal or homicidal ideation or other complicating factors. The key factor is immediate and coordinated outpatient intervention.

Most symptoms of depression will benefit from antidepressant medication coupled with counseling/psychotherapy. On rare occasions, electroconvulsive therapy (ECT) is necessary. (See the section on ECT for a discussion of ECT indications, side effects, advantages, and disadvantages.)

VARIETY OF SYMPTOMS

Different symptoms respond preferentially to different antidepressants. For example, anergia and hypersomnia respond well to medications that have stimulant properties, such as bupropion, fluoxetine, venlafaxine, desipramine, tranylcypromine, and protriptyline, whereas anorexia and insomnia respond to sedating antidepressants, such as most tricyclics. As discussed later in more detail, due to their benign side effect profile, serotonergic antidepressants are currently the first-line antidepressants for most depressive symptoms, with use of adjunctive medications to treat symptoms that do not immediately respond to serotonergic drugs (for example, insomnia and anorexia). Several lists below give information regarding approximate ranking of medication choice for various symptoms based on therapeutic effects and side effects.

DURATION OF SYMPTOMS

In general, the more chronic the duration of symptoms prior to treatment, the longer it will take for improvement and the longer the patient should stay on an effective medication to receive optimal benefit. For example, treatment of dysthymia, which is a chronic condition, usually takes a longer period of time to resolve than treatment of adjustment disorder with depressed mood or a major depression recently precipitated by a stressor.

COEXISTING CONDITIONS

Coexisting conditions such as psychotic symptoms, history of manic episodes, attention deficit disorders, post-traumatic stress disorder (PTSD), severe anxiety, etc., will require various medications in addition to antidepressants for satisfactory treatment outcome. Most patients readily report depressive symptoms, but either do not volunteer the presence of other symptoms or are not able to recognize their presence. Hence the real challenge to a specialist in psychiatry is to elicit the presence of other symptoms that complicate the treatment of depression. An antidepressant prescribed by a primary care physician should work as well as the same antidepressant prescribed by a psychiatrist. Most referrals to psychiatrists are those patients who did not respond well to antidepressants started by primary care physicians. In the majority of these cases, concurrent conditions exist, requiring adjunctive medications. It is the psychiatrist's responsibility to identify these conditions and provide treatment. The impressive safety of serotonergic antidepressants makes it convenient for primary care physicians to use them to treat uncomplicated depressions as effectively as psychiatrists.

SPECIFIC DIAGNOSTIC AND MANAGEMENT CONCEPTS

Depressive symptoms, regardless of severity, will benefit from antidepressants. Mild symptoms show almost complete resolution on fairly low doses in general. Severe symptoms improve less completely and may need high doses or combinations, in general. Both mild and severe symptoms will respond to ECT in a similar fashion. However, as discussed elsewhere, ECT is usually reserved for severe symptoms that do not respond to aggressive medication intervention for various reasons described in Chapter 6. Common symptoms, with some overlap, that respond to antidepressants are listed in Table 1.1.

Many of the symptoms in this list are highly suggestive of depression, such as suicidality, feelings of hopelessness, feelings of worthlessness, anhedonia, crying episodes, sadness, depressed mood, inappropriate guilt, etc., while others, such as aches and pains, fatigue, hypochondriacal concerns, psychomotor agitation or retardation, somatic preoccupation, anorexia, poor memory, etc., are less specific for depression. The presence of the latter group of symptoms should prompt consideration of medical etiologies, such as cancer, hormonal abnormalities, neurological disorders, and other medical problems.

Even in a patient presenting with suicidal ideation, intent, and plan, which are highly specific for depression, it is important to evaluate symptoms and understand them in the proper context. For example, it would be a clinical error to involuntarily commit a suicidal patient who refuses treatment in the context of a diagnosis of terminal cancer with severe pain and a life expectancy of several months, assuming the decision to end the person's life is based on rational thinking. Although an extreme example, this is mentioned to illustrate the clinical principle that all symptoms, including symptoms highly specific to a disorder, should still be interpreted by a clinician.

Depressive symptoms can present in varying severity, in different configurations, in changing patterns, in varying duration, and with or without precipitants. It has to be emphasized that the ideal treatment of depression, or any emotional illness, is a combination of medications (and/or ECT) and psychotherapy. Since the focus of this text is on clinical diagnosis and pharmacologic management, the adjunctive need for psychotherapy is not mentioned every time medications are discussed, in the interest of parsimony.

Depressive symptoms are predominant in the following disorders:

- Major depressive disorder
- Dysthymic disorder
- Depressive disorder, NOS

- Adjustment disorder with depressed mood
- Adjustment disorder with mixed anxiety and depressed mood
- Bipolar I disorder, depressed
- Bipolar II disorder
- Cyclothymic disorder
- Dementia with depressed mood
- Schizoaffective disorder, depressive type

TABLE 1.1. Common Symptoms That Respond to Antidepressants, with Some Overlap

Depressed mood or sadness	Helplessness
Anhedonia	Brooding
Anergia	Apathy
Decreased motivation	Decreased activity
Crying	Vague and diffuse aches and pains
Increased emotionality/ sensitivity	Guilt
Increased anger	Excessive self-criticism
Anger outbursts	Increased frustration
Increased worrying	Excessive discouragement
Anxiety	Feeling slowed down
Anxiety attacks	Unrealistic pessimism
Moodiness	Expectation of doom
Anorexia	Psychomotor agitation
Hyperphagia	Psychomotor retardation
Insomnia	Fear or phobia
Hypersomnia	Poor self-confidence
Suicidality	Low self-esteem
Hopelessness	Decreased libido
Worthlessness	Social withdrawal
Ruminative preoccupation	Emotional blunting
Decreased conversation	Somatic preoccupation
Hypochondriacal concerns	Fatigue
Decreased concentration	Decreased memory
Difficulty making decisions	Difficulty thinking
Feelings of inadequacy	

Depressive symptoms are also seen in various other disorders such as schizophrenia, personality disorders, and substance abuse. Negative or deficit symptoms of schizophrenia are frequently difficult to distinguish from a depressive disorder. If depressive symptoms are the only symptoms present, antidepressant medications are sufficient. However, if other symptoms such as anxiety, psychosis, attention deficit, and mood swings are present, appropriate treatment for the other conditions, using various other medications, is necessary in addition to antidepressant medications.

This discussion uses the term "depressive symptoms" rather than specific "depressive disorders." If depressive symptoms are present, treatment using antidepressants should be considered, regardless of the primary diagnosis. It is a common clinical observation that many schizophrenics do better with the addition of a low dose of an antidepressant medication to their antipsychotic medication. In clinical practice, virtually all patients come to the clinician because of some distress either perceived by themselves or identified by significant others who persuade or coerce the patient to seek psychiatric evaluation. Because of the stigma and the consequent ambivalence that are still associated with a psychiatric diagnosis and treatment, patients typically minimize (or even deny) their symptoms, perhaps hoping that the clinician will also concur with their subconscious wish to avoid psychiatric diagnosis and treatment. Although this is extreme among patients with psychotic disorders and among patients coerced into undergoing a psychiatric evaluation, patients with common problems such as depression and anxiety also tend to minimize, to some extent, the severity of their symptoms. The clinician, in these circumstances, must have a low threshold to identify symptoms and treat them. The presence of even one depressive symptom deserves consideration for treatment, whether or not the patient meets the criteria for a diagnosis according to *DSM-IV*. For practical purposes, the *DSM-IV* criterion that requires that symptoms should "cause clinically significant distress or impairment in social, occupational, or other important areas of functioning" is met by virtue of the patient presenting to the office or the hospital.

Let me illustrate this point with several variations of a simple presenting complaint. A wife persuades her husband to see a psychiatrist with the presenting complaint that the husband has been irritable, which in turn is causing marital conflicts. A careful psychiatric evaluation fails to reveal any other symptom, and the husband reports that he has an irritable temperament that is part of his personality. His wife reports that counseling in the past has helped improve symptoms, to some extent, temporarily. The husband does not see the need for treatment.

In this example, the husband probably does not meet the criteria for a psychiatric diagnosis that most insurance companies, Medicare, or Medicaid would accept. Yet, the clinician's task is to tactfully persuade the husband to initiate treatment by empathically confronting him as follows:

- The symptom is causing marital distress.
- The symptom is also causing psychological stress in the husband, though he may not be fully aware of it.
- There is a chance that the symptom of irritability can generalize to other interpersonal contexts, without the husband's full awareness, leading to potential problems.
- Irritability is an easily treatable symptom with medications that have very little side effects.
- Receiving counseling while on medication can yield better results than either one treatment alone.
- Successful treatment can lead to a happier marriage as well as enhanced personal happiness.

It is a common observation that many people consider symptoms such as irritability, moodiness, anger outbursts, etc., as part of their innate temperament, and hence minimize or dismiss their dysfunctional effects, especially in the interpersonal realm. Yet these are the symptoms that can cause serious problems in marriages and in the workplace, or in any context in which stable interpersonal interaction is important.

In a variation of the same example, a husband arrives at the office complaining of irritability. The patient has been able to control the irritability by employing considerable psychological resources, leaving him mentally exhausted at the end of the day. The patient seeks treatment. His wife has no complaints regarding him and is unaware of the problem.

In this scenario there is personal distress and one symptom–criteria that are not sufficient for a *DSM-IV* diagnosis–yet it is incumbent upon the clinician to offer treatment to this patient. With most patients, more than one symptom can be identified and hence the need for treatment is obvious.

Major depression in its severe form will usually include irrational beliefs, thoughts, and perceptions. Since severely depressed patients' thinking is usually irrationally negative and morbid, it is important to consider adjunctive use of low doses of antipsychotics even if obvious psychotic symptoms are not present. It is very difficult to elicit psychotic symptoms from severely depressed patients since they feel hopeless and tend to keep their thoughts to themselves, unlike manic patients whose thought processes are usually evident in their profuse verbalization and/or in their behavior. Similarly, in severely manic patients, psychotic symptoms are usually present. The difference is that it is very easy to detect psychotic symptoms in manic patients because they are unable to keep thoughts to themselves or they have difficulty controlling their behavior. Depression and mania are thought to be on a continuum, with euthymia at the midpoint of the continuum. It is fairly easy to diagnose even a hypomanic patient, but depression even at a moderate degree is less obvious.

Figure 1.1, derived from the author's clinical experience, illustrates that even mild forms of mania are associated with psychotic symptoms, whereas only severe depression is associated with significant psychotic thinking. The treatment implication is that almost all hypomanias and

FIGURE 1.1. The Relationships Between (1) Degree of Mania and Psychotic Symptoms, and (2) Degree of Depression and Psychotic Symptoms. Clinical significance is described in text.

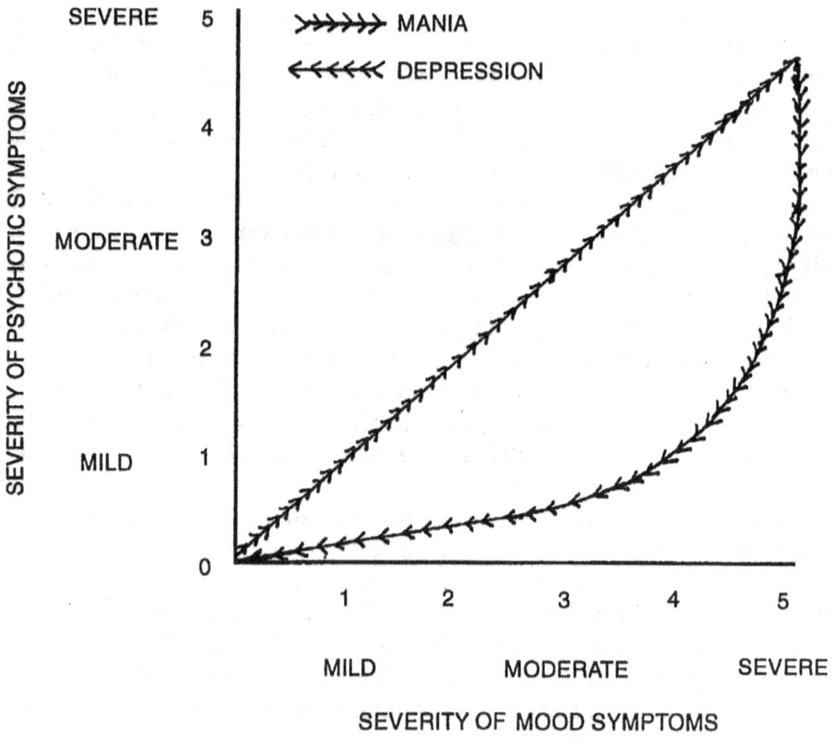

manias, as well as severely depressed patients, could benefit from varying doses of antipsychotics in the short term.

Since there is such an inward focus and regression to the point of being autistic in some cases of severe depression, the presence of psychotic symptoms, unfortunately, is sometimes missed. If such patients are started on an antidepressant, which by itself (in the absence of adjunctive antipsychotics) can at times make the psychosis worse, serious adverse consequences can result. If depression and mania are on a continuum with euthymia in the middle, and if it is readily evident that psychotic symptoms are usually present with mania, it should not be surprising that severe forms of depression are also associated with psychotic symptoms. What is striking is the difficulty in identifying the presence of psychotic symptoms in depressed patients, unless the psychosis is of moderate or greater severity. Hence, it is important to diligently look for these elusive symptoms and treat them with adjunctive antipsychotic medication. One advantage in treating primary mood disorders presenting with psychotic features is that the duration of the use of antipsychotics can usually be short-term. Once the depressive or manic episode is brought under control, the antipsychotic can be gradually tapered off while keeping the patient on an antidepressant (in the case of depression), or on a mood stabilizer (in the case of mania), on a longer-term basis.

Obsessive-compulsive symptoms, which can coexist with depression, also respond to antidepressant medications. Similarly, coexisting panic disorder, anorexia, and bulimia will respond to antidepressants.

Serotonergic antidepressants, along with bupropion, have an excellent side effect profile. They are the drug of choice among antidepressants in a modern psychiatric practice. Their effectiveness is similar to TCAs and MAOIs. However, the anticholinergic, cardiovascular, and other side effects such as weight gain and sedation associated with TCAs and MAOIs make them poor choices compared with SSRIs and bupropion. Prior to the introduction of SSRIs, the antidepressants used most often by the author were nortriptyline, imipramine, desipramine, and phenelzine, which are as effective as SSRIs, but when side effect profiles are compared, SSRIs have several advantages. TCAs are still used quite frequently in my office practice as adjunctive medications rather than as primary medications. In this role they are very useful, and sometimes necessary, in conjunction with SSRIs, as will be explained in detail in Chapter 2.

Chapter 2

Pharmacological Treatment of Depression

GENERAL MANAGEMENT CONCEPTS

All depressive symptoms are more or less equally responsive to available antidepressants; however, there are significant and substantial differences in side effect profiles that primarily determine the choice of an antidepressant for a particular patient. The exploitation of side effects for patient benefit requires a combination of science and art, the basics of which every physician who prescribes antidepressants should know. The side effect profile should not be the only consideration in choosing an antidepressant. Certain depressive symptoms respond preferentially to certain classes of antidepressants. Various effective techniques developed from the author's experience of treating thousands of depressed patients are described below. MAOIs (phenelzine, tranylcypromine, isocarboxazid) have relatively superior effectiveness in patients with atypical depressive symptoms, panic disorder, and social phobia. Less widely known is the effectiveness of serotonergic antidepressants (fluoxetine, sertraline, paroxetine, venlafaxine, and fluvoxamine) on anger and obsessive-compulsive symptoms. Clomipramine (Anafranil), which is a TCA, is indicated for treatment of obsessive-compulsive disorder. Similarly, bupropion (Wellbutrin) is considered preferable in patients with anergia, hypersomnia, and psychomotor retardation. Table 2.1 lists antidepressant choice based on various presenting symptoms. These medication characteristics will be discussed in greater detail. A ranking of antidepressants based on side effects is given in Table 2.2.

In an outpatient psychiatric and primary care practice, antidepressants are some of the most commonly prescribed medications. Thorough familiarity with the diagnosis of depression and the prescription of antidepressants is essential for physicians dealing with depression. Antidepressants are effective for treatment of depressive disorder, as well as for a variety of

TABLE 2.1. Antidepressant Choice Based on Various Presenting Symptoms

EFFECT	Depressed Mood	Crying Episodes	Irritability and Anger	Insomnia	Anorexia	Anergia	Decreased Libido	Anxiety	Obsessional Symptoms	Excessive Emotional Sensitivity
High	SSRIs TCAs MAOIs mirtazapine bupropion nefazodone trazodone	SSRIs TCAs MAOIs mirtazapine buproprion nefazodone trazodone	SSRIs TCAs MAOIs mirtazapine nefazodone trazodone	TCAs trazodone nefazodone mirtazapine	TCAs MAOIs mirtazapine	SSRIs MAOIs stimulating TCAs bupropion	buproprion nefazodone trazodone mirtazapine	TCAs MAOIs SSRIs nefazodone trazodone mirtazapine	clomipramine SSRIs	SSRIs MAOIs
Medium			bupropion	fluvoxamine	nefazodone trazodone bupropion	mirtazapine nefazodone trazodone sedating TCAs	TCAs	bupropion	nefazodone trazodone TCAs MAOIs mirtazapine	mirtazapine TCAs nefazodone trazodone bupropion
Low				SSRIs MAOIs bupropion	SSRIs		MAOIs SSRIs		bupropion	

Note: It is naive and even misleading to imply that antidepressant choice is based on a discrete symptom. In real life, symptoms present in clusters. Therefore, the antidepressant that provides the best fit is chosen to efficiently address all the symptoms. Other factors such as side effects, pharmacokinetics, and interaction potential also influence the eventual choice. Not infrequently one antidepressant can be combined with another antidepressant to obtain the desired effect. These factors and techniques are described in the text and illustrated in the clinical cases. Venlafaxine, though not truly an SSRI, is included in the SSRI group for convenience.

TABLE 2.2. Ranking of Antidepressants Based on Side Effects

LEVEL	Anti-cholinergic	Nausea, G.I. Effects	Anxiety, Tremor	Sexual Dysfunction	Anorexia	Weight Gain	Insomnia	Seizure	Sedation
Most	sedating TCAs clomipramine	venlafaxine sertraline	fluoxetine bupropion venlafaxine sertraline paroxetine fluvoxamine mirtazapine	paroxetine clomipramine fluoxetine sertraline venlafaxine fluvoxamine	fluoxetine sertraline bupropion fluvoxamine paroxetine venlafaxine	TCAs mirtazapine	bupropion MAOIs fluoxetine sertraline paroxetine	clomipramine bupropion	sedating TCAs trazodone nefazodone mirtazapine
Medium	MOAIs stimulating TCAs mirtazapine	fluvoxamine nefazodone trazodone paroxetine fluoxetine	clomipramine stimulating TCAs	MOAIs TCAs	trazodone nefazodone	MOAIs	protriptyline venlafaxine	TCAs	clomipramine stimulating TCAs
Least	bupropion trazodone nefazodone SSRIs	mirtazapine TCAs MOAIs clomipramine bupropion	sedating TCAs nefazodone trazodone	mirtazapine nefazodone trazodone bupropion	TCAs MAOIs mirtazapine	SSRIs bupropion nefazodone trazodone	mirtazapine fluvoxamine TCAs nefazodone trazodone	mirtazapine SSRIs nefazodone trazodone MAOIs	SSRIs bupropion

other psychiatric disorders such as anxiety disorder, obsessive-compulsive disorder, social phobia, bipolar disorders, deficit symptoms of psychosis, and personality disorders. Depression is usually a coexisting condition or sequela associated with these disorders. In actual clinical practice, the astute clinician searches for symptoms such as anxiety, mild obsessive-compulsive symptoms, mild paranoia, panic disorder, bipolar disorder, and various psychoses. Approximately half of patients with depression are also found to have these symptoms. The significance of this clinical observation is that for optimal treatment of a patient who is treated in the office or who is seen in the hospital, more than one diagnosis is made, in most cases. Many of the coexisting conditions may not be at the level or intensity that meets *DSM-IV* diagnostic criteria; hence, a high degree of suspicion and a detective attitude are necessary to uncover and identify associated conditions and to effectively treat them. It is important to keep in mind that psychotic, paranoid, and bipolar patients, and those with obsessive-compulsive disorder and antisocial personalities, can present with the chief complaint of depression and/or anxiety. Of all the problems mentioned above, the most critical to recognize is the presence of underlying psychosis, paranoia, and bipolar disorder. Psychotic patients can often have what is known as negative symptoms, which are also called deficit symptoms. Postpsychotic demoralization or secondary depression can also be present in patients with a primary psychotic disorder. Side effects of antipsychotic medications, such as akinesia and apathy, have depressive characteristics. At the same time if an antidepressant is prescribed to a psychotic patient without a concomitant antipsychotic medication, there is a significant risk of the patient becoming floridly psychotic and paranoid, though less depressed.

All antidepressants have the potential to precipitate or uncover mania; however, this should not be a major concern unless the patient has had manic or hypomanic episodes in the past, in which case, the risk of a switch to mania is present. In such a patient, prophylactic treatment with a mood stabilizer, in addition to an antidepressant, should be considered. The identification of a history of mania or hypomania should at least prompt the physician to monitor the patient's mental status closely if the physician chooses to treat such a patient with antidepressants alone. Lithium has mild antidepressant effects in addition to superior antimanic effects. Therefore, the physician is usually safe in adjunctively using lithium in a depressed patient with prior episodes of mania or hypomania, because lithium can augment the antidepressant effects of the antidepressant as well as provide some protection against mania. As a general rule, physicians should strive to resolve patients' problems by using the least number of medications at the lowest effective dose. Specific treatment strategies for depression and concomitant symptoms are discussed below.

ANTIDEPRESSANT CHOICE

The hierarchy of antidepressants in current psychiatric practice is the following:

- First choice–serotonergic antidepressants, bupropion, mirtazapine, and nefazodone
- Second choice–tricyclics
- Third choice–monoamine oxide inhibitors
- Fourth choice–ECT

There can be many exceptions to this general hierarchy in individual cases.

Antidepressants can be used in various combinations for different purposes, as follows:

- To augment antidepressant effects
- To treat symptoms that the primary antidepressant does not treat
- To treat nondepressive symptoms (e.g., negative symptoms, attention deficit hyperactivity disorder [ADHD], anxiety, bipolar history)
- To treat antidepressant side effects

AUGMENTATION

Several antidepressant augmenters are listed below. The success rates of these to convert a nonresponder to a responder are fairly low, probably in the order of 20 to 25 percent in the author's clinical experience.

- Lithium (serum level of 0.5 to 0.8 mEq/L)
- Thyroid supplements
- Stimulants–except with MAOIs
- Buspirone (Buspar)–except with MAOIs
- Other antidepressants that work on different neurotransmitters (except with MAOIs)
- Anticonvulsants such as carbamazepine and valproic acid
- Fenfluramine (Pondimin)–except with MAOIs
- Pindolol (Visken)

Lithium

In general, augmenters are used only after trying several antidepressants from different classes of antidepressant medications. The serum lithium level that is preferred for augmentation in conjunction with an antidepressant is usually in the range of 0.5 to 0.8 mEq/L, whereas for treatment of mania, a serum level of 0.8 to 1.3 mEq/L is desirable. The higher the serum lithium level, the greater the chances of side effects such as fine hand tremors, nausea, diarrhea, and polyuria. The sustained-release forms such as Eskalith CR and Lithobid tend to cause less gastric irritation and more diarrhea, and the regular preparation tends to cause less diarrhea but more gastric irritation. However, since gastric irritation and nausea are more common in general, and since the cost difference between regular and slow-release preparations is not great, the author routinely prescribes the relatively more expensive sustained-release forms. In most cases the following doses are sufficient to give a serum level of 0.5 to 0.6 mEq/L:

- Eskalith CR 225 mg in the morning (AM) and 450 mg at bedtime (HS)
- Lithobid 300 mg po AM and HS
- Lithium carbonate 300 mg po AM and HS

Since the elderly are more susceptible to the neurological side effects of lithium, the dosage should be even lower, in the range of 150 to 450 mg per day. Although breaking a sustained release tablet defeats the sustained release mechanism to some extent, this is not clinically significant. Lithium augmentation is particularly effective for depressed patients who have had a manic or hypomanic episode in the past, or those who have a family history of bipolar disorder. Moreover, lithium is protective in patients who have a history of mania or hypomania who present with a depressive episode. These individuals are at higher risk of a switch to mania as a result of antidepressant treatment. Hence, lithium offers advantages as a prophylactic medication and as an antidepressant augmenter in bipolar patients presenting with depression. (Refer to the section on lithium for details on lithium side effects and management.)

Thyroid Supplements

Thyroid augmentation using levothyroxine or T4 (Synthroid) at doses of 25 to 50 mcg per day or liothyronine or T3 (Cytomel) at doses of 10 to 40 mcg per day can be employed. A baseline thyroid profile, if not obtained as part of the initial depression workup, should be obtained prior to starting thyroid supplements. Side effects such as osteoporosis and symptoms of thyrotoxicosis are possible with thyroid excess. Therefore, the dosage used for thyroid augmentation should not be high enough to cause suppression of TSH. Thyroid supplementation is also believed to decrease frequency of dysphoric episodes in rapid-cycling bipolar disorder.

Stimulants

Antidepressant effects can be augmented by the addition of stimulants, in treatment-resistant cases. The usual effective doses are the following:

- Dextroamphetamine (Dexedrine) 5-10 mg twice a day (BID)
- Dexedrine spansule capsule 10-15 mg AM
- Methylphenidate (Ritalin) 5-20 mg BID
- Ritalin SR 20 mg AM
- Pemoline (Cylert) 37.5-75 mg daily

If significant anergia, hypersomnia, poor concentration, or ADD symptoms are present and are not responsive to antidepressant treatment, including trial on bupropion (Wellbutrin), consideration should be given to using stimulants adjunctively, since these symptoms are particularly responsive to stimulants. Stimulants should preferably be given prior to 6 p.m. to minimize interference with sleep. They are relatively contraindicated in patients who are at risk for substance abuse. Stimulants should not be given with MAOIs. Initially start at low doses and increase gradually if needed.

Buspirone (Buspar)

Buspirone at a dose of 10 to 15 mg BID or three times a day (TID) added to an antidepressant regimen has the potential to augment antidepressant effects, especially if depression is accompanied by prominent anxiety symptoms. Buspirone should not be used with MAOIs. Buspirone may improve symptoms of PTSD, such as startle response, flashbacks, anger outbursts, and hypervigilance. Patients presenting with PTSD usually have some depressive symptoms and hence commonly require treatment using an antidepressant.

Other Antidepressants

An antidepressant of one class may be combined with an antidepressant from another class for purposes of augmentation to convert a nonresponder to a responder. Various combinations are given below.

Serotonergic Antidepressants and Tricyclic Antidepressants

– fluoxetine 20-80 mg AM		desipramine 25-50 mg HS
– sertraline 50-200 mg AM	+	nortriptyline 25 mg HS
– paroxetine 20-60 mg AM		imipramine 25-50 mg HS
		amitriptyline 25-50 mg HS
		doxepin 25-50 mg HS
– fluvoxamine 50-200 mg HS	+	protriptyline 10-20 mg AM
– nefazodone 200-400 mg HS	+	protriptyline 10-20 mg AM
– trazodone 200-400 mg HS	+	protriptyline 10-20 mg AM
– bupropion 75-150 mg AM	+	serotonergic antidepressants at noon
– bupropion 75-150 mg AM	+	TCA at half the usual dose at bedtime (equivalent to imipramine 50-150 mg HS)

Selected TCAs and MAOIs

– nortriptyline 25-50 mg HS		
– amitriptyline 50-100 mg HS	+	phenelzine 15-30 mg AM and noon
– doxepin 50-100 mg HS		tranylcypromine 10 mg AM and noon
– trimipramine 50-100 mg HS		
– trazodone 50-200 mg HS (not a TCA)		

In general, the dose of the primary antidepressant should be less than the maximum dose, and the antidepressant added to the existing (primary) antidepressant should be at low doses to minimize risk from interaction effects related to hepatic enzyme inhibition and increased side effects. The antidepressant that has greater risk for adverse effects is added to the ongoing antidepressant at low doses. For example, since bupropion is known for increased risk of seizures, it is added at low doses to another antidepressant given at moderate doses. Hence, bupropion should not be given at the maximum dose of 450 mg per day along with another antidepressant because of the increased risk of seizure due to combined effects. Combinations of antidepressants should be attempted cautiously with very low starting doses, and gradual and smaller dosage increments. This is particularly true when combining MAOIs with TCAs, which can lead to serotonergic or hyperthermic crisis. For this reason, combining MAOIs to TCAs is only infrequently done for treating the most treatment-resistant cases. If MAOIs and TCAs are to be combined, patients should be kept on a moderate dose of a TCA first, and then an MAOI at very low doses should be added to the ongoing TCA with gradual increase in the dose of the MAOI, as clinically necessary. Another option is to start both MAOI and TCA at very low doses and increase both very gradually in smaller-than-usual increments. TCA should not be added to a patient already on an MAOI because of greater risk of hyperthermic or serotonergic reaction. Amitriptyline, nortriptyline, doxepin, and trimipramine tend to cause hyperthermic or serotonergic reaction less frequently, compared to other TCAs. However, the risk is not zero; some individuals may be more susceptible to adverse effects than others. MAOIs should not be combined with serotonergic antidepressants, clomipramine, bupropion, or buspirone, because of increased risk of interaction.

Anticonvulsants

Carbamazepine (Tegretol) at 300 to 600 mg per day in divided doses or divalproex sodium (Depakote) at 500 to 1,000 mg per day in divided doses occasionally is effective as an augmenting medication, particularly in depressed patients with prior history of mania or hypomania, or if depression is characterized by extreme mood changes, or in patients with dysphoric mania or bipolar II disorder. Labile affect and dysphoria associated with central nervous system (CNS) lesions may also respond to anticonvulsants. Effects of liver enzyme induction by carbamazepine on other medications should be considered when the combination involves carbamazepine. For example, carbamazepine can decrease the serum levels of antipsychotics, TCAs, oral contraceptives, and warfarin, among others, and can increase the neurological side effects of lithium, probably necessitating a decrease in the lithium dose.

Fenfluramine (Pondimin)

Fenfluramine is an appetite suppressant with serotonin release and reuptake blocking properties. It is a central nervous system depressant in therapeutic doses. Fenfluramine is available in 20 mg scored tablets. Because of its sedating effects it should not be administered with sedating antidepressants. It is contraindicated with MAOIs or within 14 days of discontinuing an MAOI, due to risk of serotonergic crisis.

Occasional improvement in depression and anxiety symptoms have been observed when low doses of fenfluramine were administered with

SSRIs. Typically it is given at bedtime at a 10 to 20 mg dose when used as an antidepressant augmenter. If obesity is a coexisting condition, the administration of fenfluramine two hours prior to the evening meal may provide the added anorexigenic effect. Its serotonin-enhancing effects can interact with the serotonergic effects of SSRIs, leading to serotonin excess and resultant serotonin syndrome in rare cases (see Chapter 5 for a brief discussion of serotonin syndrome). Because of this, the author typically starts the patient on fenfluramine 10 mg (half of a 20 mg tablet), and if this dose is tolerated well for a week the dose is increased to 20 mg. Since the dosage used by the author for augmentation purposes is 20 mg, which is a very low dose, side effects and interaction problems have not occurred in the majority of patients. The recommended dosage range for use as an anorexiant is 20 to 40 mg TID. The *PDR* should be consulted for further pharmacological information. Since experience in the adjunctive use of fenfluramine is limited and since it can precipitate agitation in some patients, its cautious use should be limited to treatment-resistant patients. Moreover, because of the rare incidence of primary pulmonary hypertension due to fenfluramine treatment, it is currently considered a poor choice as an antidepressant augmentor.

Pindolol (Visken)

A recent report described the use of pindolol for antidepressant augmentation (Blier and Bergeron, 1995). Pindolol is a nonselective beta-adrenergic antagonist with serotonin reuptake blocking properties. The addition of pindolol 2.5 mg TID to ongoing SSRI antidepressant therapy produced rapid improvement in depression in most patients without alterations in blood pressure or pulse. Given its intrinsic serotonergic activity, concurrent administration with MAOIs is best avoided pending further studies and documented clinical experience.

DISCONTINUATION OF ANTIDEPRESSANTS

Although antidepressants are not addictive and hence can be technically discontinued abruptly, it is clinically prudent to taper them off slowly over a period of two to three weeks, if possible, unless termination of antidepressant treatment is due to side effects or toxicity, in which case discontinuation may be abrupt. Sudden discontinuation of antidepressants can cause nightmares, nausea, dizziness, headaches, and anxiety. This discontinuation syndrome is most pronounced for antidepressants with fairly short half-lives. The shorter the half-life of the antidepressant, the earlier the symptoms will emerge after discontinuation and the greater the severity. These symptoms are not serious or dangerous, and will usually subside on their own in four to six days. Table 2.3 gives the approximate time it takes for discontinuation syndrome to emerge after stopping various common antidepressants. For phenelzine, the discontinuation syndrome can be intense with severe anxiety, nightmares, and even confusion bordering on psychosis, in some cases; hence, a gradual taper is highly recommended when discontinuing patients from phenelzine.

With a slow taper, much of the patient discomfort associated with discontinuation syndrome can be avoided. If patients are warned of this possibility, they are more likely to tolerate these symptoms better, without panicking. The discontinuation syndrome can be minimized by switching the patient to another compatible antidepressant rapidly. For example, an SSRI can be started on the second or third day after stopping another SSRI or TCA; obviously, low starting doses are recommended to avoid the risk of interaction problems. Switching when a MAOI is involved must follow the guidelines briefly described in Chapter 4 on the use of phenelzine and tranylcypromine.

TABLE 2.3. Latency Period for Emergence of Antidepressant Discontinuation Syndrome

Antidepressant	Number of Days after Abruptly Stopping Antidepressant for Discontinuation Symptoms to Emerge	Usual Severity
venlafaxine	1-2 days	moderate
nefazodone	1-2 days	mild
paroxetine	2-3 days	moderate
fluvoxamine	2-3 days	mild
sertraline	3-5 days	mild
fluoxetine	7-10 days	very mild
imipramine	2-5 days	mild
desipramine	2-5 days	mild
nortriptyline	2-5 days	mild
clomipramine	2-5 days	mild
protriptyline	4-7 days	mild
phenelzine	1-3 days	severe
tranylcypromine	1-3 days	moderate

Chapter 3

Adjunctive Medications to Treat Symptoms That Do Not Respond to Antidepressant Treatment

DEPRESSION, LOSS OF APPETITE, AND WEIGHT LOSS

Loss of appetite and weight loss are commonly seen with depression and are also common side effects of serotonergic antidepressants, the first-line antidepressants in modern clinical practice because of their comparatively benign side effect profile. When a serotonergic antidepressant is started in a patient who is already anorectic, the weight loss may be undesirable, especially if the patient's baseline weight is in the optimal range. It should be noted that in most cases antidepressant-induced loss of appetite and weight loss are temporary and tend to plateau within two to three months of starting the medication. However, in some individuals, loss of appetite or weight loss are not desired or may persist beyond a desirable point. In these individuals, a serotonergic antidepressant can be combined with a TCA for appetite stimulation. Moreover, this combination may even enhance the antidepressant effects to some extent. Since the TCA dose needed to accomplish this is very low, side effects are usually tolerable. Some examples are listed below:

– Serotonergic antidepressant at therapeutic dose	+	amitriptyline 10 to 25 mg HS
		doxepin 10 to 25 mg HS
	+	nortriptyline 10 to 25 mg HS
– Bupropion at therapeutic dose		imipramine 10 to 25 mg HS
		desipramine 10 to 25 mg HS

Incidentally, the anorectic side effects of SSRIs and bupropion can be and have been exploited to help obese patients lose weight. With TCAs and MAOIs, weight gain rather than weight loss is the concern. Lithium, carbamazepine and valproic acid also can cause an increase in appetite. Although cyproheptadine (Periactin) is commonly used to increase appetite, it is not recommended in combination with serotonergic antidepressants, since its antiserotonin action can interfere with antidepressant activity except when used intermittently to reverse the sexual dysfunction caused by SSRIs. It should be noted that fluoxetine, paroxetine, and sertraline can lead to significant inhibition of the hepatic metabolism of TCAs and thereby can increase the plasma TCA levels. Since low doses of TCAs are typically employed when a combination regimen is prescribed, these interactions should not cause concerns regarding toxicity related to adverse interaction effects, except in the hepatically impaired and in the elderly.

DEPRESSION AND INSOMNIA

Since most TCAs have sedating properties in varying degrees, they are effective when insomnia is a symptom. Trazodone (Desyrel), mirtazapine (Remeron), and nefazodone (Serzone) also have similar effects. However, serotonergic antidepressants (except perhaps fluvoxamine) in the initial several weeks of treatment do not facilitate sleep; in fact, they may even cause insomnia. For this reason, they are typically prescribed for morning intake when initiated. Since most depressed patients suffer from insomnia and since serotonergic antidepressants are currently the first-line antidepressants, adjunctive medication is usually necessary. Effective combinations are:

– Serotonergic antidepressants (at therapeutic dose)	+	trazodone 50-150 mg HS
– Serotonergic antidepressants	+	benzodiazepines (lorazepam 0.5 mg HS) (temazepam 15 mg HS) (zolpidem 5-10 mg HS) (clonazepam 0.5 mg HS) (estazolam 1-2 mg HS) (quazepam 7.5-15 mg HS) (flurazepam 15 mg HS)

– Serotonergic antidepressants	+	sedating TCAs (amitriptyline 10 to 25 mg HS) (doxepin 10 to 25 mg HS) (trimipramine 25 mg HS)

In Cases of Severe Insomnia

– Serotonergic antidepressants	+	benzodiazepine
	+	trazodone 50-150 mg HS
– Serotonergic antidepressants	+	benzodiazepine + TCAs

All MAOIs can cause insomnia, in which case benzodiazepines are preferred as hypnotics. Benzodiazepines, however, are associated with problems such as tolerance and the risk of dependence. Therefore, they should be used only short term, and should be avoided in patients at risk for substance abuse. If benzodiazepine hypnotics are used long term, they are best used on an "as-needed" basis. For those who have chronic insomnia, the addition of trazodone or low doses of TCAs can help keep the dose of benzodiazepine hypnotics low. However, there are some patients who need a benzodiazepine hypnotic for the long term because other sleep aids are either ineffective or insufficient.

DEPRESSION AND ANERGIA

Antidepressants in most cases improve anergia along with other symptoms of depression, but occasionally anergia persists after resolution of other symptoms. Several antidepressants, including bupropion, fluoxetine, sertraline, protriptyline, desipramine, and tranylcypromine, are particularly effective if anergia is a prominent symptom. If monotherapy with one of these antidepressants fails to improve other symptoms of depression, it may be used adjunctively in a combination treatment regimen in an effort to obtain improvement of anergia as well as other symptoms of depression. The use of MAOIs in combination therapy is risky; it is best avoided. As in all cases, combinations are used only when a single medication cannot efficiently treat all of the symptoms. Examples of various combinations effective for improvement of anergia are as follows:

– Serotonergic antidepressants	+	bupropion 75 to 100 mg BID
– Tricyclic antidepressants	+	dextroamphetamine 5 to 10 mg BID
		methylphenidate 5 to 10 mg BID

DEPRESSION AND ANXIETY

Depression and anxiety often coexist. In most such cases effective treatment of depression using an antidepressant medication eventually controls anxiety. Occasionally, anxiety symptoms persist despite adequate treatment of the depression. Serotonergic antidepressants and bupropion can cause anxiety and restlessness, especially in the first several weeks of treatment; hence, adjunctive use of benzodiazepines may be necessary on an as-needed basis. Only rarely does a patient need standing antianxiety medications, in which case buspirone (Buspar) is the drug of choice. Since buspirone's antianxiety effect is fairly mild, it may not be sufficient for patients with intense anxiety. However, buspirone can eliminate the need for or help decrease the dose of benzodiazepines, if the anxiety is mild. Since buspirone has a one- to two-week latency period and is not acutely effective for anxiety, patients should be instructed to take buspirone regularly and to expect a delay of several weeks for onset of action. The recommended benzodiazepine dosage is as follows:

- Lorazepam 0.5 mg BID-TID as needed (PRN)
- Alprazolam 0.25 to 0.5 mg TID PRN
- Clonazepam 0.25 to 0.5 mg BID PRN (lowest strength tablet is a scored 0.5 mg tablet)

Clonazepam, in particular, should be withdrawn gradually because of a tendency to cause withdrawal seizures. Their potential for tolerance makes benzodiazepines less effective when taken regularly for several months, necessitating dosage escalation to maintain efficacy.

DEPRESSION AND DECREASED LIBIDO

Decreased libido is a common symptom of depression. Unfortunately, most of the antidepressants also cause a decrease in libido as a medication side effect. In addition, antidepressants interfere with sexual functioning by inhibiting orgasm and ejaculation, and by inhibiting pleasurable bodily sensation. Impotence, though less common, may also be a side effect. Serotonergic antidepressants and MAOIs are particularly implicated in causing sexual dysfunction, with TCAs having intermediate effects and antidepressants such as bupropion, trazodone, nefazodone, and mirtazapine having the least deleterious effects on sexual functioning. Further details on each of these drugs are given in Chapter 4.

Since serotonergic antidepressants are the first-line antidepressants currently, it is to be expected that sexual side effects will be common. Given such a high incidence of sexual side effects associated with serotonergic medications, why are they used as the first-line medications? Why not use bupropion, nefazodone, and trazodone as the first-line medications? In general, serotonergic antidepressants are as effective as TCAs and MAOIs but are devoid of the anticholinergic, antihistaminic, cardiovascular, and hypotensive side effects. In the author's experience, bupropion, nefazodone, and trazodone have only intermediate efficacy in severe depression, though they are excellent choices for treatment of mild to moderate depression. Trazodone as a single medication needs to be given at high doses (for example at 400 to 500 mg per day) for antidepressant efficacy. At this dosage, sedation and orthostatic hypertension can become excessive, limiting its usefulness. To some extent, nefazodone shares similar problems. With bupropion the dosage ceiling of 450 mg per day, a strict interdose interval requirement, as well as the necessary TID schedule at the higher dosage range, affect compliance and usefulness in severe depressions where high doses are typically needed. (A sustained-release form of bupropion currently pending FDA approval could eliminate this drawback, and its clinical profile is summarized in Chapter 4.)

There is no point in trying to sustain or improve sexual functioning at the expense of effectively treating the more disabling symptoms of depression. Bupropion, nefazodone, mirtazapine, and trazodone are effective in treating mild to moderate depressions seen in office settings, depending on presenting symptoms and individual tolerance, and hence should be considered among the first-line antidepressants. (Descriptions of individual clinical profiles of each of these antidepressants are discussed in Chapter 4.) There are several medications available to treat sexual dysfunction; however, the effectiveness of these medications is low:

– Primary antidepressant	+	yohimbine 5.4 mg TID
		amantadine 100 mg BID-TID
		bupropion 100 mg at noon or 75 mg AM and at noon
		bethanechol 25 mg BID-TID or two hours before coitus
		cyproheptadine 4 to 8 mg two hours before coitus
		trazodone 50 to 150 mg HS
		nefazodone 100 to 200 mg HS

methylphenidate 10 to 20 mg two hours before coitus

dextroamphetamine 5 to 15 mg two hours before coitus

pemoline 37.5 to 75 mg daily

Patients who are concerned about sexual dysfunction due to depression or due to antidepressant side effects should be advised that since the chance of success with any one of these adjunctive medications is low, they should persevere and be willing to tolerate the frustration inherent in the systematic sequential trial of several of these medications. If the patient is cooperative and the physician is diligent, at least some improvement in sexual functioning can be achieved with the addition of one of the medications listed above. Obviously, it is preferable for the patient to be switched to an antidepressant that has no sexual side effects such as mirtazapine. Unfortunately, this is not possible in most cases of severe depression, thereby leaving the physician to resort to the use of adjunctive medications. If the depression is mild to moderate and if sexual dysfunction is a concern, try bupropion, mirtazapine, nefazodone, trazodone, or TCAs. Drug "holidays" or "vacations" intended to restore sexual functioning during these holidays may be mostly ineffective when taking drugs that have fairly long half-lives unless the drug-free period is for more than several days. Furthermore, there is a risk of emergence of withdrawal symptoms or relapse if the drug has a short half-life. However, for patients with mild symptoms, drug holidays might temporarily improve sexual functioning without significantly affecting the drug's efficacy.

DEPRESSION AND PSYCHOTIC SYMPTOMS

Depressive and psychotic symptoms occur together in varying degrees of intensity in a variety of conditions, including major depression with psychotic features, schizoaffective disorder, and bipolar disorder. "Delusional depression" and "psychotic depression" are still commonly used names for major depression with psychotic features. As emphasized throughout the text, regardless of the diagnostic terminology in current use, treatment is directed toward the symptoms. Hence, if psychotic symptoms are present, they should be treated. In general, if psychotic symptoms are severe in intensity, the dosage of medication needed will probably be higher than if the psychotic symptoms are mild.

Since the presence of mild psychotic symptoms is difficult to diagnose and as a result is often missed even by psychiatrists, a detailed discussion is warranted. Most severe depressions are associated with irrational thinking: irrational guilt, irrational pessimism, the desire to be punished, somatic complaints, and an extreme sense of despair and hopelessness that has no basis in reality. Such patients should be treated with low doses of antipsychotics for the first several weeks in addition to full antidepressant doses. Suicide based on irrational thinking is a serious risk during the initial treatment phase in patients with severe depression, even when psychotic symptoms are not obvious. The presence of suicide risk outweighs any concerns regarding antipsychotic side effects, especially when low doses for one to three weeks are used in most cases. Hence, the prudent clinical approach in treating a severely depressed patient is to err on the side of caution, and to have a low threshold for using low doses of antipsychotics temporarily if irrational thinking is present or suspected, even if the symptoms do not reach obvious psychotic intensity. Suicides and homicides of loved ones are at times committed by patients with severe depression and untreated underlying psychosis that is well-guarded by the patient. These patients' initial presentation may indicate only severe depression. The antipsychotic, when used, should be rapidly tapered off as the depression is lifted, and the patient should continue on the antidepressants. In patients with obvious psychotic symptoms, the duration of antipsychotic treatment and the dose are usually greater. Some of these patients may need to stay on an antipsychotic medication chronically.

The favorable side effect profile of olanzapine and risperidone should make them the first-line antipsychotics of choice in current psychiatric practice. For mild psychotic symptoms, the effective dose of risperidone could be as low as 0.5 mg daily. In elderly patients and in brain-injury cases, even 0.25 mg (one-quarter of a 1 mg tablet) may be sufficient. Psychotic symptoms associated with predominantly depressive symptoms can be managed on risperidone 0.5 to 2 mg per day, along with full antidepressant doses. Olanzapine dose range for mild psychotic symptoms associated with depressive disorders is 2.5 to 5 mg, preferrably given at bedtime. For moderate to severe psychotic symptoms, olanzapine dosage range is 5 to 20 mg HS. Refer to Chapter 11 for detailed clinical profiles of all currently available antipsychotics.

Extreme hostility with tendencies to externalize blame should be treated as a psychotic symptom for clinical purposes, though eventually serotonergic antidepressants should control anger and hostility, enabling antipsychotics to be tapered off. Once the anger is controlled, most patients are able to benefit from psychotherapy, thereby gaining insight and increased self-awareness.

DEPRESSION AND ADULT ATTENTION DEFICIT DISORDER

When depression and attention deficit disorder (ADD) are present in a patient, a combination of an antidepressant and a stimulant medication may become necessary. Bupropion and venlafaxine are sometimes effective in treating both conditions. Many adult ADD patients who respond well to stimulants are also depressed, with symptoms such as decreased frustration tolerance, increased irritability, and moodiness. Typical combinations for treatment are the following:

– Serotonergic antidepressants	+	methylphenidate SR 20 mg AM or BID
		dextroamphetamine 5-15 mg BID
		pemoline 37.5 mg-112.5 mg daily

If bupropion and stimulants are used, the dose of bupropion should not exceed 300 mg per day in three divided doses because of the increased risk of seizures posed by the combination.

Some of the adult ADD symptoms such as poor concentration, distractibility, poor attention span, impatience, poor memory retention, difficulty completing tasks, and restlessness are also symptoms that can occur with depressive disorder, anxiety disorder, and manic episodes. In some cases it is difficult to make a diagnosis based on clinical evaluation alone. In these cases, a trial on stimulants is warranted. Although stimulants have a nonspecific positive effect on cognitive functions in most individuals, the effect on people with ADD is marked, both cognitively and behaviorally; for those with other disorders, stimulants usually cause behavioral effects such as restlessness, insomnia, anxiety, and anorexia.

A history of substance abuse is a relative contraindication for treatment using stimulants that have high abuse potential. In these patients, pemoline, bupropion, clonidine, guanfacine, desipramine, imipramine, venlafaxine, or tranylcypromine should be considered.

DEPRESSION AND HISTORY OF MANIA

Depressed patients who have a history of mania or hypomania usually need treatment using a combination of antidepressants and mood stabilizers. The most common mood stabilizer is lithium, followed by valproic acid, lamotrigine, carbamazepine, and gabapentin. Verapamil, clonazepam, and clonidine are sometimes helpful. Combinations of an antidepressant and a mood stabilizer are frequently used because most patients with a manic or hypomanic episode, organic mood disorder, dysphoric mania, or schizoaffective disorder will eventually need an antidepressant to treat depressive symptoms. More than one mood stabilizer can be used if one medication is not sufficient to control symptoms. Common combinations of mood stabilizers are as follows:

- Lithium + Carbamazepine
- Lithium + Valproic acid
- Lithium + Clonazepam
- Lithium + Verapamil
- Carbamazepine + Verapamil
- Lithium + Lamotrigine
- Lithium + Gabapentin

Drug interaction and increased side effects should be kept in mind. Slower-than-usual dosage increments and more frequent laboratory monitoring of serum levels are recommended when combinations are used, especially when one or more medications have a narrow therapeutic range, as is the case with lithium.

It should be noted that carbamazepine, being a tricyclic compound, theoretically has the potential to cause a serotonergic crisis when coadministered with MAOIs. However, in the author's experience of treating several patients on an MAOI-carbamazepine combination, no hyperthermic or serotonergic crises have been observed. Patients tolerated the combination well and it was found clinically effective in most cases. Obviously when any combination involving an MAOI is used, low starting doses and smaller-than-usual dosage increments are typically employed.

Chapter 4

Practical Clinical Profiles of Antidepressant Medications: Advantages and Disadvantages

INTRODUCTORY STATEMENTS

All antidepressants and stimulants in current clinical use are discussed with a clinical focus. A summary of advantages and disadvantages is listed for each antidepressant. Cost analyses and cost comparisons are given for the more expensive SSRIs. Practical strategies for the management of antidepressant side effects are described in Chapter 5. For the elderly and medically ill, dosage should be reduced by one-third to one-half of the usual starting and maintenance doses recommended for healthy adults. In general, for the elderly, a longer interval between dosage escalation and smaller dosage increments are also prudent.

BUPROPION (WELLBUTRIN)

Bupropion is a norepinephrinergic antidepressant with mild dopaminergic properties and a half-life of approximately ten hours. It is metabolized by the liver and primarily excreted by the kidneys. The dosage range is between 100 mg and 450 mg. The maximum single dose is 150 mg and the maximum total daily dose is 450 mg. It is available in 75 mg and 100 mg tablets. Though it is not scored, it can be easily divided using a pill splitter to obtain lower doses. Several elderly patients have shown adequate response at a dose as low as 50 mg daily.

Bupropion is particularly effective for patients presenting with symptoms such as anergia, apathy, psychomotor retardation, poor concentration, anhedonia, loss of interest in activities that were once enjoyable, and depressed mood. It is also a good choice for patients who have depression associated with bipolar disorder, hypomania, and cyclothymia, since it may not increase "cycling" as frequently as other antidepressants, and for depressed patients with attention deficit symptoms.

If the highest single dose of 150 mg is used, a dosing interval of six hours is recommended to decrease the risk of seizure due to peak drug levels that can lower the seizure threshold. Since bupropion decreases the seizure threshold at twice the rate of other antidepressants, the single maximum dose limit of 150 mg and daily total maximum limit of 450 mg should be strictly followed. The estimate of seizures reported in the *PDR* is 4 per 1,000 for bupropion and approximately 2 per 1,000 for other antidepressants. Bupropion is started in outpatients at 75 to 100 mg po AM and at noon for one week. If there is no adequate response, the dosage is increased to 100 mg po AM, at noon, and at 5 p.m. for one week. If side effects such as anxiety, headache, or insomnia develop, symptomatic treatment is appropriate. For example, for anxiety, lorazepam 0.5 mg po up to TID, or alprazolam 0.25 mg to 0.5 mg po up to TID may be used. For insomnia, lorazepam 0.5 mg po hs, zolpidem 5 mg to 10 mg po hs, or temazepam 15 mg to 30 mg po hs may be tried.

If, after one week, there is no adequate response to bupropion 100 mg po TID, and if side effects are not significant, the dosage may be increased to 150 mg po TID with specific advice to take the doses with a minimum six-hour interval between doses. The last dose should be taken before 6 or 7 p.m. to decrease the chance that bupropion will interfere with sleep. When side effects become intolerable and cannot be managed, further dosage increase should not be attempted and consideration should be given to discontinuing the medication.

Since bupropion is not available in generic form at the time of this writing, a patient who takes 150 mg po TID will need to take two 75 mg tablets to get a 150 mg dose, needing a total of six tablets a day. At 60 cents a pill, the total daily cost will be approximately $3.60, and the monthly cost at approximately $108.

A history of seizures and bulimia/anorexia are contraindications to prescribing bupropion. Patients taking bupropion should be made aware of seizure precautions, dosage limits, and the necessity of avoiding alcohol. They should also be instructed to avoid activities that could decrease seizure threshold, such as sleep deprivation. The fact that the patient was instructed on the above precautions should be noted on the chart. Though seizure by itself is not a serious incident–it may even improve depression–it can be dangerous and fatal, depending on the context in which it occurs. If the patient is not warned of the dosage limits and of the relatively higher risk of seizure while taking bupropion, the physician may be held liable, should injury occur due to seizure. If they forget to administer a dose, many patients will double the next dose to catch up. A patient taking bupropion 100 mg po BID, TID, or QID should be *specifically* advised *not* to take two tablets together to "catch up," since a 200 mg dose exceeds the single dose maximum of 150 mg. Bupropion has been successfully used for treatment of attention deficit hyperactivity disorder (ADHD) at generally lower doses compared to the dosage for treatment of depression. Its energizing and antidepressant properties might possibly be exploited to assist patients coping with nicotine withdrawal in the context of participation in a multidisciplinary smoking cessation program. The sustained-release formulation of bupropion is probably a safer option for this purpose, compared to the regular (immediate-release) formulation.

Bupropion is remarkably devoid of any deleterious effects on libido or sexual performance. Given the high prevalence of sexual side effects associated with serotonergic antidepressants and MAOIs, and the moderate prevalence with TCAs, bupropion has a distinct advantage in this respect. I have found occasional success in partially restoring sexual function and libido in patients by adding a low dose of bupropion (at doses of 75 to 100 mg po BID) to a serotonergic antidepressant. However, the success rate of this intervention is not high. Bupropion can also be adjunctively added at low doses if the primary antidepressant fails to improve anergia. It should be remembered that the addition of bupropion has the potential to decrease seizure threshold, especially if the patient is on a TCA, which can independently decrease seizure threshold relatively more than serotonergic medications. Hence, the dose of bupropion should not exceed 200 mg per day in divided doses, and the dose of the primary antidepressant should not be at the maximum dose, when combination treatment is attempted, in the author's opinion. Adjunctive use of bupropion with clomipramine (Anafranil) should be attempted cautiously since clomipramine by itself decreases seizure threshold appreciably.

Summary of Advantages and Disadvantages of Bupropion

Advantages

- Effective for atypical depression or mild to moderate depression
- Does not cause sexual dysfunction
- Low anticholinergic side effects
- Low cardiovascular side effects

- Relatively low GI side effects
- Can be used for treatment of ADHD
- Effective for anergia, hypersomnia, apathy, and psychomotor retardation
- Possibly does not increase "cycling" in bipolar depression
- May be occasionally effective in partially restoring sexual function in patients who have sexual dysfunction due to antidepressant treatment
- FDA pregnancy category B

Disadvantages

- Need for strict dose adherence because of seizure risk
- Need for multiple dosing can affect compliance
- Relatively higher incidence of headaches
- Relatively higher incidence of insomnia and anxiety
- Contraindicated in patients with a history of seizure or who are predisposed to seizures or in patients with bulimia/anorexia
- Relatively high cost since several pills are required

BUPROPION SUSTAINED-RELEASE (WELLBUTRIN SR)

A sustained-release formulation of bupropion is expected to be introduced as 100 and 150 mg dose tablets in December 1996. The sustained-release form has a more convenient BID schedule compared to the currently available immediate-release form which has a TID-QID dosing schedule, making it very inconvenient for most patients to adhere to. Furthermore, the immediate-release form carries a seizure risk slightly higher than that of TCAs. The sustained-release tablet is expected to overcome these problems. BID schedule recommended for the sustained-release form requires a minimum interval of eight hours between doses. The maximum single dose for the sustained-release formulation is 200 mg, and maximum daily dose is 200 mg BID (total 400 mg). Compared to the immediate-release form, the sustained-release form provides lower peak bupropion plasma levels and less variability in peak and trough steady-state bupropion plasma concentration. Therefore, the seizure risk of the sustained-release formulation is expected to be lower than that of the immediate-release form of bupropion, and might even bring the seizure risk down to the lower levels typically associated with TCAs.

The starting dose may be either 150 mg AM or 100 mg BID. The dose may be increased to 150 mg BID and, if necessary, eventually to 200 mg

BID after one to two weeks on a fixed dose. Various dosing regimens are possible within the general dosing guidelines mentioned previously, depending on individual patient needs and characteristics. Some dosing examples are given below.

Bupropion SR dose	Possible clinical applications
100, 150, or 200 mg AM	Elderly, adjunctive use in a combination regimen, mild depression, ADHD, medically ill patients
150 mg BID or 200 mg BID	major depression, dysthymia, ADHD

The dose of the sustained-release form is comparable to the immediate-release form dose except that the maximum recommended sustained-release dose is 200 mg BID (total 400 mg per day), whereas the maximum recommended immediate-relase dose is 150 mg TID (total 450 mg per day). The side effects reported for the sustained-release formulation are dry mouth, tremor, sweating, and tinnitus. Based on the experience with immediate-release formulation of bupropion and that of sustained-release formulations of other medications, transient side effects such as headache, nausea, hypermotility of the GI tract, and insomnia if the second dose is taken close to bedtime are possibilities. However, widespread clinical use is necessary to completely identify the side effect profile of the sustained-release formulation or any new drug. Combining sustained-release and immediate-release forms is not recommended due to the probability that an immediate-release form could increase the peak plasma bupropion in a patient also taking the sustained-release form, thereby nullifying the improved safety profile of the sustained-release form with regard to seizure risk.

In summary, the sustained-release form is an improvement over the immediate-release form because of decreased seizure risk due to lower peak bupropion plasma levels and a more convenient BID schedule which should result in better patient compliance. The medication cost is expected to be comparable to the immediate-release form.

Summary of Advantages and Disadvantages of Bupropion Sustained-Release

Advantages

– Effective for depression, particularly if anergia, hypersomnia, apathy, or psychomotor retardation is present

- Can be used for treatment of ADHD
- Does not cause sexual dysfunction
- Low anticholinergic side effects
- Low cardiovascular side effects
- Possibly does not increase cycling in bipolar patients
- May be occassionaly effective in partially alleviating antidepressant induced sexual dysfunction, and possibly as an aid to smoking cessation
- FDA pregnancy category B

Disadvantages

- BID dosing, though an improvement over the immediate-release form, can still affect patient compliance to some extent
- At the higher dose range, insomnia, anxiety, and headache can potentially be side effects, although these were not frequent in premarketing trials
- Seizure risk at 200 mg BID was not studied in premarketing trials; theoretically, the seizure risk of sustained-release formulation is expected to be lower than that of the immediate-release formulation even at the highest recommended sustained-release dose
- Contraindicated in patients with a history of seizures or bulimia/anorexia

FLUOXETINE (PROZAC)

Fluoxetine is a serotonergic antidepressant with antianxiety and anti-obsessive-compulsive effects. It has a half-life of two to three days, and is 95 percent plasma protein bound. The active metabolite norfluoxetine has a half-life of six to eight days. It is metabolized by the liver and excreted by the kidneys. It is available in 10 mg and 20 mg capsules and in liquid form.

The dosage range is from 10 mg to 80 mg, although most patients respond between a 20 mg and 60 mg dose. In rare instances, a dose of 100 mg has been necessary for effectiveness. All of the serotonergic medications are much safer than TCAs in overdose. Fluoxetine is as effective as TCAs, and its side effects are more tolerable than those of TCAs. It has minimal anticholinergic and cardiovascular side effects. The common side effects associated with fluoxetine are nausea, anxiety, insomnia, loss of appetite, sexual dysfunction, mild jaw and neck muscle stiffness, and headaches. Paradoxically, it is used for treatment of intractable headaches. All of the side effects except sexual dysfunction tend to improve over a few weeks. There are fairly successful and simple interventions to deal with all of the common side effects; each of these will be explained later.

Fluoxetine has proven to be particularly effective in patients with anger outbursts, irritability, moodiness, crying spells, excessive emotional sensitivity, obsessive or compulsive characteristics, irrational fears, hypochondriasis, anergia, hypersomnia, anxiety attacks, and hyperphagia. In obsessive-compulsive disorder, the doses tend to be at the higher range, usually 60 mg to 80 mg per day. Fluoxetine is typically started at 20 mg po AM after breakfast because an evening dose interferes with sleep in most patients. Patients should be informed of possible short-term nausea, anxiety, insomnia, heartburn, and sexual dysfunction. They should be assured that, in the majority of patients, most of these side effects subside in seven to ten days. If side effects persist, there are simple and effective medication interventions. In some patients, fluoxetine causes mild sedation and yawning, in which case it may be given at bedtime.

In generalized anxiety disorder, fluoxetine is usually given in low doses, at 5 mg to 20 mg daily. The liquid form is very convenient when an intermediate dose or a dose lower than 10 mg is indicated. Anxiety and an akathisia-like symptom can be initial side effects of fluoxetine, for which short-term adjunctive prescription of benzodiazepines may be needed. Fluoxetine can also be effective in patients with hypochondriasis and somatization disorders, which have anxiety and obsessive features as underlying symptoms.

Summary of Advantages and Disadvantages of Fluoxetine

Advantages

- Lack of TCA/MAOI side effects
- Effective for depression, OCD, anxiety, bulimia/anorexia, etc.
- Does not produce weight gain in most patients
- Mild to moderate energizing effects
- Good safety profile for patients with cardiovascular problems
- Long half-life is advantageous should patients forget to take medication occasionally
- Once-a-day administration
- Side effects are usually mild and tend to subside over time

- Tends to cause fewer GI side effects compared to other serotonergic medications
- Safety in overdose

Disadvantages

- Causes insomnia and weight loss in some patients
- Long half-life makes it difficult to switch to other medications, e.g., switching to an MAOI requires a five- to six-week wait
- Causes sexual dysfunction (decreased libido, orgasmic and ejaculatory inhibition, and erectile difficulties) in about 60 percent of patients
- High cost of medication due to a lack of availability of higher dosage strength; many patients need two to three 20 mg capsules per day, costing $100 to $150 per month
- Initial negative publicity related to a number of unsuccessful lawsuits (both criminal defense and product liability) claiming that fluoxetine induced suicidal and/or homicidal behavior, causing resistance in some patients which is sometimes difficult to overcome despite reassurance (however, lately the patient resistance has largely subsided and should not be a concern for the prescribing physician)
- High protein binding causes displacement of other medications with high protein binding, and vice versa (although in most cases, this is not clinically significant)

SERTRALINE (ZOLOFT)

Sertraline is a serotonergic antidepressant that is effective and FDA-approved for treatment of depression and obsession-compulsive disorder. FDA approval for treatment of panic disorder is pending. It can also be used for treatment of other conditions, such as anxiety disorder and bulimia/anorexia. Sertraline and its active metabolites have a combined half-life of approximately one to three days. It is about 98 percent protein bound. Sertraline is metabolized by the liver and excreted by the kidneys. It can be given once a day, usually in the morning with breakfast, to minimize possible GI irritation and insomnia.

Sertraline has side effects similar to fluoxetine and other SSRIs. However, in the author's experience, it tends to cause nausea and dyspepsia slightly more often than fluoxetine, paroxetine, nefazodone, and fluvoxamine. Therefore, the author's practice is to recommend antacids or H_2 blockers during the first week of sertraline treatment. Anxiety and insomnia as initial side effects are also seen, but probably less frequently compared to fluoxetine. Other side effects such as decreased libido, ejaculatory and orgasmic inhibition, insomnia, and slight decrease in appetite are similar to fluoxetine. It should be used with caution in patients taking terfanadine, astemizole, or cisapride due to hepatic enzyme inhibition leading to potential for QT prolongation. Loratadine (claritin) does not cause significant interaction with sertraline.

It is available in scored tablets in 50 mg and 100 mg strength. The usual dosage range is 50 to 200 mg, with the maximum recommended dose being 200 mg. The majority of patients tend to respond optimally at 100 mg, given as a one-time dose in the morning with breakfast to minimize GI side effects and insomnia. Those with generalized anxiety disorder tend to respond at lower dose, such as the 25 to 50 mg range, and those with obsessive-compulsive disorder tend to need dosages in the upper ranges such as 200 mg, with most depressions responding in the midrange at 100 to 150 mg. Several of the patients who the author had to treat at 300 mg were patients with obsessive-compulsive disorder. Patients who responded at the 300 mg dosage tolerated the medication without significant side effects, except decreased libido and anorgasmia, which can occur at any dosage range.

The cost advantage of sertraline, since it is available in scored tablets at 50 mg and 100 mg dosages is significant when compared to fluoxetine. The cost of a sertraline 100 mg pill is $60 per month, whereas fairly equivalent doses of fluoxetine at 40 mg (consisting of two 20 mg capsules) will cost about $100 per month, a cost savings of approximately $40 per month at current prices. Those who do well on sertraline 50 mg daily can realize further cost savings by obtaining 100 mg tablets and dividing them.

Any medication in tablet form can be similarly divided, in individual cases, if cost saving can be achieved, except for some of the slow-release preparations in which breaking a tablet can possibly affect the controlled-release function.

Summary of Advantages and Disadvantages of Sertraline

Advantages

- Effective for depression, anxiety, obsessions, compulsions, bulimia, etc.
- Better side effect profile compared to TCAs and MAOIs
- Once-a-day dosing

- Cost advantages as described above
- Flexibility of scored tablet
- Patients with cardiovascular problems are not affected
- Side effects are usually mild and tend to subside over time
- Safety in overdose

Disadvantages

- Slightly higher incidence of nausea and dyspepsia, compared to fluoxetine, but less than venlafaxine (Effexor)
- Sexual dysfunction similar to all other serotonergic medications (approximately 60 percent of patients)
- High protein binding causes displacement of other medications with high protein binding and vice versa (this is not clinically significant in most cases)

PAROXETINE (PAXIL)

Paroxetine is a serotonergic antidepressant with a half-life of 20 hours and 95 percent plasma-protein binding. It is available as tablets in scored 20 mg and unscored 10, 30, and 40 mg strength. The dosage range is between 10 mg and 60 mg. Most people respond to dosages in the 30 mg to 40 mg range. It has no active metabolites. Paroxetine has been found to be effective for the treatment of depression, anxiety disorders, obsessive-compulsive disorder, and bulimia. It is formally approved by the FDA for treatment of depression, obsessive-compulsive disorder, and panic disorder.

Paroxetine can be administered once a day, usually with breakfast to minimize possible GI irritation. It is a more potent serotonin reuptake inhibitor than either fluoxetine or sertraline. In clinical experience, paroxetine tends to have relatively less GI irritation compared to sertraline. The incidence of anxiety as a side effect is less compared to fluoxetine or sertraline. Hence, it is well-suited for patients with anxiety disorder, panic disorders, and obsessive-compulsive disorder, although all serotonergic antidepressants have excellent antianxiety effects. Insomnia as a side effect is also relatively less frequent. However, relatively greater incidence of sexual side effects such as decreased libido and inhibited orgasm are seen with paroxetine in clinical experience, compared to all other antidepressants, with the possible exception of clomipramine (Anafranil) and MAOIs. This is a subtle clinical distinction and therefore may not be pronounced enough to be considered as a factor in choosing among various SSRIs.

Since paroxetine's half-life is only 20 hours, patients could experience relapse of depression and anxiety, with increased likelihood of withdrawal symptoms such as nausea, GI upset, dizziness, and headaches if even a few doses are missed. Therefore, the patient should be instructed to remember to take the medication daily. Rarely, patients experience emergence of depression and anxiety symptoms approximately 12 to 16 hours after the morning dose, in which case, half or one-third of the morning dose can be administered in late afternoon, which usually controls this problem effectively. When withdrawing from paroxetine, patients should be instructed to taper off by gradually decreasing doses over a period of five to eight days to minimize withdrawal symptoms. If the medication must be stopped abruptly for any reason, reassure the patient that the withdrawal symptoms may be uncomfortable but are not serious. These symptoms generally subside in three to five days. Symptomatic treatment using benzodiazepines or antinausea medications–depending on the specific withdrawal symptom–may help.

The availability of paroxetine tablets in four different strengths should enable flexible dosing and some cost savings for patients. At a cost of $2 per pill, a patient taking paroxetine 30 mg daily–which is fairly equivalent to 40 mg of fluoxetine (Prozac) and 100 mg of sertraline (Zoloft)–will have to spend approximately $60 per month, making paroxetine comparable to sertraline but less expensive than fluoxetine.

Paroxetine is usually started at 20 mg every morning, preferably after breakfast, with a 10 mg increase every two weeks, up to 60 mg to achieve maximum response. For some patients, the dose must be increased to 80 mg (preferably given as one 40 mg dose in the morning and at noon), although 60 mg is the maximum recommended by the drug manufacturer. As with all medications, if intolerable side effects emerge and if they cannot be adequately managed, paroxetine should be discontinued in favor of trying another medication.

Summary of Advantages and Disadvantages of Paroxetine

Advantages

- Effective for depression, anxiety disorders, obsessions, compulsions, eating disorders, and other SSRI indications
- Lack of TCA/MAOI side effects
- No significant weight gain
- No significant GI side effects
- Less incidence of anxiety as a side effect
- Does not commonly cause insomnia
- Safer in overdose, compared to TCAs, bupropion, and MAOIs
- No active metabolites

- Flexible and convenient once-a-day dosing in scored tablet form (the 10, 30, and 40 mg pills are not scored, but can be easily divided)
- Does not have significant cardiovascular side effects
- Fairly short half-life enables more expeditious switch to other medications
- Clinically significant drug interactions due to hepatic enzyme inhibitors or induction are rare

Disadvantages

- Slightly higher incidence of sexual dysfunction (estimated 65 to 70 percent), compared to other SSRIs (estimated 60 to 65 percent) based on the author's clinical observations. This difference may not be statistically significant
- Greater protein binding can displace other drugs that are highly protein bound (although not clinically significant in most cases)
- Short half-life tends to lead to rapid reemergence of depressive/anxiety symptoms and/or emergence of withdrawal symptoms if patient misses medication for several days or abruptly stops taking medication

VENLAFAXINE (EFFEXOR)

The antidepressant venlafaxine is a serotonin and norepinephrine reuptake inhibitor with a half-life of approximately five hours and plasma protein binding of about 28 percent. It is available as scored tablets in quite a range of doses at 25 mg, 37.5 mg, 50 mg, 75 mg, and 100 mg. Its serotonergic and norepinephrinergic actions make it truly a "broad-spectrum" antidepressant much like imipramine. In clinical practice, venlafaxine appears to be as effective as imipramine, other TCAs, and MAOIs in the treatment of depression. However, the significant advantage of venlafaxine, compared to TCAs and MAOIs, is the lack of TCA side effects. It tends to cause mild elevation in blood pressure; hence, regular blood pressure monitoring is recommended for those who have hypertension or borderline hypertension, especially in the initial three to four weeks of beginning treatment and after each dose increase.

The effective dosage range is between 75 mg and 300 mg in two or three divided doses. The maximum recommended dose is 375 mg per day in divided doses. Venlafaxine weakly inhibits reuptake of dopamine at the higher dosage range although the clinical significance of this phenomenon is not clear. The author has no experience in treating patients at higher than the maximum dosage of 375 mg per day in divided doses.

The theoretical advantage of venlafaxine is its broad spectrum activity and hence the likelihood that it will treat depression that is mediated by serotonin as well as norepinephrine. There is a claim that venlafaxine tends to energize patients due to its activity on the norepinephrine neurotransmitter system. From the author's clinical experience in treating in excess of 100 patients on venlafaxine so far, with some of them at 375 mg a day, the energizing effects are comparable to other energizing serotonergic medications such as fluoxetine and sertraline. In this respect, theoretical expectation and clinical experience correlate only to a limited extent. The incidence of nausea and dyspepsia seems to be slightly higher compared to other serotonergic antidepressants, with the incidence of sexual side effects similar to other SSRIs. Prophylactic administration of antacids or H_2 blockers during the first week of venlafaxine therapy could reduce the incidence of GI side effects.

The scored tablet and multiple-strength format allow flexible dosing, enabling some cost advantages for the patient, especially at the lower dosage range, where a 100 mg strength tablet at a cost of approximately $1.25 can be divided for twice-a-day dosing. Venlafaxine at a dose of 200 mg per day will cost approximately $57 per month, as compared to a fairly equivalent dose of fluoxetine at 40 mg per day costing $100 per month, sertraline at 100 mg daily costing approximately $60 per month, and paroxetine at 30 mg daily costing approximately $60 per month, thus making venlafaxine one of the least expensive of the new generation of antidepressants. Since most patients respond at 150 mg per day or less and since scored tablets up to 100 mg strength are available, the cost savings is even greater.

Venlafaxine is usually started at 25 mg three times a day with meals, to minimize gastrointestinal side effects. This can be prescribed as 25 mg po TID or 50 mg one-half tablet po TID. Higher starting doses increase the chance of GI side effects. Further dose increases at a rate of 75 mg per week may be attempted every week until satisfactory clinical response is seen or side effects interfere with treatment, up to the maximum dose of 375 mg per day in divided doses.

Since venlafaxine tends to work somewhat faster, if no improvement is found on a steady dose in a week, a further dose increase of 50 to 75 mg per week may be attempted. There are a few patients who may respond at very low doses such as 25 mg to 50 mg taken as a one-time dose. Venlafaxine does not frequently cause insomnia and in a fair number of cases, has been found to improve sleep, making a bedtime dose appropriate. Since venlafaxine binds protein at only 28 percent, it does not alter the serum levels of other drugs that are highly protein bound; this is an advantage compared to other serotonergic drugs, all of which are highly protein bound.

Since venlafaxine has a short half-life, multiple dosing is needed. This characteristic increases the chances of emergence of withdrawal symptoms on abrupt discontinuation of the medication. Gradual tapering over five to seven days is recommended. Greater patient motivation is required for compliance with multiple dosing schedules.

Summary of Advantages and Disadvantages of Venlafaxine

Advantages

- Broad spectrum of activity
- Effective in treatment of depression, atypical depression, anxiety disorders, obsessive-compulsive disorder, bulimia, etc.
- Low protein binding, offering increased safety in use with patients on medications that are highly bound to plasma protein
- Possible faster onset of action
- Cost advantage and dosing flexibility; at low dosage ranges, venlafaxine is the least expensive of the serotonergic antidepressants, making it the "best buy" in the author's cost comparison
- Lack of TCA/MAOI side effects
- No significant weight gain
- No active metabolites
- Safer in overdose, compared to TCA/MAOI or bupropion
- Short half-life enables faster switch to other medications such as MAOIs
- Clinically significant drug interactions due to hepatic enzyme inhibitors or induction are rare

Disadvantages

- Nausea and dyspepsia are common initial side effects
- Tendency to cause mild increase in blood pressure in some patients
- Need for multiple dosing requires greater patient motivation
- Short half-life can lead to reemergence of depression/anxiety symptoms or emergence of withdrawal symptoms if several doses are missed or medication is abruptly discontinued
- Sexual side effects similar to SSRIs

FLUVOXAMINE (LUVOX)

Fluvoxamine is a serotonergic antidepressant approved for treatment of obsessive-compulsive disorder, with a half-life of 16 hours and protein binding at 80 percent. It may also be used for treatment of depression, anxiety disorders, and eating disorders. Fluvoxamine is available in scored tablets of 50 mg and 100 mg strengths. It is contraindicated in patients taking terfenadine (Seldane), Cisapride (Propulsid) or astemizole (Hismanal), due to rare risk of cardiac arrhythmia resulting from QT prolongation.

Fluvoxamine has all of the advantages of serotonergic antidepressants, with a similar side effect profile; however, there are some differences that are clinically important. Since insomnia is not a common side effect, it may be started in the evening or at bedtime as a once-a-day 50 mg or 100 mg dose. Anxiety as a side effect is relatively less frequent than with other serotonergic antidepressants, and gastrointestinal side effects are similar to other SSRIs. Sexual dysfunction tends to be somewhat less compared to other SSRIs, estimated at 40 percent in the author's clinical experience. It has been effective in the treatment of obsessive-compulsive disorder in some patients who did not respond satisfactorily to clomipramine (Anafranil), fluoxetine (Prozac), or other SSRIs, suggesting that it is a useful option among SSRIs for treatment of obsessive-compulsive disorder. Hence, overall efficacy is estimated to be similar to fluoxetine, sertraline, and paroxetine for treatment of obsessive-compulsive disorder. The maximum dose recommended is 300 mg per day, in divided dosages. It is started at 50 mg or 100 mg at bedtime, with a 50 mg increase, as needed, every two weeks until the maximum dose of 300 mg is reached. The average effective dose is 100 to 200 mg per day. The availability of scored tablets in 50 mg and 100 mg strengths offers flexibility of dosing and possible cost savings especially at lower doses. For example, it will cost a patient approximately $85 per month on fluvoxamine 150 mg daily, compared to sertraline (Zoloft) 100 mg daily costing $60 per month, fluoxetine (Prozac) 40 mg costing $100 per month, paroxetine (Paxil) 30 mg costing $60 per month, and venlafaxine (Effexor) 100 mg costing $40 per month.

Summary of Advantages and Disadvantages of Fluvoxamine

Advantages

- Effective for treatment of obsessive-compulsive disorder (the only FDA-approved use in the United States at present), depression, anxiety disorders, and bulimia

- Lack of TCA side effects
- Fairly safe in overdose (as with all SSRIs)
- Comparatively low incidence of sexual dysfunction (estimated at 40 percent, which is still significant, but lower than other SSRIs)
- Flexible dosing and possible cost saving, due to scored-tablet format in 50 mg and 100 mg strengths
- Low incidence of insomnia, anxiety, and weight gain as side effects
- No active metabolites
- Does not have significant cardiovascular side effects
- Once-a-day bedtime dosing convenient for most patients

Disadvantages

- Causes GI side effects similar to most SSRIs
- Current FDA approval only for obsessive-compulsive disorder (although this does not prevent physicians from using it for other conditions such as depression, anxiety, bulimia, etc.)

MIRTAZAPINE (REMERON)

Mirtazapine is an antidepressant with noradrengergic and serotonergic pharmacological actions, introduced in the United States in August 1996. Its presynaptic α_2 (Alpha-2) adrenoreceptor antagonism stimulates release of norepinephrine and serotonin. It has a half-life of approximately 30 hours, making it suitable for once-daily dosing. Plasma-protein binding is estimated at 85 percent. It is eliminated by hepatic metabolism and excreted by the kidneys; therefore, dosage adjustment may be necessary for the hepatically and renally impaired. Mirtazapine is available in scored 15 mg and 30 mg tablets. The effective dosage range recommended by the manufacturer is 15 to 45 mg, preferably given at bedtime.

The side effect profile of mirtazapine is different from that of SSRIs and TCAs. Common side effects include sedation, increased appetite, weight gain, dizziness, orthostatic hypotension, malaise, apathy, anxiety, and agitation. Most patients eventually develop tolerance to the side effects. Two out of 2,796 patients in premarketing clinical trials exposed to mirtazapine developed agranulocytosis, and a third patient developed severe neutropenia, yielding a crude incidence of severe neutropenia of one per one thousand patients. Mirtazapine should be discontinued if signs of infection such as flu-like symptoms, sore throat, fever, chills, fatigue, or stomatitis develop along with a low WBC count. Although the incidence of agranulocytosis associated with mirtazapine is extremely low, it is relatively contraindicated with clozapine because of potential for additive risk of suppression of bone marrow. WBC monitoring is not routinely recommended for patients taking mirtazapine.

Mirtazapine does not cause significant sexual dysfunction. Its sedative effects could be exploited in patients who have anxiety and insomnia when given at bedtime. However, the author's limited clinical experience with mirtazapine so far has indicated that approximately 50 percent of patients had difficulty tolerating mirtazapine due to daytime sedation, a "drugged" feeling, activation at night time, and restlessness when the mediation was started with the first dose at 15 mg daily as suggested by the drug manufacturer. Hence the author's current practice is to start mirtazapine at 3.75 mg (1/4 tablet) or 7.5 mg (1/2 tablet) at HS for the first four days before gradually increasing the dose. For the treatment of anxiety, a low starting dose of 3.75 mg BID may be better tolerated. Since antidepressants may take from two to four weeks for response, it is prudent to wait a minimum of two weeks in an outpatient setting prior to increasing the dose beyond 15 mg daily, which is considered a low therapeutic dose. In partial responders, addition of a low dose of an SSRI such as fluoxetine 10 to 20 mg, paroxetine 10 to 20 mg, or sertraline 25 to 50 mg AM may be effective in some patients. If activation is predominant in a particular patient, mirtazapine may be switched to AM schedule. A 14-day drug washout interval is required between administration of mirtazapine and MAOIs. Additional clinical experience will provide more definitive information as to the drug's effectiveness, tolerability, and patient acceptance in an outpatient practice environment. The price of mirtazapine 30 pills (15 mg or 30 mg) is approximately $60 which compares favorably with the price of SSRIs.

Summary of Advantage and Disadvantages of Mirtazapine (Remeron)

Advantages

- Effective for depression; possibly effective for anxiety at a low dose
- Once-a-day dosing
- Lack of sexual dysfunction
- Flexibility of a scored tablet
- Safer than TCAs in overdose
- Not a significant inhibitor of cytochrome P450 enzymes
- Does not affect cardiac conduction at therapeutic doses

Disadvantages

- Sedation, somnolence, dizziness, and activation possibly excessive unless starting dose is 7.5 mg or less; tolerance to side effects may take several weeks*
- Patient tolerance somewhat less compared to SSRIs; tolerance comparable to TCAs (secondary amines); better tolerated than tertiary amines*
- Rare incidence of agranulocytosis (estimated at 1.1 per 1,000 patients); need to warn patients of this risk and to report signs of infection can affect patient acceptance

TRAZODONE (DESYREL)

Trazodone is an antidepressant with serotonin receptor blocking properties and modest inhibition of serotonin reuptake. It has a half-life of about five hours. Trazodone is effective for treatment of depression, anxiety, and other conditions that typically respond to antidepressants. At low doses given at bedtime, its sedative effects can be exploited to improve sleep. In clinical experience, its antidepressant effects are not as impressive as SSRIs or TCAs. However, it is very commonly used as an adjunctive medication at low doses for insomnia, chronic pain, aggression, anxiety, post-traumatic stress disorder, and obsessive-compulsive disorder.

It is available in 50, 100, 150, and 300 mg tablets. The usual effective dosage range for treatment of depression is between 300 mg and 500 mg per day, given in divided doses with the major portion given at bedtime. The maximum daily dose is 600 mg, given in divided doses. Most patients tend to need 400 mg or more per day for antidepressant effect. As the dose is increased, the frequency of side effects such as sedation, orthostatic hypotension, and dizziness can also increase. For treatment of insomnia and as an adjunctive medication, the dosage range is 50 to 150 mg, given at bedtime for insomnia, and in divided doses for other purposes.

For treatment of depression, trazodone is started at 50 mg, three times a day, with daily increments of 50 mg until a total daily dose of 300 mg is reached. Further increases are made weekly at a rate of 100 mg per week up to a maximum dose of 600 mg per day in multiple doses. The dose is

---

*These observations are primarily based on the author's limited clinical experience of treating approximately 40 patients using mirtazapine at the time of this writing.

reduced by half in the elderly and medically ill. Since cardiac arrhythmia can be a concern at high doses, an EKG is recommended if doses greater than 400 mg per day are prescribed. Male patients should be warned of the very rare incidence of priapism which, if not diagnosed and treated early, can lead to impotence. Trazodone can antagonize the antihypertensive effects of clonidine (Catapres).

Summary of Advantages and Disadvantages of Trazodone

Advantages

- Effective in treatment of mild to moderate depression
- Excellent as an adjunctive medication for insomnia and for other conditions as indicated, at low doses
- Medication of choice for treating insomnia in patients with risk of substance abuse
- Low cost due to generic availability
- Safety in overdose
- Low anticholinergic side effects
- No significant weight gain
- Low incidence of sexual dysfunction

Disadvantages

- Antidepressant effect is only modest in most patients with severe depression
- Side effects of sedation and orthostatic hypotension can be dose-limiting

NEFAZODONE (SERZONE)

Nefazodone is an antidepressant with several actions at the synapse. It is an inhibitor of serotonin reuptake, and a serotonin receptor blocker. To a lesser extent, it inhibits norepinephrine reuptake. Thus, it shares some of the neurotransmitter dynamics of trazodone (Desyrel) and venlafaxine (Effexor). Although nefazodone is formally approved by the FDA for treatment of depression, it has broader clinical applications as do all antidepressants; for example, to treat anxiety, phobic and obsessive-compulsive disorders, posttraumatic stress disorder, etc. It tends to cause sexual dysfunction less frequently compared to SSRIs. As with other SSRIs, it is devoid of anticholinergic side effects and has very low cardiovascular toxicity. Nefazodone potentiates the effects of alprazolam (Xanax) and triazolam (Halcion) by increasing their blood levels; hence, the dosage of the latter two medications should be reduced by one-half to one-third if nefazodone is added. The hepatic metabolism of terfanadine (Seldane), astemizole (Hismanal), and cisapride (Propulsid) can be inhibited by nefazodone, leading to potential toxicity and prolongation of QT interval. Therefore, nefazodone is contraindicated with these drugs. Loratadine (Claritin) does not cause significant interaction with nefazodone.

It has a half-life of approximately six hours and is highly plasma-protein bound. Available dosages are 100, 150, 200, and 250 mg tablets. Typical effective dosage range is between 300 and 500 mg in divided doses, with the major portion preferably given at bedtime. The maximum dose is 600 mg per day. A dose of 300 mg or less may be given in one bedtime dose if daytime sedation or insomnia is a problem.

Clinical experience based on prescribing nefazodone to both inpatients and outpatients has revealed that its effectiveness in treating severe depression and anxiety is comparable to a range between that of SSRIs and trazodone. Its mildly sedating property and relatively low interference with sexual functioning as seen in clinical practice so far are clear advantages over SSRIs and MAOIs, particularly for treating mild to moderate depression. The estimate of sexual dysfunction associated with nefazodone is at 15 percent in the author's clinical experience, compared to 60 percent associated with SSRIs. When sexual dysfunction occurs with nefazodone, the severity is also less. The most frequently reported side effects of nefazodone are somnolence, nausea, dizziness, asthenia, lightheadedness, dry mouth, constipation, blurred vision, and confusion. Postural hypotension can occur in susceptible patients, such as patients with cardiovascular or cerebrovascular disease, or patients taking antihypertensive medication. Most of the side effets subside during the first one to two weeks of nefazodone therapy. Since nefazodone is fairly new, additional clinical experience will further clarify nefazodone's therapeutic and side effect profile in relation to established antidepressants.

The cost for a patient on nefazodone 200 mg twice a day for one month is approximately $40, compared to fluvoxamine (Luvox) 150 mg daily costing $85 per month, venlafaxine (Effexor) 100 mg twice a day costing $57 per month, paroxetine (Paxil) 30 mg daily costing $60 per month, sertraline (Zoloft) 100 mg daily costing $60 per month, and fluoxetine (Prozac) 40 mg daily costing $100 per month. Nefazodone offers significant cost advantages compared to SSRIs and bupropion, as evident from the comparative cost analysis given here.

Although the manufacturer's recommendation is to start patients at 100 mg twice a day, given the frequent complaint of nausea, the author's suggestion is to start nefazodone at 50 mg three times a day with meals to minimize GI side effects, in spite of the slight decrease in bioavailability when taken with food. After about five days, the dose may be doubled to 100 mg three times a day with meals. After the patient is tolerant of the possible GI side effects, the dosing schedule may be changed to twice a day, with the major dose given at bedtime. Dosage increases over 300 mg are usually achieved at a rate of 100 mg increments per week, up to a maximum of 600 mg per day in two to three divided doses, unless side effects interfere. For the elderly and medically ill, dosage should be reduced by half.

Summary of Advantages and Disadvantages of Nefazodone

Advantages

- Effective for treatment of mild to moderate depression and anxiety
- Lack of TCA side effects
- Significantly less incidence of sexual dysfunction, compared to SSRIs
- Safety profile similar to SSRIs
- Relatively low cost (a "best buy")
- May aid sleep when given at bedtime
- Low incidence of weight gain

Disadvantages

- Nausea, sedation, and dizziness can be initial side effects
- Need for multiple dosing schedule
- High protein binding causes displacement of other drugs that are protein bound (although this is not clinically significant in most cases)

IMIPRAMINE (TOFRANIL)

Imipramine is a tricyclic antidepressant that inhibits serotonin and norepinephrine reuptake, with a half-life of 24 hours. It is available in doses of 10, 25, and 50 mg tablets, in parenteral form for IM use, and as Tofranil PM capsules containing imipramine pamoate in doses of 75, 100, 125, and

150 mg for once-a-day administration. Since imipramine hydrochloride and pamoate have fairly long half-lives and are fairly sedating, either may be used as a one-time dose at bedtime. The hydrochloride form is available in generic form, making it less expensive compared to the pamoate form. Imipramine is the gold standard for comparing the efficacy of other antidepressants due to its broad spectrum biochemical action (fairly equal inhibition of serotonin and norepinephrine reuptake) and its proven efficacy over many years of clinical use. It is probably the most studied of all the antidepressants. Imipramine shares all of the typical side effects of tricyclic antidepressants.

For hospitalized patients, treatment is initiated at 25 mg two or three times a day, with a daily increase of 25 mg each day until a dose of 150 mg per day in divided doses is reached. Thereafter, dosage may be increased by 50 mg every seven days, up to a total of 300 mg per day unless side effects emerge. For outpatients, treatment is begun at 25 mg twice a day, with 25 mg increments every three to four days, and the patient is monitored in the office weekly until improvement is noted. Most patients respond at 75 to 150 mg, given as a one-time dose at bedtime.

If insomnia is a major problem, all of the dose may be administered at bedtime. For the elderly or for children, half of the dosage range given above is used for initiation, with smaller and more gradual dosage increases subsequently.

Imipramine can be used for depression, anxiety, phobia, eating disorders, social phobia, pain syndrome, panic disorders, attention deficit hyperactivity disorder, stage 4 parasomnias (such as nocturnal enuresis and sleepwalking), nightmares, and urinary incontinence. Imipramine should be discontinued gradually over four to six days, especially if the total daily dose exceeds 200 mg, to minimize uncomfortable withdrawal symptoms associated with discontinuation. Imipramine can be used as an adjunctive medication along with serotonergic antidepressants and bupropion (Wellbutrin) at low doses, such as 10 to 25 mg given as a bedtime dose for antidepressant augmentation, insomnia, anorexia, and for gastrointestinal discomfort (associated with serotonergic drugs).

Since imipramine and various TCAs are substrates for various isoenzymes in the cytochrome P-450 system, and since most serotonergic drugs inhibit P-450 enzymes, the dosage of TCAs, antipsychotics, and benzodiazepines should be lowered if used concurrently. Fairly reliable plasma levels of the active parent compound imipramine and the active metabolite desipramine are available. The therapeutic plasma level of imipramine (imipramine and desipramine) is estimated to be between 200 and 250 ng/ml. It is not necessary to obtain TCA blood levels routinely simply because blood levels are available. TCA blood levels may be obtained in the following circumstances:

- Diagnosing and monitoring toxicity
- Monitoring compliance and confirming noncompliance
- Arriving at the lowest effective dosage in patients at greater risk for adverse effects (the elderly, children, and medically ill)

Summary of Advantages and Disadvantages of Imipramine

Advantages

- Broad spectrum antidepressant with proven efficacy
- Moderate sedation may help patients with insomnia
- Well-studied and still widely used
- Effective for a variety of conditions as listed
- Low cost due to generic availability
- Fairly reliable blood level available

Disadvantages

- Anticholinergic and cardiac side effects
- Lethal in overdose
- Weight gain (problem in most patients)
- Sedation is usually excessive at the higher dosage range
- Not well-tolerated by the elderly and medically ill (at high doses)
- Greater risk of interaction with over-the-counter medications and alcohol, compared to serotonergic drugs
- Affects cardiac conduction at high doses

AMITRIPTYLINE (ELAVIL)

Amitriptyline is a tricyclic antidepressant with a half-life of 24 hours, used for treatment of depression, anxiety, pain syndromes, eating disorders, panic disorder, attention deficit hyperactivity disorder, and stage 4 parasomnias. It has pronounced anticholinergic and sedative effects; thus, it is preferably given at bedtime. It is available in parenteral form for IM use and in tablet form in 10, 25, 50, 100, and 150 mg strengths. Anticholinergic side effects, sedation, and hypotensive effects make it hazardous for use in the elderly and in children. Its norepinephrine reuptake blockage is moderate, and serotonin reuptake blockage is fairly strong.

Its appetite stimulant properties can be exploited for the purpose of counteracting the anorexia found in depression or other conditions, and for treating the anorectic side effects of serotonergic drugs by giving it at 10 to 25 mg doses as an adjunctive medication at night. The author has employed amitriptyline in treating anorexia due to various causes, such as cancer chemotherapy, pain, gastrointestinal problems, depression, and due to medications, with good results. In most cases, a dose of 10 mg is sufficient. It also has additional desirable effects of aiding sleep and reducing gastrointestinal discomfort without producing excessive daytime sedation or significant anticholinergic effects–as long as low doses are employed. It is seldom used in the IM form. Since the introduction of serotonergic medication, it is only occasionally used as the primary antidepressant. When used as an antidepressant, it is started at 25 mg po two times a day, with daily increases of 25 mg until a dose of 150 mg is reached. Further increases of 50 mg per week up to 300 mg per day may be made if needed. The dosage is reduced by half in the elderly and in children.

Despite the desirable appetite stimulant effects in patients with anorexia nervosa or bulimia nervosa, its use as a primary medication in these patients is not recommended because the dramatic increase in appetite and weight is frightening to these patients who stop the medication or compensate by increasing purging behavior. The strategy for the pharmacological management of eating disorder patients is described in Chapter 13.

Summary of Advantages and Disadvantages of Elavil

Advantages

- Effective antidepressant
- Effective for a wide variety of conditions, as listed
- Low cost due to generic availability
- Excellent adjunctive medication at subtherapeutic doses (10 to 50 mg per day)

Disadvantages

- High anticholinergic, sedative, and cardiac side effects
- Lethal in overdose
- Weight gain is fairly common
- Not well-tolerated by the elderly and medically ill (at high doses)
- Greater risk of interaction with over-the-counter medications and alcohol, compared to serotonergic medications
- Affects cardiac conduction at high doses

DOXEPIN (SINEQUAN)

Doxepin is a tricyclic antidepressant with a half-life of 20 hours, available in liquid form and in 10, 25, 50, 75, 100, and 150 mg capsules. The usual dosage range for treatment of depression is between 100 and 200 mg, with a maximum dose of 300 mg per day, with all or most of it given at bedtime to enhance sleep and to minimize daytime sedation. It has pronounced anticholinergic and antihistaminic (H_1 and H_2 blocking) effects. It inhibits uptake of norepinephrine and serotonin moderately.

Treatment of inpatients is typically started at 25 mg twice or three times a day and increased by 25 mg daily up to 150 mg per day. Further titration is made at a rate increase of 50 mg per week, up to a maximum dose of 300 mg per day, unless side effects emerge. In outpatients, the dosage increase is instituted much more gradually. In the elderly and children, the dosage is reduced to one-half the adult dosage.

Doxepin is used infrequently as a primary antidepressant for the treatment of depression, having given way to the new generation antidepressants such as the serotonergic drugs and bupropion. However, it is excellent as an adjunctive medication in the dosage range of 10 to 50 mg given as a bedtime dose for insomnia, anorexia (due to medication side effects or other causes), gastrointestinal irritation, and chronic pain syndrome. It can be used for all conditions for which amitriptyline is used. Weight gain, anticholinergic side effects, and sedation are significant at high doses.

Summary of Advantages and Disadvantages of Doxepin

Advantages

- Effective antidepressant
- Effective for multiple indications, as listed
- Low cost due to generic availability
- Liquid and tablet form
- Excellent as an adjunctive medication at subtherapeutic doses (10 to 50 mg at bedtime)

Disadvantages

- High anticholinergic, sedative, and cardiac side effects
- Lethal in overdose
- Weight gain
- Poorly tolerated by the elderly and medically ill (at high doses)

- Greater risk of interaction with over-the-counter medications and alcohol, compared to new-generation antidepressants
- Affects cardiac conduction at high doses

TRIMIPRAMINE (SURMONTIL)

Trimipramine is a tricyclic antidepressant that has a half-life of approximately 12 hours. It inhibits reuptake of both norepinephrine and serotonin, but the potency is less compared to imipramine. It has high anticholinergic and sedative properties. Its indications, dosage, and side effects are similar to amitriptyline. It is available as 25, 50, and 100 mg capsules.

Summary of Advantages and Disadvantages of Trimipramine

Advantages

- Effective antidepressant
- Effective for multiple indications (as amitriptyline)
- Low cost due to generic availability

Disadvantages

- Moderately high anticholinergic, sedative, and cardiac side effects
- Lethal in overdose
- Weight gain
- Poorly tolerated by the elderly and medically ill (at high doses)
- Greater risk of interaction with over-the-counter medications and alcohol, compared to serotonergic medications
- Limited dosage strength options available, compared to other TCAs
- Affects cardiac conduction at high doses

DESIPRAMINE (NORPRAMIN)

Desipramine, an active metabolite of imipramine, is a tricyclic antidepressant with a strong degree of blockage of norepinephrine reuptake. It is available in 10, 25, 50, 75, 100, and 150 mg tablets. It provides fairly reliable blood level, with antidepressant effects expected above a plasma level of 125 ng/ml. The usual effective adult dosage range is 100 to 200 mg per day, with a maximum dose of 300 mg per day. Since it has a half-life of approximately 24 hours, once-a-day dosing at bedtime is possible. It has very low anticholinergic and sedative effects compared to other tricyclics, making it safer for use with the elderly, medically ill, and with children. Cardiac side effects are similar to those caused by other tricyclic medications. The indications and uses are varied, as with imipramine.

It is usually started in dosage ranges similar to that of imipramine. Due to its predominant norepinephrinergic effects, it may have stimulating properties. However, in clinical practice, it is the author's observation in general that SSRIs have greater stimulating effects. Though reliable plasma level is available, it should be obtained only if clinically necessary. Routine blood level monitoring unnecessarily increases the cost of health care.

Summary of Advantages and Disadvantages of Desipramine

Advantages

- Effective antidepressant
- Effective for various uses (as with the parent compound, imipramine)
- Low anticholinergic, sedative, and hypotensive effects
- Low cost due to generic availability
- Excellent to augment the effect of serotonergic antidepressants and possibly convert a nonresponder to a responder (dosage range 25 to 50 mg)
- Reliable plasma level available

Disadvantages

- Lethal in overdose
- Weight gain
- Greater risk of interaction with over-the-counter medications and alcohol, compared to serotonergic medications
- Affects cardiac conduction

NORTRIPTYLINE (PAMELOR, AVENTYL)

Nortriptyline, an active metabolite of the parent compound amitriptyline, is a tricyclic antidepressant with a half-life of about 30 hours. It is available in 10, 25, 50, and 75 mg capsules, and in liquid form for oral use. The usual effective dosage range is between 75 and 150 mg. It is started at 25 mg twice a day, with a 25 mg increase every two to three days, until a dose of 100 mg per day is reached. Further dosage increase, if needed, is at a rate of 25 mg per week up to a maximum dosage of 150 mg per day. Nortriptyline is believed to have a "therapeutic window" consisting of plasma level between 50 and 150 ng/ml. Levels below 50 ng/ml and above 150 ng/ml are said to have decreased efficacy for treatment of depression and other conditions.

Nortriptyline can be used for other indications, as in the case of amitriptyline and imipramine. It has relatively low anticholinergic, sedative, and hypotensive side effects, making it especially suitable for use in the elderly, the medically ill, and children. Since it has moderately high reuptake inhibition of norepinephrine compared to serotonin, it is an excellent adjunctive medication at low doses for use with serotonergic medications as an augmenter. It can also be used as an appetite stimulant or as a mild sleep aid.

Although it has low anticholinergic activity, nortriptyline can still cause constipation, dry mouth, blurry vision, tachycardia, orthostatic hypotension, and prolongation of cardiac conduction in some individuals at average to high doses.

Although it has a therapeutic "window" of plasma level, it is not recommended that blood levels be obtained routinely or repeatedly, except in the following circumstances:

- Suspicion of toxicity
- Monitoring compliance or confirmation of noncompliance
- To arrive at the lowest effective dose in patients at risk for adverse effects (the elderly, the medically ill, and children)

The use of nortriptyline as a primary antidepressant is decreasing in favor of the new generation of antidepressants; however, adjunctive use at low doses is quite effective.

Summary of Advantages and Disadvantages of Nortriptyline

Advantages

- Effective antidepressant
- Effective for other uses (as with imipramine)
- Effective as an augmenter with serotonergic drugs to convert a non-responder to a responder
- Low anticholinergic, sedative, and hypotensive side effects
- Low cost due to generic availability
- Capsule and liquid form
- Reliable plasma level available

Disadvantages

- Lethal in overdose
- Weight gain
- Affects cardiac conduction in high doses (as with all TCAs)
- Greater risk of interaction with over-the-counter medications and alcohol (compared with new generation antidepressants)

MAPROTILINE (LUDIOMIL)

Maprotiline is a tetracyclic antidepressant with a half-life of approximately 40 hours and a fairly strong norepinephrinergic property. It is available in 25, 50, and 75 mg tablets. The usual effective therapeutic dosage range is between 75 and 150 mg in divided doses, with a maximum of 225 mg per day in divided doses. Since maprotiline appreciably lowers seizure threshold at high doses, its use has been infrequent. It is contraindicated in patients at risk for seizure.

Maprotiline is used for treatment of depression and various other conditions, as with any other TCAs. Given its seizure risk liability, and given the availability of numerous other antidepressants, which have better side effect profiles, maprotiline is no longer in frequent use as a primary antidepressant.

Summary of Advantages and Disadvantages of Maprotiline

Advantages

- Effective antidepressant
- Effective for other uses (as with imipramine)
- Low cost due to generic availability

Disadvantages

- Lethal in overdose
- Decreases seizure threshold more than other antidepressants (except possibly clomipramine and bupropion) at equivalent doses
- Moderate anticholinergic, sedative, and hypotensive side effects
- Affects cardiac conduction at high doses
- Poorly tolerated by the elderly and medically ill (at high doses)
- Greater risk of interaction with over-the-counter medications and alcohol, compared with serotonergic medications

PROTRIPTYLINE (VIVACTIL)

Protriptyline is a norepinephrinergic tricyclic antidepressant with stimulating effects. It has a half-life of about three days. It is available in 5 and 10 mg tablets. The usual effective antidepressant dosage range is 30 to 40 mg given as a one-time dose, with a maximum dose of 60 mg per day. It is typically started at a dose of 10 mg two times a day, with daily increases of 5 mg until a total daily dose of 40 mg is reached. The dosage is then increased at a rate of 5 mg per week up to 60 mg per day unless side effects interfere. In outpatients, dosage is increased more slowly. In the elderly and medically ill, half the dosage range cited above is recommended.

Protriptyline is indicated for treatment of depression and for other conditions for which TCAs are employed. In addition, its stimulating properties may be exploited for treatment of central or mixed sleep apnea and narcolepsy. In narcolepsy it can secondarily improve cataplexy, sleep paralysis, and hypnogogic hallucinations, by virtue of increasing REM latency and decreasing REM intensity and duration. Although the effects on sleep are characteristic of all TCAs, protriptyline's stimulating effects may improve daytime alertness in people who have narcolepsy. It has moderate anticholinergic and fairly low hypotensive and appetite stimulant effects. Its long half-life is suitable for once-a-day dosing.

Summary of Advantages and Disadvantages of Protriptyline

Advantages

- Effective antidepressant
- Effective for various other uses, as listed
- One of the few TCAs with stimulating effects
- Low sedating and hypotensive side effects
- Less weight gain, compared to other TCAs

Disadvantages

- Lethal in overdose
- Moderate anticholinergic side effects
- Affects cardiac conduction at high doses
- Poorly tolerated by the elderly and medically ill (at high doses)
- Greater risk of interaction with over-the-counter medications and alcohol (as compared with new-generation antidepressants)

AMOXAPINE (ASCENDIN)

Amoxapine, an effective antidepressant, has several metabolites that have mild antipsychotic properties. It has a half-life of about ten hours. Amoxapine is primarily norepinephrinergic. It has relatively fewer anticholinergic and sedative side effects, compared to imipramine.

Due to its dopamine receptor (D2) blocking effects, it can produce all the adverse effects commonly associated with typical antipsychotics, such as extrapyramidal symptoms (EPS), dyskinesia, and neuroleptic malignant syndrome. It can significantly lower seizure threshold in high doses.

It is available in 25, 50, 100, and 150 mg tablets. The usual effective therapeutic dosage range is between 150 and 300 mg per day in multiple doses, with the major portion given at bedtime. The maximum daily dosage is 600 mg. Amoxapine can be started at 25 mg twice or three times a day and increased by 25 mg daily until a dose of 200 mg per day is reached. Thereafter, the dose is increased at a rate of 50 mg increments per week, up to 600 mg per day in divided doses, unless side effects emerge. In the elderly and medically ill, half the cited dosage range is used. In outpatient settings, the dosage increase is instituted more gradually.

There are some practical advantages of using amoxapine for patients with depressive and psychotic symptoms, in terms of efficiency and economy, because of its built-in antipsychotic effects. However, in most cases of primary depression with psychotic features, one of the goals of treatment is to gradually withdraw or decrease the antipsychotic medication after the acute psychotic symptoms are controlled and, if possible, to maintain the patient on the antidepressant medication. Amoxapine does not allow independent titration of the antidepressant and the antipsychotic. If a patient is depressed or anxious and has no need for antipsychotic medication, it is not desirable to expose the patient to antipsychotic drugs indefinitely. For these reasons, the author's preference is not to use amoxapine except in the very rare case where amoxapine is uniquely effective and desirable for clinical reasons.

Summary of Advantages and Disadvantages of Amoxapine

Advantages

- Effective antidepressant
- Effective and economical for treating depression with mild psychotic symptoms
- Low cost due to generic availability
- Fairly low anticholinergic, sedative, and hypotensive side effects

Disadvantages

- Lethal in overdose
- Lowers seizure threshold in high doses
- Metabolites possess antipsychotic activity and associated neuroleptic side effects
- Slows cardiac conduction at high doses
- Poorly tolerated by the elderly and medically ill (at high doses)
- Greater risk of interaction with over-the-counter medications and alcohol, compared to new-generation antidepressants

CLOMIPRAMINE (ANAFRANIL)

Clomipramine is a tricyclic antidepressant approved and primarily used for treatment of obsessive-compulsive disorder. It has relatively more potent serotonergic effects compared to its norepinephrinergic properties. Although its FDA approval is for treatment of obsessive-compulsive disorder, it can be used as an antidepressant and an antianxiety medication, as can all TCAs. It has a half-life of 30 hours, and is 95 percent protein-bound. Clomipramine is available in 25, 50, and 75 mg capsules. Treatment is started at 25 mg BID with 25 mg increments every two to three days until a dose of 150 mg is reached. Thereafter, dosage is increased by 25 mg per week if needed, up to a maximum dose of 250 mg per day in divided doses.

Clomipramine, being a tricyclic antidepressant, has significant anticholinergic and other typical tricyclic side effects. In addition, it tends to lower seizure threshold more than other antidepressants. Hence, the maximum recommended dose of 250 mg per day should not be exceeded. While all antidepressants–except perhaps MAOIs and SSRIs–lower seizure threshold, in the author's experience the incidence of generalized seizures precipitated by clomipramine is higher than any antidepressant, including bupropion (Wellbutrin), at comparable dosage range. Therefore, the author has a conservative approach of not exceeding clomipramine 225 mg per day and not exceeding 150 mg per dose to keep the seizure risk low. As in the case of bupropion, patients on clomipramine should be educated about the increased seizure risk and strictly cautioned not to exceed dosage limits. If a patient who is at increased risk for seizures for any reason needs to be on clomipramine, prophylactic anticonvulsant treatment should be considered. The caution regarding slightly increased seizure risk is given by the author only in cases in which the dosage exceeds 150 mg per day; the clinician must maintain a balance between encouraging and reassuring the patient and frightening the patient by listing side effects that are rare and of no practical significance. The common side effects of clomipramine are dose-dependent in a fairly linear fashion. They are dry mouth, blurry vision, constipation, increased heart rate, sedation, weight gain, and increased sweating. Most of these side effects subside over a period of two to three weeks, although sweating and sedation tend to persist. TCAs can exacerbate narrow-angle glaucoma. The patient can also develop postural hypotension and slowing of cardiac conduction. Central nervous system side effects include sedation, lethargy, and a central anticholinergic syndrome particularly in elderly patients on high doses. Sexual dysfunction such as decreased libido, erectile difficulties, and inhibited orgasm are also fairly common, estimated at 60 to 70 percent. Sexual dysfunction associated with clomipramine is higher than with other TCAs.

Summary of Advantages and Disadvantages of Clomipramine

Advantages

- The most effective medication for obsessive-compulsive disorder
- Effective for depression and anxiety
- Less weight gain, compared to other TCAs

Disadvantages

- Lethal in overdose
- Significantly lowers seizure threshold at high doses
- Moderate anticholinergic side effects
- Affects cardiac conduction at high doses
- Greater risk of interaction with over-the-counter medications and alcohol, as compared with new-generation antidepressants
- Poorly tolerated by the elderly and medically ill (at high doses)

PHENELZINE (NARDIL)

Phenelzine is an irreversible inhibitor of monoamine oxidase and, similar to imipramine, is an effective antidepressant for treatment of depressive symptoms, anxiety disorders, phobias, and for a variety of other symptoms. Phenelzine may be used with antipsychotics, mood stabilizers, and benzodiazepines. Since it does not lower seizure threshold as much as other antidepressants, it may be safer in patients at risk for seizure. Phenelzine has a half-life of about three hours. It is available as 15 mg tablets. The typical dosage range for treatment of depression is between 45 and 75 mg per day in divided doses, usually given as morning and noon doses. The maximum dose is 90 mg per day, although some patients are able to tolerate a higher dose. Treatment is started at 15 mg twice a day, with an increase of 15 mg every two days until a dose of 60 mg per day is reached. Further increases are at a rate of 15 mg per week if needed, up to a maximum dose of 90 mg per day unless side effects interfere. For the elderly and medically ill, the dosage is increased more gradually because of commonly observed orthostatic hypotension.

Although phenelzine is a very effective antidepressant, it is used infrequently in clinical practice because of serious dietary and medication interactions that can cause hypertensive and hyperthermic crises and the consequent requirement of adhering to strict diet and of avoiding medications that can interact with monoamine oxidase inhibitors.

Since phenelzine irreversibly inhibits monoamine oxidase, it takes approximately 14 days after stopping phenelzine for the enzyme to resynthesize, requiring adherence to dietary and concomitant medication precautions for about two weeks after stopping.

Hypertensive crisis, characterized by hypertension, occipital headache, nausea, sweating, vomiting, palpitations, tachycardia, and restlessness, can occur when a patient on an MAOI treatment consumes food containing high concentrations of tyramine or is exposed to sympathomimetic medications such as stimulants and various over-the-counter cold, allergy, and decongestant medications containing ingredients such as ephedrine, phenylephrine, pseudoephedrine, phenylpropanolamine, oxymetazoline, and other adrenergic agents. Concurrent use of cocaine or stimulants can lead to serious hypertensive crisis. It is a prudent practice for patients to carry either nifedipine (Procardia) 10 mg for sublingual administration or chlorpromazine (Thorazine) 25 mg for po administration, for emergency use in case of an accidentally induced hypertensive crisis. Nifedipine capsules can be squeezed and the contents placed under the tongue for rapid absorption. The most effective intervention is to administer phentolamine 5 mg intravenously by slow push. Foods to be avoided due to high tyramine content are aged cheese, liver, red wines, beer, pickled fish, yeast extracts, dry sausage, salami, bologna, smoked meat, raspberries, soy sauce (in large amounts), sauerkraut, meat extracts, and fava beans. Cottage cheese, cream cheese, ricotta cheese, sour cream, and yogurt should not cause food interaction problems. MAO enzymes break down tyramine, which has sympathomimetic actions. The inhibition of MAO enzymes by MAOIs results in an increase in tyramine level and its sympathomimetic actions, leading to hypertensive crisis. In general, it is better to avoid all alcoholic beverages, both because of alcohol's potential for interaction with MAOIs and because of its adverse central nervous system effects.

A serotonergic crisis characterized by hyperthermia, delirium, agitation, hypotension or hypertension, confusion, and muscle twitches can occur when an MAOI interacts with meperidine (Demerol), serotonergic antidepressants, TCAs, and dextromethorphan, which is an ingredient in various over-the-counter antitussives. Morphine, codeine, and fentanyl are safer drugs to use in patients on MAOIs. Serotonergic crisis usually requires hospitalization and supportive measures for proper management. A serotonin antagonist, such as cyproheptadine (Periactin), at doses of 4 to 8 mg three times a day may help mild to moderate cases. Patients taking MAOIs should carry a wallet card or wear a bracelet indicating MAOI use.

Common side effects of phenelzine are orthostatic hypotension, weight gain, sedation, sexual dysfunction, insomnia, anticholinergic effects, and myoclonic jerks. Orthostatic hypotension can be managed by increasing salt intake or adding regular coffee to the diet, or in more severe cases by use of fludrocortisone (Florinef) at a dose of 0.1 to 0.2 mg daily. If weight gain is a problem, switching to tranylcypromine (Parnate) can help. Trazodone (Desyrel) at low doses, as well as standard hypnotic drugs, may be used for treatment of insomnia. Attempts to treat sexual dysfunction have low success rates; however, the following may be tried:

- Yohimbine (Yocon) 5.4 mg three times a day (monitor closely for interaction)
- Cyproheptadine (Periactin) 4 to 8 mg BID or two to three hours before coitus
- Bethanechol (Urecholine) 25 mg TID or two hours before coitus

Since MAOIs can act as a pyridoxine (vitamin B6) antagonist, prophylactic administration of pyridoxine at doses of 50 to 100 mg daily should be considered.

In addition to use for depression, MAOIs can be used for various psychiatric problems, such as social phobia, post-traumatic stress disorder, panic disorder, etc. From a practical standpoint, MAOIs are infrequently used even for their primary indication of depression since the advent of SSRIs; thus, it should be obvious that for secondary indications, although MAOIs may be effective, their use is rare, and is usually reserved for conditions for which other medications have not proven effective.

Summary of Advantages and Disadvantages of Phenelzine

Advantages

- Effective antidepressant
- Effective for various anxiety disorders, particularly panic disorder and phobic disorders
- Does not lower seizure threshold as much as TCAs
- Fewer cardiac side effects compared to TCAs (except orthostatic hypotension)

Disadvantages

- Hypertensive crisis risk necessitates dietary restrictions and avoidance of various medications
- Serotonergic crisis risk requires the prohibition of various medications
- Orthostatic hypotension, weight gain, and sexual dysfunction fairly common
- Irreversible inhibition of MAO; 14 days to clear
- Can elevate liver enzymes
- Lethal in overdose, similar to TCAs

TRANYLCYPROMINE (PARNATE)

Tranylcypromine, a reversible MAOI, is an effective antidepressant that is also useful in the treatment of anxiety, panic, and phobic disorders. It has fewer anticholinergic and more stimulant properties than phenelzine; hence, it may be particularly effective in treatment of "retarded" depression or depression characterized by significant anergia, hypersomnia, psychomotor retardation, or apathy. Tranylcypromine is available as a 10 mg tablet. It tends to cause less weight gain compared to TCAs and other MAOIs. It has a half-life of 2.5 hours. The average effective dose range is between 20 and 40 mg per day in divided doses, the maximum dose being 60 mg per day. The usual starting dose is 10 mg in the morning and at noon. The dose is increased to 30 mg per day in divided doses after two to three days. Further increases are made at a rate of 10 mg every one to two weeks, up to a maximum dose of 60 mg in divided doses.

Tranylcypromine tends to initiate antidepressant effects somewhat faster than phenelzine and TCAs. Since it is a reversible inhibitor of monoamine oxidase, the enzyme action is usually restored in about five to seven days after stopping the medication, after which other medications can be started. However, the drug manufacturer recommends a 14-day interval between stopping tranylcypromine and starting another antidepressant. A 14-day interval is usually necessary to begin MAOI treatment after stopping most TCAs and serotonergic medications. Exceptions are for fluoxetine (Prozac) and for protriptyline (Vivactil), which, due to their long half-lives, require five-week and three-week intervals respectively, prior to starting MAOIs. The interval between stopping an MAOI and starting another antidepressant depends upon the characteristic and dosage of the MAOI. For example, irreversible MAOIs such as phenelzine (Nardil) and isocarboxazid (Marplan) at moderate to high doses require a two-week period for the monoamine oxidase enzyme to resynthesize, whereas at low doses, a 10-day interval is usually sufficient since the extent of inactivation of the enzyme is probably not complete at low doses. On the other hand, reversible MAOIs such as tranylcypromine (Parnate) may require only a seven-day interval prior to starting a TCA or serotonergic medication. Antidepressants with a fairly short half-life such as trazodone, venlafaxine, nefazodone, and bupropion may require only a seven- to ten-day interval prior to starting MAOIs.

Risk of hypertensive and serotonergic crises due to interaction with tranylcypromine is similar to phenelzine, requiring the same precautions regarding dietary and medication interaction as described in relation to phenelzine.

In current clinical practice, tranylcypromine, as in the case of other MAOIs, is used only when other less complicated medications (such as TCAs, serotonergic drugs, and bupropion) fail to control the symptoms; however, it remains an important option for patients with treatment-resistant depression.

Summary of Advantages and Disadvantages of Tranylcypromine

Advantages

- Effective antidepressant
- Effective for other conditions for which MAOIs are used
- Stimulating effect is beneficial in "retarded" depression
- Low anticholinergic and sedative effects
- Faster acting than most antidepressants
- Reversible inhibition of monoamine oxidase enzyme affords an interval of seven days between stopping tranylcypromine and starting another antidepressant (14-day interval preferred to assure safety)
- No significant weight gain
- Does not lower seizure threshold as much as TCAs

Disadvantages

- Risk of hypertensive and serotonergic crises, requiring strict dietary and medication interaction precautions
- Orthostatic hypotension fairly common, but less than phenelzine
- Lethal in overdose, similar to TCAs
- Insomnia is a common side effect

General Precautions Regarding MAOIs

MAOIs are contraindicated for administration with all serotonergic medications and most TCAs. A two-week interval should elapse between stopping phenelzine and beginning a TCA or a serotonergic medication, and a one-week interval is required between stopping tranylcypromine and starting another antidepressant. However, when stopping a TCA or a serotonergic medication and starting an MAOI, different time intervals apply, depending on the half-life of the medication being stopped. For example, due to the long half-life of fluoxetine and its active metabolites, an interval of five to six weeks is necessary. With shorter half-life medications such as paroxetine, fluvoxamine, and venlafaxine, a shorter interval of eight to ten days may be sufficient before beginning treatment using MAOIs.

Generally, concurrent administration of all antidepressants and MAOIs is contraindicated. However, in my clinical experience, low doses of amitriptyline (Elavil), nortriptyline (Pamelor), and trazodone (Desyrel) have been added to MAOIs with good results and without any complications. It is safer to add the other medications to a stable dose of MAOI, rather than adding the MAOI in a patient who is already receiving one of the mentioned medications. MAOIs may be used with antimanic medications, including carbamazepine (Tegretol), which in clinical experience has been found to be safe and effective by the author. Close patient monitoring, especially blood pressure monitoring, is required when a combination involving an MAOI is used.

MAOIs are currently used as a last resort in most cases, because of their dietary restrictions and risk of serious interaction with numerous over-the-counter medications, other prescription medications, and drugs of abuse. Hence, they are, for the most part, contraindicated in patients who are at risk for impulsive behavior, alcohol and drug abuse, medical problems, and who are generally unreliable. Needless to say, many psychiatric patients fall into this category.

In addition to following the interval guidelines when switching a patient from an MAOI to another antidepressant, the starting dose of the antidepressant should be one-half of the usual recommended starting dose.

This is particularly important when a patient starts an SSRI or clomipramine after being on an MAOI. The low starting dose of the new antidepressant should serve as a test dose to minimize the danger of serotonin syndrome. The low dose may be given for two to three days before increasing to the usual starting dose. If the patient tolerates the test dose well, further dose increases can be more rapid.

Usual Starting Dose	Starting Dose After MAOI, or for an Extremely Restless or Anxious Patient
– fluoxetine 20 mg AM	– fluoxetine 10 mg AM
– sertraline 50 mg AM	– sertraline 25 mg AM
– paroxetine 20 mg AM	– paroxetine 10 mg AM
– venlafaxine 37.5 mg BID-TID	– venlafaxine 25 mg BID
– fluvoxamine 50 mg BID	– fluvoxamine 25 mg BID
– clomipramine 25 mg BID	– clomipramine 25 mg HS

Mild serotonin syndrome can be controlled by benzodiazepines. Severe serotonin syndrome usually requires emergency management in a hospital setting.

The advent of serotonergic medications has given more options to the psychiatrist, thereby drastically reducing the frequency of use of MAOIs in modern psychiatric practice. It must be noted that MAOIs have excellent antidepressant and antianxiety properties that are particularly effective for patients with the so-called atypical depression, consisting of symptoms such as rejection sensitivity, hyperphagia, hypersomnia, anxiety, and dysphoria. However, serotonergic medications and bupropion (Wellbutrin) are much safer as first-choice medications for atypical depression as well as for depression and anxiety in general.

DEXTROAMPHETAMINE (DEXEDRINE)

Dextroamphetamine is a central nervous system stimulant medication with dopaminergic and norepinephrinergic properties, primarily used for treatment of attention deficit hyperactivity disorder (ADHD) in children and for narcolepsy. Other uses include augmentation of antidepressants (except MAOIs) and treatment of antidepressant-induced sexual dysfunction. It is a schedule II drug and has a half-life of about ten hours. Methamphetamine is similar to dextroamphetamine in pharmacology, indications, side effects, and dosage. Dextroamphetamine is available in 5 mg tablets and in sustained release capsules at 5, 10, and 15 mg capsules. Methamphetamine is available in 5 and 10 mg tablets, and sustained release tablets in 5, 10, and 15 mg strengths. The usual effective dosage range in children ages six and older is 5 to 20 mg daily, in divided doses. Some children may need up to 40 mg per day. The medication is started at 5 mg twice a day, with weekly increases by 5 mg, up to a maximum dose of 40 mg per day, unless side effects intervene. The sustained release forms may be given as a once-a-day dose in the morning, after the maintenance dose is established.

When used to augment antidepressant effects in adults, the usual dosage range is 10 to 20 mg in the morning or in divided doses. The dosage range is the same for treatment of sexual dysfunction. The addition of stimulants to antidepressant medication should be considered in treatment-resistant cases where various antidepressant trials along with more standard augmenters such as lithium, thyroid hormone, buspirone, etc., have failed.

Similarly, stimulants may be considered for treatment of antidepressant-induced sexual dysfunction if a switch to another antidepressant that does not cause sexual dysfunction is not an option due to clinical reasons, and if simpler interventions such as the addition of bethanechol (Urecholine), amantadine (Symmetrel), and cyproheptadine (Periactin), are not effective.

The side effects of stimulants include anxiety, restlessness, insomnia, tachycardia, headache, anorexia, hypertension, and arrhythmia. Since amphetamines antagonize the antihypertensive property of methyldopa (Aldomet, Aldoclor, Aldoril), they should not be administered together. Mild, temporary growth retardation is reported on rare occasions in children taking amphetamines.

Amphetamines should not be prescribed for patients at risk for drug abuse because of its potential for abuse or for causing dependence. Ironically, it is not uncommon to see attention deficit problems in patients who have substance abuse problems, especially stimulant abuse. ADHD may well be one of the risk factors contributing to the development of substance abuse. Whether or not to use stimulants for treating a patient with ADHD who also has a history of drug abuse is a clinical dilemma because these patients are at high risk for abusing prescription stimulants. The author tends to try medications with less potential for abuse to treat such patients. Options include bupropion (Wellbutrin), desipramine (Norpramin), fluoxetine (Prozac), protriptyline (Vivactil), venlafaxine (Effexor), and tranylcypromine (Parnate). Tranylcypromine can even serve a disulfiram-like deterrent function in motivated and compliant patients against abusing stimulants and alcohol, because the danger of hypertensive reaction works as a deterrent. Use of any MAOI, including tranylcypromine, in patients with risk of drug abuse should be attempted cautiously. Refer to the section on MAOIs for details. Pemoline (Cylert), which has the least abuse potential among stimulants, may be an option in compliant, reliable, and motivated ADHD patients with a history of drug abuse.

METHYLPHENIDATE (RITALIN)

Methylphenidate is a short-acting stimulant primarily used for treatment of ADHD and narcolepsy. It can also be used for augmentation of antidepressants and for treating antidepressant-induced sexual dysfunction. It is a schedule II drug with a half-life of 1.5 hours. It is available as 5, 10, and 20 mg tablets and as 20 mg sustained-release tablets. The usual effective dosage range for treatment of ADHD in children older than the age of six years is between 10 and 20 mg per day in divided doses or as a morning dose of 20 mg of the sustained-release form. Some children and adults may need up to 60 mg per day in divided doses for optimal effect. Patients are started at 5 mg in the morning and at noon, with an increase to 10 mg twice a day after one week, if needed. Further increase is in weekly 10 mg increments, up to a maximum of 60 mg per day, unless side effects interfere. Once the effective dose is determined, patients may be switched to the sustained-release form. The dose for antidepressant augmentation is between 5 and 10 mg twice a day. The dosage for treatment of antidepressant-induced sexual dysfunction is also similar. Side effects and precautions are the same as for dextroamphetamine.

PEMOLINE (CYLERT)

Pemoline is a central nervous system stimulant primarily used for the treatment of ADHD. It has the advantage of being classified as a schedule IV drug. Pemoline has a half-life of about 12 hours, and hence can be given once a day, unlike dextroamphetamine and methylphenidate. Its onset of clinical response is slow compared to amphetamines, usually taking one to two weeks for effects. It is available as 18.75, 37.5, and 75 mg tablets, and 37.5 mg chewable tablets. The usual effective dosage range for children older than six years is 37.5 to 75 mg daily, given as a one-time dose in the morning. The maximum dose is 112.5 mg per day. It is usually started at 37.5 mg, with weekly increments of 18.75 mg as needed. The dosage for treating antidepressant-induced sexual dysfunction and for antidepressant augmentation is between 18.75 and 75 mg per day.

Side effects include elevated liver enzymes, insomnia, anxiety, anorexia, headaches, and nausea. Monthly liver function test monitoring for the first four months is prudent.

Compared to amphetamines, the abuse potential of pemoline is low; still, the same cautions as discussed with regard to amphetamines should apply when prescribing pemoline to patients with a history of substance abuse. Its efficacy for partially reversing the sexual dysfunction caused by SSRIs and TCAs is less than that of schedule II stimulants, in the author's experience.

Chapter 5

Common SSRI and Other Antidepressant Side Effects and Their Management

SEROTONIN SYNDROME

Serotonin syndrome occurs due to excessive serotonin levels in the circulatory system. The syndrome can vary in severity from mild to severe. Severe symptoms consist of hyperthermia, agitation, delirium, sweating, anxiety, hypotension or hypertension, confusion, and muscle twitches. Extremely severe reactions can lead to convulsions, coma, and even death. Serotonin syndrome commonly occurs when SSRI or a serotonergic TCA interacts with an MAOI, meperidine, or any of several kinds of decongestants. Sec the section on MAOIs for details regarding interaction involving MAOIs.

In general, SSRIs and clomipramine should not be started at higher than the usual starting dose, regardless of whether or not the patient had taken an MAOI, because some patients are very sensitive to the serotonergic effects of SSRIs and require several days of adaptation before they can tolerate higher doses.

If a patient is judged to require a higher than usual starting dose for a specific clinical reason, the prudent strategy is still to start at the usual starting dose and then to increase the dose rapidly so that if the patient happens to be sensitive to increased serotonin levels, the possible serotonin syndrome is likely to be mild and easily manageable. (See Table 5.1.) For instance, if a patient who is fairly sensitive to serotonin is started on fluoxetine 60 mg, the chances of a severe reaction are high, whereas the reaction in response to a starting dose of fluoxetine 20 mg or less is likely to be mild. Rapid dosage increase is safer than starting a new patient on high doses because the physician has no way of knowing which patient has excessive sensitivity to SSRIs. Some patients have mild serotonin

TABLE 5.1. Usual Starting Dose of SSRIs

	Usual Starting Dose
Fluoxetine	20mg AM
Sertraline	50mg AM
Paroxetine	20mg AM
Venlafaxine	37.5 mg BID-TID
Fluvoxamine	50mg BID
Clomipramine	25mg BID

syndrome consisting of anxiety, headache, restlessness, and diaphoresis even on usual starting doses of SSRIs and clomipramine. In most cases, these side effects subside over one to two weeks, or with treatment using benzodiazepine or clonidine. Some patients are extremely sensitive to serotonergic medications. SSRIs have overall superior safety in overdose and in terms of side effects. However, they are potent medications. Hence, the author's recommendation is not to start SSRIs or clomipramine at higher than usual starting doses even if the presenting depressive symptoms are severe and the physician is aiming for a quick response. In fact, some patients who are extremely restless and anxious to begin with may need to be started on one-half of the recommended starting dose. Serotonin syndrome also rarely occurs due to coadministration of trazodone, nefazodone, buspirone, over-the-counter decongestants, fenfluramine, and possibly pindolol, in patients already on fairly high doses of one of the SSRIs. Mild serotonin syndrome can be managed by use of benzodiazepines and decreasing the dose of or eliminating the offending medication. Severe serotonin syndrome may require management in the hospital.

ADRENERGIC DECONGESTANTS AND SEROTONIN SYNDROME

Various adrenergic decongestants in cold and allergy preparations can on rare occasions interact with SSRIs and cause symptoms such as increased anxiety, restlessness, agitation, diaphoresis, headaches, and hypertension or hypotension. Patients may be advised to try the first dose of a decongestant when they are home or in an environment where they are able to assist themselves or seek help should a reaction occur, as opposed to taking the first dose just before driving or jogging. If the first dose is tolerated well, then it is safer to continue decongestants as needed. Treatment can include one or more of the following:

- Use a benzodiazepine for temporary relief of symptoms (e.g., lorazepam 0.5 to 1 mg po).
- Prescribe cyproheptadine 4 to 8 mg po.
- Prescribe clonidine 0.1 mg po or guanfacine 1 mg po if hypotension is not present.
- Switch to an SSRI with less serotonin selectivity (e.g., switch to fluoxetine or fluvoxamine instead of paroxetine or sertraline [Refer to the list that follows for ranking of serotonin selectivity of common SSRIs]).
- Avoid adrenergic decongestants, if possible, and use antihistamines.
- Taper off the SSRI and consider a TCA.

Ranking of SSRIs Based on Selectivity of Serotonin Reuptake Inhibition

• Highest	paroxetine
	sertraline
	clomipramine (TCA)
	fluvoxamine
• Lowest	fluoxetine

SEXUAL DYSFUNCTION

Sexual dysfunction due to antidepressants includes decreased libido, erectile dysfunction, inhibited orgasm, inhibited ejaculation, and diminution of pleasurable body sensation in response to intimate touch. In clinical experience, one of the above-mentioned side effects occurs in approximately 60 percent of patients on SSRIs, making it the most common, but probably the most underreported, side effect. One has to specifically ask patients about this side effect in order for them to report it. There is some tolerance to this side effect over time, but complete normalization to baseline sexual functioning is rare while patients are on SSRIs. The incidence of sexual dysfunction related to TCAs and MAOIs is about 25 percent, except for clomipramine at 60 percent.

The severity of sexual dysfunction is for the most part dose-related, and hence decreasing the dose may improve sexual functioning, but this may also affect antidepressant efficacy. Patients should be cautioned not to be alarmed if any of the sexual side effects emerge. Surprisingly, most patients adjust to the sexual dysfunction and are not too bothered by it, probably accepting this side affect as a trade-off. If patients are unable to tolerate sexual dysfunction, the options are a change of medication or a trial of one of the medication interventions to treat the dysfunction.

Switching the patient to one of the other SSRIs is not very effective because all of those medications, such as paroxetine (Paxil), venlafaxine (Effexor), fluoxetine (Prozac), sertraline (Zoloft), and fluvoxamine (Luvox), also cause sexual dysfunction. Nefazodone, bupropion, mirtazapine, and trazodone have significantly lower incidence and severity of sexual dysfunction as a side effect. The incidence of sexual dysfunction associated with fluvoxamine is slightly lower compared to other SSRIs.

Various low efficacy medication interventions may be tried to treat sexual dysfunction. Bupropion at 75 to 150 mg as a one-time dose at noon or 75 mg po in the morning and at noon may be tried in conjunction with fluoxetine or one of the other SSRIs. In the author's experience, a 20 percent success rate has been observed when bupropion is added. Because of bupropion's tendency to decrease seizure threshold, the dosage of bupropion is kept low. A word of caution, however: bupropion should not be combined with clomipramine, which by itself tends to lower seizure threshold.

A second low probability intervention is the addition of methylphenidate (Ritalin) at a 5 mg or 10 mg dose two to three hours prior to sexual activity, or dextroamphetamine (Dexedrine) 5 to 10 mg at noon, though insomnia can be a problem. Another option is cyproheptadine (Periactin) at 4 mg to 12 mg two to three hours before coitus. However, since cyproheptadine has antiserotonin effects, frequent use may block the main effects of the serotonergic medication and can precipitate sudden emergence of the symptoms controlled by the primary medication, such as depression, anxiety, obsession, or compulsion. Other medications with low probability of success are pemoline (Cylert) 37.5 mg daily, bethanechol (Urecholine) at 25 mg po TID, bromocriptine (Parlodel) at 0.625 to 1.25 mg po BID, amantadine (Symmetrel) 100 mg po BID, and yohimbine (Yocon) 5.4 mg po TID.

In any case, patients should be reassured that sexual dysfunction is caused by the medication and is not because of the loss of love or caring on their part. They should also be informed that sexual functioning will return to baseline when the responsible medication is eventually discontinued.

It should be mentioned that sexual side effects of SSRIs can be exploited for the benefits of patients with premature ejaculation, nymphomania, and for control of dysfunctional behavior involving sexual fixation, compulsions, or perversions. They can be an aid to those who are required or wish to maintain celibacy, especially if sexual desires become overwhelming.

GASTROINTESTINAL SIDE EFFECTS

Gastrointestinal side effects include nausea, dyspepsia, eructation, loose bowel movements, dysgeusia, bloating, and flatulence. These affect about 30 percent of patients, and fortunately most of these side effects subside gradually in one to three weeks as patients continue taking the medication. If a patient has dyspepsia to begin with, the author recommends prophylactic treatment for one to two weeks by concurrent administration of H2 blockers such as ranitidine (Zantac) 150 mg po BID, cimetidine (Tagamet) 300 mg po BID, nizatidine (Axid) 150 mg po BID, or famotidine (Pepcid) 20 mg po BID. Antacids and antigas over-the-counter medications may also be tried on an as-needed basis. If patients have gastrointestinal side effects as well as insomnia and/or loss of appetite, an excellent adjunctive medication is doxepin (Sinequan) 10 mg to 25 mg at bedtime. Taking the medication with or after food intake can also help. Constipation, which is a common side effect of TCAs and MAOIs, is not seen with serotonergic medications.

LOSS OF APPETITE

Mild loss of appetite leading to weight loss of approximately 2 to 5 percent is seen in some patients taking SSRIs. However, most patients develop a tolerance to the loss of appetite; hence, weight loss does not continue for more than three to four months. This is in contrast to TCAs, which cause an increase in appetite with approximately 5 to 10 percent weight gain. In some patients the weight gain continues as long as the patient is on the TCA and can be substantial, depending on the length of time on the medication. Patients who are already anorectic present a problem when considering fluoxetine and most serotonergic medications because of the potential for further weight loss. An effective strategy to deal with this problem is prescribing nortriptyline 10 mg, imipramine 10 mg, amitriptyline 10 mg, or doxepin 10 mg at bedtime.

Moderate anorexia as a side effect may be an advantage in patients who present with hyperphagia, which can be one of the symptoms of depression, especially that of atypical depression. (Atypical depression is such a common syndrome in outpatient practice that it should hardly be called "atypical" anymore.) Clinical experience reveals that much of the anorectic effect of fluoxetine is seen in the higher dosage ranges, such as 40 mg to 80 mg. Patients report that their craving for sweets and carbohydrates, as well as compulsive binging are better controlled on SSRIs.

INSOMNIA

Initial, middle, and terminal insomnia are seen in patients taking fluoxetine and serotonergic medications, although it is somewhat less prevalent with fluvoxamine (Luvox) and nefazodone (Serzone). Insomnia must be treated for overall patient comfort and for fast recovery from the primary symptoms. Management includes administration of benzodiazepines for a brief period of time. For initial insomnia, zolpidem (Ambien) 5 mg to 10 mg, lorazepam 0.5 mg to 1 mg, and alprazolam 0.25 mg to 0.5 mg are effective. For middle and terminal insomnia, lorazepam 0.5 mg to 1 mg, temazepam 7.5 mg to 30 mg, clonazepam 0.5 mg to 1 mg, and flurazepam 15 mg to 30 mg are effective. The author's first-choice medication for insomnia is trazodone (Desyrel) 50 mg to 150 mg. Trazodone has the advantage of being nonaddictive, with no appreciable tolerance or abuse potential. Other options, especially in patients in whom abuse is a concern, include medications such as amitriptyline 10 mg to 25 mg, doxepin 10 mg to 25 mg, imipramine 10 mg to 25 mg, nortriptyline 10 mg to 25 mg, hydroxyzine 25 mg to 50 mg, and diphenhydramine 25 mg to 50 mg at bedtime.

ANXIETY AND AGITATION

Paradoxically, SSRIs can cause anxiety and restlessness in approximately 15 percent of patients, especially during the first one to two weeks of initiating treatment. This may represent a very mild form of serotonin syndrome. This side effect tends to subside on its own, usually in two to three weeks; therefore, in most cases, education and reassurance are all that is needed. In some cases in which anxiety and restlessness are more persistent and may represent a form of akathisia, symptomatic treatment using low-dose benzodiazepines is effective. For example, lorazepam 0.5 mg po BID or TID, alprazolam 0.25 mg to 0.5 mg po TID, or clonazepam 0.5 mg po BID for two to three weeks on an as-needed basis is helpful. Clonidine 0.1 mg po BID-TID or guanfacine 1 mg po HS or BID may also be tried.

Very rarely, SSRIs can cause severe agitation and restlessness that may constitute mild to moderate serotonin syndrome, requiring immediate discontinuation of the medication and treatment using benzodiazepines. Hence, patients should be monitored closely during the first several months of treatment and should be instructed to call the physician if any unusual symptoms or problems emerge. Patients may be switched to another SSRI that may not cause restlessness. Other options include lowering the dose of the SSRI and/or prescribing a benzodiazepine for as-needed use. Rarely, TCAs and MAOIs can also cause this side effect.

HEADACHE

While SSRIs are sometimes used to treat chronic headaches, they can cause headaches as a side effect, which usually subsides in two to three weeks. If symptomatic treatment of the headache through the use of acetaminophen, aspirin, or nonsteroidal anti-inflammatory drugs is not effective, the particular SSRI may have to be discontinued and the patient switched to another SSRI. Most sedating TCAs and MAOIs improve headaches.

SEDATION

Mild sedation and somnolence are also seen in a small percentage of patients for whom administration of the medication at night may resolve the problem.

MUSCLE TIGHTNESS

Muscle tightness, especially of the posterior neck and jaw muscles, as well as bruxism, are occasionally seen. These side effects tend to subside over time. Gradual dosage increase is suggested in these patients. Benzodiazepines can be used on an as-needed basis for control of muscle tightness.

SWEATING AND TREMORS

Both sweating and tremors may be effectively controlled on beta blockers such as propranolol 10 mg TID, propranolol LA 60 to 120 mg daily, or atenolol 50 mg daily. Benzodiazepines are also helpful. Clonidine 0.1 mg BID or guanfacine 1 to 2 mg HS is sometimes effective. If sweating and tremors are marked, discontinuation of the medication may be necessary.

MANIA

Any antidepressant in therapeutic doses has the potential to precipitate mania, primarily in patients who are predisposed to it by virtue of having an undiagnosed bipolar disorder, which in most cases presents with a first episode of depression. Management consists of reducing the dosage of the antidepressant or discontinuing it, depending on the severity of the manic episode. Immediate treatment of the manic episode must be initiated.

PSYCHOSIS

Antidepressants can trigger manifestation of psychotic symptoms in susceptible individuals, requiring immediate recognition of the problem and the addition of antipsychotic medication. Most patients with underlying psychosis have depressive symptoms such as low-grade dysphoria, excessive emotional sensitivity, social withdrawal, demoralization, apathy, and blunted affect–all of which may represent the so-called negative or deficit symptoms of chronic psychosis. Antidepressants can improve the above-listed symptoms, but can precipitate florid psychosis if antipsychotics are not used concurrently.

ANTICHOLINERGIC SIDE EFFECTS

Anticholinergic side effects are frequently manifested while taking tricyclic antidepressants. Common anticholinergic side effects are constipation, dry mouth, blurred vision, urinary hesitation, urinary retention, tachycardia, exacerbation of narrow-angle glaucoma, and, in severe cases, paralytic ileus. Typically, these side effects improve over a period of two to three weeks. Highly anticholinergic antidepressants such as amitriptyline, trimipramine, doxepin, protriptyline, imipramine, clomipramine, and maprotiline cause a greater degree of these side effects compared to desipramine, nortriptyline, and amoxapine, which have relatively low anticholinergic properties. SSRIs, trazodone, nefazodone, mirtazapine, and bupropion have extremely low anticholinergic effect. The anticholinergic effects of MAOIs are fairly low, with phenelzine having greater anticholinergic effects compared to tranylcypromine. A slow dosage increase gives time to develop tolerance to the anticholinergic side effects. If anticholinergic side effects persist, a less anticholinergic antidepressant should be considered. However, if the patient needs to continue an antidepressant that is causing anticholinergic side effects, there are various management options, described as follows.

Constipation

Constipation may respond to increased fluid intake; increasing bulk by consuming high-residue foods such as fruits, vegetables, and fiber; and by using bulk laxatives and stool softeners. The following over-the-counter products may also remedy the symptom:

Bulk-Forming Drugs:

methylcellulose (Citrucel)
phyllium (Metamucil)
calcium polycarbophil (Fiberall, Fibercon)

Laxatives/Stool Softeners:

bisacodyl (Dulcolax)
docusate sodium (Colace)

Enemas may occasionally be necessary to relieve constipation if simpler interventions fail. Treatment using bethanechol (Urecholine) 10 to 25 mg TID is effective in some patients.

Dry Mouth

Effective interventions include frequent rinsing, sucking ice cubes or hard candy, chewing sugarless gum, or using bethanechol 10 to 25 mg po TID.

Urinary Hesitation or Retention

Bentanechol 10 to 25 mg TID can be used. Severe urinary retention may require using a urinary catheter to empty the bladder and discontinuing the offending medication, especially in patients who have prostatic hypertrophy.

Blurred Vision

Blurred vision is more noticeable with near objects, as in reading. Pilocarpine 1 percent solution, one drop every six hours during waking hours, is effective in severe cases.

Hypotension

Postural hypotension is a common side effect of sedating TCAs and MAOIs and, to a limited extent, trazodone and nefazodone. Patients should be advised to be cautious when getting up from a lying or sitting position, or after bending down. Adequate fluid intake and supplemental sodium intake (in the absence of congestive heart failure) should be of help. If hypotension is marked, it is preferable to switch to another antidepressant.

Cardiac Conduction

TCAs can prolong cardiac conduction and can cause heart block. They should, therefore, be avoided in patients who have heart block. TCAs can also produce tachycardia and various electrocardiogram (EKG) changes, including widening of QRS and increase of PR interval. Rare sudden death has occurred, probably due to cardiac arrhythmias.

Weight Gain

Weight gain is very common in patients taking TCAs and phenelzine. Fenfluramine (Pondimin) is a serotonergic anorexiant that is occasionally effective in suppressing appetite. It may be used at doses of 20 mg BID one to two hours before meals. Possible risk of serotonergic crisis should preclude its use with MAOIs. See Chapter 2 for clinical guidelines regarding concurrent use of antidepressants and fenfluramine.

Narrow-Angle Glaucoma

TCAs can precipitate narrow-angle glaucoma and can lead to vision damage. Eye pain could be a symptom that should arouse immediate suspicion that glaucoma may be present. An eye examination should be scheduled without delay, as eye pain in glaucoma is a true medical emergency with vision loss as a possible consequence.

Seizure

All antidepressants lower the seizure threshold to varying degrees. Clomipramine and bupropion lower seizure threshold more than others, with SSRIs and MAOIs having the least effect on seizure threshold. If high doses of clomipramine and bupropion are necessary or if a patient is at risk for seizure, consideration should be given to adding an anticonvulsant for prophylaxis.

Table 5.2 lists various medications and dosages for treatment of common antidepressant side effects.

TABLE 5.2. Adjunctive Medication Menu for Treatment of Common Symptoms or Side Effects (in mg)

Insomnia	Dyspepsia	Anorexia	Anxiety	Sexual dysfunction
lorazepam 0.5-1 temazepam 7.5-30 zolpidem 5-10 alprazolam 0.25-1 clonazepam 0.5-1 diazepam 5-10 chlordiazepoxide 10-25 flurazepam 15-30 triazolam 0.125-0.25 estazolam 1-2 oxazepam 15-30 quazepam 7.5-15 clorazepate 3.75-15 trazodone 50-100*** nefazodone 50-100 amitriptyline 10-25 doxepin 10-25 imipramine 10-50 nortriptyline 10-25 diphenhydramine 25-50 hydroxyzine 25-50 chloral hydrate 500-1,000	ranitidine 150 BID famotidine 20 BID nizatidine 150 BID antacids PRN doxepin 10-25 HS	doxepin 10 amitriptyline 10 imipramine 10 nortriptyline 10 desipramine 10 trimipramine 25	lorazepam 0.5 BID-TID alprazolam 0.25-0.5 TID clonazepam 0.5 BID-TID Any other benzodiazepine for 1 to 2 weeks, until anti-depressant effects begin	yohimbine 5.4 TID cyproheptadine 4-8** two hours before coitus amantadine 100 BID-TID bupropion 100-150 AM or noon* bethanechol 25 BID-TID methylphenidate 5-10 two hours before coitus dextroamphetamine 5-10 two hours before coitus trazodone 50-100*** nefazodone 100-200 bromocriptine 1.25 pemoline 37.5-75 daily

* Note seizure precautions in text
** Can precipitate depression
*** Rare incidence of priapism

Chapter 6

Electroconvulsive Therapy

Electroconvulsive therapy (ECT) is a remarkably effective treatment for depression. It can also be employed for the treatment of functional catatonia and mania. Psychotic depression is by far the most common indication for ECT. Although it can be used as a first-line treatment, it is typically used in clinical practice only after pharmacotherapeutic approaches have failed. A small percentage of patients do not respond satisfactorily to any of the wide variety of antidepressants currently available.

ADVANTAGES AND DISADVANTAGES

ECT is very safe when administered with anesthesia. It is administered in a hospital setting, generally during an inpatient hospitalization. Outpatient ECT is usually given for maintenance treatment, rather than for the initial ECT course.

Despite its effectiveness in all forms of depression, catatonia, and mania, it is used as a last resort when the following conditions exist: the patient cannot tolerate medication for whatever reason, the patient is a nonresponder to medication, or the symptoms or the consequences of symptoms are so severe that the patient cannot wait for medication to begin to work. Relative contraindications include increased intracranial pressure, recent myocardial infarction (within two to four months), severe hypertension, pheochromocytoma, recent intracerebral hemorrhage, severe pulmonary disease, and severe congestive heart failure. ECT for a patient with these conditions should be undertaken only with appropriate precautions and medical backup. The presence of an Axis II personality disorder or other Axis III conditions should not, by themselves, be a contraindication for ECT. It is estimated that approximately 60 percent of patients with treatment-resistant depression will respond to ECT.

It is important to note that ECT is quite costly. For example, ten treatments of ECT with a 21-day hospital stay at a nonpreferred rate cost approximately $25,000 to $30,000 with itemized billing in a private facility. A ten-course outpatient ECT costs $7,000 to $10,000 with itemized nonpreferred billing (costs are less with preferred contract arrangements). Given these costs, it behooves the practitioner in today's managed care environment to utilize pharmacotherapy whenever possible.

ECT is particularly effective for rapid treatment of psychotic depression and catatonia, which do not respond to medication intervention. It is a reasonable question to ask why ECT is not the treatment of first choice before a trial on medication when ECT is safe and effective. The reasons for using ECT as a last resort in current psychiatric practice, are as follows:

- Public stigma is still significant, requiring substantial justification for its use.
- ECT is labor intensive because of the use of hospital facilities, recovery room, services of anesthesiologists and nurses, and auxiliary services.
- Anesthesia is required.
- Treatment typically requires three weeks of hospitalization for approximately eight to ten treatments. (Maintenance ECT does not require hospitalization.)
- Nearly all patients who receive ECT will still need to be maintained on an antidepressant or mood stabilizer since ECT by itself is not a permanent cure for depression.
- In practice, even in so-called emergency cases, there is usually a delay of two to three days before ECT is actually started. (Delays are due to the time it takes to obtain the required labs, X-rays, EKG, anesthesia consult, patient and/or family education and consent, schedule of other consults as necessary, need for guardianship or permission by the court for treating severely regressed or catatonic patients who may be unable to give informed consent, etc.) In contrast, medication or a combination of medications, can usually be started immediately.
- Initiation of medication treatment is much more expedient, convenient, and at least at the onset, much less expensive.
- Newer antidepressants, which have recently become available, have fewer side effects and are better tolerated by the elderly and the medically ill.
- Risperidone and olanzapine, which have rapid effects and fewer extrapyramidal symptoms (EPS), are available for use in psychotic depression.

- There is higher initial expense because of the following fees: psychiatrist, anesthesiologist, hospital recovery room, procedure room, medications, transportation, treatment, inpatient hospital room, various consultants, and various lab tests during the entire hospitalization.
- Clozapine, which can effectively treat intractable psychotic depression and schizoaffective disorder, depressed type, is available.
- Memory loss, although temporary in most cases, can be prolonged in some cases. Eventually, memory function is expected to return to baseline for the great majority of patients except for memory of the seizure episode itself. Unfortunately, the side effect of temporary memory loss is exaggerated by various nonmedical anti-ECT movements. This results in frightening the public and discrediting ECT.

Bilateral ECT is more effective than nondominant hemisphere (usually right) unilateral ECT; however, bilateral ECT produces greater memory impairment, confusion, and headache. Bilateral ECT, therefore, is used when fast response is desired for clinical reasons, and is usually switched to unilateral ECT after the first two or three treatments. Bilateral ECT is also employed when unilateral ECT is ineffective. Current practice is to use brief-pulse right unilateral ECT in the majority of cases. Multiple unilateral ECT treatments (usually two) in one session is another alternative to bilateral ECT in patients needing a quick response.

As emphasized throughout this text, medications and procedures treat specific symptoms and signs, not diagnoses. This concept applies to ECT also. For example, it is generally held that schizophrenia does not respond to ECT. However, it must be remembered that schizophrenia is a heterogeneous condition with considerable overlap of affective symptoms, either primary or secondary. ECT is effective in treating the affective symptoms of schizophrenia or other conditions. It does not improve thought disorders. Similarly, it is the general consensus that ECT is not indicated for symptoms of personality disorders.

In some of the ECT protocols, the presence of a personality disorder is a contraindication for ECT. Many of the component symptoms of borderline personality disorder, however, are affective in nature, with strong depressive and hypomanic characteristics. These affective symptoms can be successfully treated by ECT. The presence of borderline personality disorder symptoms should alert the clinician to treatment-responsive affective symptoms. Unfortunately, any difficult, treatment-resistant, complicated, or hostile patient is labeled "borderline" and considered a poor responder to treatment if not altogether untreatable. There are numerous instances of so-called borderline personality disorder patients who respond well to antidepressants, mood stabilizers, antipsychotics (including clozapine), or combinations of the above medications to the point that the personality disorder is no longer evident. There is every reason to believe that these patients would have responded equally well to ECT. Schizophreniform disorder and schizoaffective disorder, both of which have considerable affective overlap, also respond to ECT, depending on the extent of affective symptoms.

The issue is not whether or not ECT is safe and effective. It is clearly a safe and effective treatment modality. The real issue is *when* to use ECT. Should it be the first-line treatment for all depression and for other indications since it is safe and effective? In the era of TCAs and MAOIs, the side effects were not tolerated well by the elderly and the medically ill for whom ECT would be routinely considered. However, with the advent of serotonergic drugs, venlafaxine, nefazodone, bupropion, and mirtazapine, this is no longer the case. Elderly and medically ill individuals tolerate these medications well for the most part. The availability of risperidone and olanzapine has also allowed more medication options with fewer side effects. Clozapine, which has been available since 1990, is a superior medication for treatment-resistant psychosis with or without affective components. New indications for valproate and carbamazepine as primary or adjunctive medications in the treatment of rapid cycling bipolar disorder, dysphoric mania, and schizoaffective disorder have substantially increased the medication options available for conditions that previously were fairly difficult to treat and hence needed ECT for a response.

Still, there are some patients for whom medications do not work. In some cases, ECT has converted medication nonresponders to responders, in addition to treating their symptoms. After ECT has been completed, patients should be placed on medications (depending on the condition for which ECT was given) for prophylactic purposes, unless maintenance ECT is provided. Without prophylactic medications or maintenance ECT, the relapse rate in six months to one year is expected to be high.

Advantages of ECT

- It is safe and effective when appropriately used in selected cases.
- ECT has a fairly rapid and impressive response. In terms of speed of recovery and return to full functioning, ECT may be superior to medication in some severely depressed patients.
- Modified ECT, as practiced today, has a low rate of side effects and complications.
- It is effective in patients who cannot tolerate medications (e.g., the severely medically ill, women in their first trimester of pregnancy),

in patients in whom very rapid response is necessary for clinical reasons, and in medication nonresponders.
- A course of ECT could convert a medication nonresponder to a responder.
- ECT truly can be a "life saver" in severely depressed and extremely suicidal or medically ill patients and in patients with severe catatonia for whom other treatment options are not effective or not possible.

Disadvantages of ECT

- The public stigma is still present.
- Hospitalization, in most cases, or hospital-based services are necessary.
- It is labor intensive (psychiatrist, anesthetist, nurses, technicians).
- Memory loss (for the treatment period), confusion, and headaches are side effects (usually temporary).
- It is initially expensive (patients without generous third-party coverage cannot afford it, unless they are wealthy).
- The procedure is, by nature, invasive (not literally invasive, but in the sense that anesthesia is necessary, and brain cells are stimulated by externally applied electrical current, triggering seizure activity).
- It is not a permanent cure: to maintain improvement and to prevent relapse, patients have to take medication on completion of ECT, or receive periodic maintenance ECT.
- It is not 100 percent effective. Although ECT is generally very effective, not all patients respond (as is true of all treatment approaches).
- In most cases there is a delay of two to three days before treatment is started.
- ECT remains an easy target for militant groups and opportunistic politicians looking for "causes."

Chapter 7

Anxiety Disorders: Practical Diagnostic and Management Guidelines

GENERAL CONSIDERATIONS

Anxiety disorders are among the most common emotional problems seen by a physician or mental health professional. Anxiety is a component of virtually all psychiatric presentations. Anxiety disorder as a primary diagnosis constitutes approximately 10 to 20 percent of primary psychiatric diagnoses in an outpatient practice setting. Antianxiety medications are known as minor tranquilizers; they are also called sedatives because of their sedating effects. The treatment of anxiety typically uses a variety of antianxiety medications, the most common group of which is the benzodiazepines, which have sedative action. Among benzodiazepines, the most widely used as primary antianxiety medications are alprazolam (Xanax), diazepam (Valium), chlordiazepoxide (Librium), lorazepam (Ativan), oxazepam (Serax), and clonazepam (Klonopin). Benzodiazepines are relatively safe in overdose. Other antianxiety medications such as phenobarbital, meprobamate, and various barbiturates have fallen out of favor in modern clinical practice; hence, if an antianxiety medication is necessary, benzodiazepines are the medications of choice. Choosing a benzodiazepine among the many that are available depends on various factors, including pharmacological characteristics such as half-life, method of metabolism, onset of action, duration of action, and purpose. These and other factors will be explained further.

Despite the improved safety and efficacy of benzodiazepines, their role in psychiatry and medicine should be adjunctive, limited, and short-term in treatment of anxiety and other disorders. This is for several important reasons, the most salient of which are (1) the availability of serotonergic antidepressants and tricyclics which, offer many advantages in long-term treatment of anxiety; (2) the significant addiction potential of all benzodiazepines; and (3) development of tolerance when used regularly. Although tricyclic antidepressants are effective for long-term control of anxiety, the presence of considerable side effects such as sedation, dry mouth, constipation, blurry vision, cardiac problems, hypotension, weight gain, and urinary problems associated with tricyclics make TCAs relatively difficult for patients to tolerate. Hence, justifiably, physicians were reluctant to prescribe TCAs in the past for treatment of anxiety when alternatives, consisting of a variety of benzodiazepines that did not have the TCA side effects, were available. With the introduction of serotonergic antidepressants such as fluoxetine (Prozac), sertraline (Zoloft), paroxetine (Paxil), venlafaxine (Effexor), fluvoxamine (Luvox), mirtazapine, and nefazodone (Serzone), this situation has recently changed dramatically. It is obvious that the physician has a duty to help the patient without making the patient either dependent on the drug or on the physician. A prescription for greater than one month of a fairly fast-acting and short half-life benzodiazepine at high doses will inadvertently do exactly this. It is by far a clinical fallacy, not supported by clinical experience, that those who truly have an anxiety disorder such as panic disorder or obsessive-compulsive disorder do not become dependent on benzodiazepines. The central nervous system is at a high risk of physiological dependence when exposed to the drug, and hence dependency has nothing much to do with the nature of the disorder, although some individual variation in addiction liability exists within limits. Hence, ideally all antianxiety drugs should be used only as adjunctive medications in the vast majority of patients. It is well-known that a fair number of physicians, including psychiatrists, tend to prescribe antianxiety drugs as the primary medication for anxiety disorders such as generalized anxiety disorder, panic disorder, and phobic disorder. It is the author's opinion, based on extensive and successful clinical experience, that serotonergic antidepressants are a much superior choice as the primary medications for all anxiety disorders in the great majority of patients who have anxiety symptoms.

Benzodiazepines, on rare occasions, can cause disinhibition and memory loss, especially anterograde amnesia, leading to behavioral dyscontrol. Caution is recommended in their use with children, adolescents, and the elderly, who may be more prone to these effects. Approximate benzodiazepine half-life, common dosage range, and dose equivalence are listed in Table 7.1.

Since the newer antidepressants do not have TCA side effects, they may be used as first-line choices for long-term treatment of anxiety. The author

TABLE 7.1. Benzodiazepines: Approximate Half-Life, Common Dosage Range, and Dose Equivalency

Generic Name	Common Brand Name	Approximate Half-Life in Hours	Common Dosage Range (mg)	Equivalent Dose (mg)
lorazepam	Ativan	12	0.50 - 1.0 BID	1.0
alprazolam	Xanax	11	0.25 - 1.0 BID	0.5
clonazepam	Klonopin	30	0.50 - 1.0 BID	0.5
diazepam	Valium	50	5.00 -10.0 BID	5.0
chloriazepoxide	Librium	70	5.00 -25.0 BID	15.0
oxazepam	Serax	12	10.00 -15.0 BID	15.0
temazepam	Restoril	12	7.50 -30.0 HS	15.0
quazepam	Doral	50	7.50 -15.0 HS	7.5
flurazepam	Dalmane	90	15.00 -30.0 HS	15.0
prazepam	Centrax	70	5.00 -10.0 BID	5.0
clorazepate	Tranxene	60	3.75 - 7.5 TID	7.5
triazolam	Halcion	3	0.125 - 0.25 HS	0.125
estazolam	Prosom	14	1.00 - 2.0 HS	1.0
*zolpidem	Ambien	2.5	5.00 -10.0 HS	10.0

*Although a non-benzodiazepine hypnotic, can cause dependence, tolerance, and withdrawal, similar to benzodiazepines.

feels that there are many advantages in using antidepressants, particularly the newer antidepressants, for primary treatment of anxiety disorders, and in using benzodiazepines adjunctively for short-term treatment on an as needed basis. Various clinical reasons for this opinion are discussed in the following text.

Since benzodiazepines have several advantages over the older sedatives, they are commonly used in clinical practice. They are best used for short-term purposes because of the potential for dependence and tolerance, and because side effects such as depression and cognitive impairment are seen with long-term use. If an anxiety disorder or anxiety symptom is expected to need treatment for more than several weeks, it is generally prudent to use an antidepressant as the primary medication. Among antidepressant categories, the author's preference for SSRIs is not because they are more effective, compared to older antidepressants. They are not. The major advantage of SSRIs is their improved side effect profile. Their less-frequent dosing schedule is an added advantage that enhances compliance. All antidepressants are effective for the treatment of anxiety disorders and should be the primary medication for their treatment for the following specific reasons:

- Long-term effectiveness
- Ability to treat and prevent anxiety
- Lack of addiction potential
- Lack of tolerance
- Lack of need for dosage escalation
- Ability to decrease or limit the dose of benzodiazepines when used adjunctively
- Ability to improve commonly associated depressive symptoms
- Ease of discontinuation

Although TCAs, MAOIs, and serotonergic antidepressants are equally effective, serotonergic medications are preferred because of their favorable side effect profile and safety in overdose. Because there is some confusion among physicians regarding this point, it needs some elaboration and re-emphasis. The misunderstanding that serotonergic antidepressants are more effective than TCAs or MAOIs is widespread among physicians and non-physician mental health professionals. It is true that each class of antidepressants can be more effective than another class for a particular individual. For example, some of the difficult depressions that have not responded to fluoxetine, sertraline, paroxetine, venlafaxine, fluvoxamine, and nefazodone have responded to older medications such as imipramine, phenelzine (Nardil), tranylcypromine (Parnate), and clomipramine (Anafranil). It should be emphasized that the popularity and acceptance of serotonergic medications is because they have far fewer side effects when compared to TCAs and MAOIs. For example, the elderly, children, and medically ill patients tolerate SSRIs and bupropion much better than TCAs and MAOIs. Yet, there are many patients who cannot tolerate serotonergic medications, but do well on TCAs or MAOIs without any appreciable side effects. No one medication is well-tolerated by everyone. Medication effectiveness, side effect vulnerability, and tolerability are highly individual matters.

Since antidepressants do not work immediately and have a lag time of one to three weeks for response, it is usually necessary to use a benzodiazepine for treatment of acute anxiety during the first several weeks until the antidepressant becomes effective. Some patients who get only partial relief of symptoms from antidepressants will need adjunctive treatment using benzodiazepines. However, the combination of an antidepressant and a benzodiazepine will make it possible to keep the dose of the benzodiazepine lower than the dose that would be needed without the antidepressant. It is the very rare patient who cannot tolerate any of the antidepressants and as a result must rely on a benzodiazepine alone. For instance, the author can recall only 2 out of more than 500 cases of anxiety disorders for whom none of the antidepressants, including TCAs, MAOIs, and serotonergic drugs could be tolerated, necessitating maintenance on a benzodiazepine. In most cases of severe anxiety or panic disorder, a combination of an antidepressant with as-needed adjunctive use of benzodiazepines is necessary and effective. In moderate cases of anxiety disorder, antidepressants alone may be sufficient, except for the first few weeks when a benzodiazepine is used intermittently. If a particular patient requires scheduled daily doses of a benzodiazepine, the benzodiazepine dosage can be lowered when an antidepressant medication is concurrently given. Moreover, the need for benzodiazepine dosage escalation to maintain efficacy can usually be prevented or restrained using this strategy. Since anxiety and insomnia respond fairly well to all benzodiazepines, it is generally preferable to prescribe generic drugs for these indications for enhancing cost-effectiveness.

Anxiety Disorders Classification

- Generalized anxiety disorder
- Panic disorder
- Panic disorder with agoraphobia
- Agoraphobia
- Obsessive-compulsive disorder
- Adjustment disorder with anxious mood
- Specific phobia
- Social phobia

Following are *DSM-IV* diagnostic criteria for various anxiety disorders.

GENERALIZED ANXIETY DISORDER

Generalized anxiety disorder (GAD) criteria according to *DSM-IV* are as follows:*

A. Excessive anxiety and worry (apprehensive expectation), occurring more days than not for at least six months, about a number of events or activities (such as school or work performance).

---

*Italicized text is reprinted with permission from the *Diagnostic and Statistical Manual of Mental Disorders*, Fourth Edition. Copyright 1994 American Psychiatric Association.

B. The person finds it difficult to control the worry.

C. The anxiety and worry are associated with three (or more) of the following six symptoms (with at least some symptoms present for more days than not for the past six months). Note: Only one item is required in children.

1. *Restlessness or feeling keyed up or on edge*
2. *Being easily fatigued*
3. *Difficulty concentrating or mind going blank*
4. *Irritability*
5. *Muscle tension*
6. *Sleep disturbance (difficulty falling or staying asleep, or restless, unsatisfying sleep)*

D. The focus of the anxiety and worry is not confined to features of an Axis I disorder, e.g., the anxiety or worry is not about having a panic attack (as in panic disorder), being embarrassed in public (as in social phobia), being contaminated (as in obsessive-compulsive disorder), being away from home or close relatives (as in separation anxiety disorder), gaining weight (as in anorexia nervosa), having multiple physical complaints (as in somatization disorder), or having a serious illness (as in hypochondriasis), and the anxiety and worry do not occur exclusively during post-traumatic stress disorder.

E. The anxiety, worry, or physical symptoms cause clinically significant distress or impairment in social, occupational, or other important areas of functioning.

F. The disturbance is not due to the direct physiological effects of a substance (e.g., a drug of abuse, a medication) or a general medical condition (e.g., hyperthyroidism) and does not occur exclusively during a mood disorder, a psychotic disorder, or a pervasive developmental disorder.

General anxiety, or free-floating anxiety, is perhaps the most fundamental and basic of all the symptoms in psychiatry. While it is fairly easy to choose from among the antianxiety medications available for symptomatic control of anxiety, the more important task of the clinician is to identify the etiology of anxiety and provide definitive treatment. For example, if anxiety is generated due to underlying paranoia or obsession, both antianxiety medication and an antipsychotic or an antiobsessional medication may be necessary.

Generalized anxiety disorder (GAD) as a primary diagnosis is used infrequently, in fact only in the rare case where a more fundamental diagnosis cannot be found. Anxiety symptoms are associated with practically all psychiatric disorders. Effective treatment of the primary psychiatric disorder eventually will cause anxiety symptoms to subside completely. In such cases, separate treatment of anxiety using antianxiety medication is not necessary in the long term.

There are a small number of patients in whom typical GAD symptoms are present without evidence of symptoms of any other psychiatric disorder. Even in these patients, low doses of serotonergic antidepressants, TCAs, and MAOIs should be the primary medication, with adjunctive and intermittent use of benzodiazepines, for reasons already discussed.

Medication Treatment of GAD

The primary medications that are the most effective and the least problematic for long-term treatment of GAD are antidepressants. Among antidepressants, the newer SSRI antidepressants are preferred as the drugs of choice for treatment of anxiety disorders.

Fluoxetine (Prozac)

Fluoxetine at low doses, such as 5 to 20 mg per day, is effective. Fluoxetine is available in liquid form, enabling flexible dosing especially at the lower dosage ranges (1 to 20 mg). It is also available as 10 mg capsules. Patients with GAD or panic disorder do not generally tolerate high doses; hence, very low doses of 5 or 10 mg should be tried first for two to three weeks prior to increasing the dose. Since fluoxetine tends to cause mild akathisia-like symptoms in some patients and could cause short-term insomnia, adjunctive use of a benzodiazepine such as lorazepam (Ativan) at 0.5 mg po BID, alprazolam (Xanax) 0.25 to 0.5 mg po TID, or clonazepam (Klonopin) 0.5 mg po BID, may need to be prescribed on an as-needed basis.

Sertraline (Zoloft)

Sertraline (Zoloft) at low doses of 25 to 50 mg po AM is also an option for treatment of anxiety. Sertraline is available in scored tablet form, and can be easily divided to obtain lower dose forms. Sertraline can effectively treat generalized anxiety disorder and panic disorder at the low end of the dosage range. Sertraline is also effective for obsessive-compulsive disorder at a higher dosage range, such as 200 mg daily, which is the maximum dosage recommended by the drug company. Side effect profiles for all serotonergic drugs are similar and are discussed in Chapter 5.

Paroxetine (Paxil)

Paroxetine is another option as a primary medication for treatment of generalized anxiety disorder and panic disorder at a low dosage range of 10 to 30 mg per day and for obsessive-compulsive disorder at a higher dosage range of 40 to 80 mg per day. Paroxetine, like all serotonergic medications, can cause temporary anxiety as an initial side effect, but in my experience, it tends to have remarkable antianxiety effects when taken for more than two weeks. However, since its half-life is relatively short, abrupt discontinuation can lead to a syndrome consisting of dizziness, nausea, vomiting, and anxiety, which may last up to a week; hence, gradually tapering over a period of seven days is recommended. Such is not the case with fluoxetine because of its long half-life, providing built-in tapering in cases where medication is stopped abruptly.

Venlafaxine (Effexor), Fluvoxamine (Luvox) and Nefazodone (Serzone)

Venlafaxine, fluvoxamine, mirtazapine, and nefazodone can also be used for treatment of anxiety. See the antidepressant section for clinical profiles of these medications. Individual benzodiazepines and dosages are described separately at the end of this chapter. See Table 7.1 for approximate dose equivalencies of benzodiazepines, dosage range, and half-life.

Propranolol (Inderal) and Clonidine (Catapres)

Propranolol and clonidine are medications that can be used as adjunctive drugs for management of anxiety. Propranolol is a beta-adrenergic receptor blocker that suppresses some of the peripheral manifestations of anxiety. Tremors, tachycardia, hypertension, sweating, etc., can be controlled by propranolol, as well as other beta-blockers, at low doses. Propranolol dosage for use as an adjunctive medication in anxiety disorders ranges from 10 to 40 mg TID, or a long-acting preparation of 60 to 120 mg once a day. Moreover, beta blockers can be used as one of the adjunctive medications for sedatives and alcohol withdrawal. Propranolol does not, however, have crosstolerance with sedatives or alcohol and hence will not protect the patient from the primary withdrawal symptoms such as seizures and delirium. It should not be used as the sole agent for detoxification purposes.

Clonidine can be used as an adjunctive medication for treatment of anxiety disorders and for treatment of symptoms of sedative or alcohol withdrawal, as well as nicotine or opioid withdrawal. It is an antihypertensive medication that can also be used for treatment of attention-deficit hyperactivity disorder, Tourette's syndrome, akathisia, and mania. The dosage is 0.1 mg BID, with gradual increases as needed to a maximum of 0.2 mg BID. It is available as 0.1, 0.2, and 0.3 mg tablets. It is also available in a transdermal patch form or Catapres TTS-1, 2, and 3, which delivers clonidine 0.1 mg, 0.2 mg, and 0.3 mg daily, respectively. Multiple patches can be used as needed. The patch is applied once a week. It has a half-life of approximately 12 hours. Common side effects include sedation, fatigue, hypotension, dry mouth, constipation, and dizziness. Tricyclic antidepressants can neutralize the antihypertensive effect of clonidine. Transdermal preparation can cause local skin reaction at the site of application.

PANIC DISORDER

Panic disorder is characterized by panic attacks that occur suddenly. Criteria for a panic attack are listed below.*

A discrete period of intense fear or discomfort, in which four (or more) of the following symptoms developed abruptly and reached a peak within ten minutes:

1. *Palpitations, pounding heart, or accelerated heart rate*
2. *Sweating*
3. *Trembling or shaking*
4. *Sensations of shortness of breath or smothering*
5. *Feeling of choking*
6. *Chest pain or discomfort*
7. *Nausea or abdominal distress*
8. *Feeling dizzy, unsteady, lightheaded, or faint*

---

*Italicized text is reprinted with permission from the *Diagnostic and Statistical Manual of Mental Disorders*, Fourth Edition. Copyright 1994 American Psychiatric Association.

9. Derealization (feelings of unreality) or depersonalization (being detached from oneself)
10. Fear of losing control or going crazy
11. Fear of dying
12. Paresthesia (numbness or tingling sensations)
13. Chills or hot flashes

Panic disorder can occur with or without agoraphobia. The criteria for panic disorder according to DSM-IV are as follows:

A. Both 1 and 2:

1. Recurrent unexpected panic attacks
2. At least one of the attacks has been followed by one month (or more) of one (or more) of the following:
a. Persistent concern about having additional attacks
b. Worry about the implications of the attack or its consequences (e.g., losing control, having a heart attack, "going crazy")
c. A significant change in behavior related to the attacks

B. Either the absence or the presence of agoraphobia

C. The panic attacks are not due to the direct physiological effects of a substance (e.g., a drug of abuse, a medication) or a general medical condition (e.g., hyperthyroidism)

D. The panic attacks are not better accounted for by another mental disorder, such as social phobia (e.g., occurring on exposure to feared social situations), specific phobia (e.g., on exposure to a specific phobic situation), obsessive-compulsive disorder (e.g., on exposure to dirt in someone with an obsession about contamination), post-traumatic stress disorder (e.g., in response to stimuli associated with a severe stressor), or separation anxiety disorder (e.g., in response to being away from home or close relatives).

Panic disorder is a form of anxiety disorder, and is best treated by using antidepressants. Of all the categories of antidepressants, serotonergic antidepressants should be the drug of choice because of their efficacy, safety, and favorable side effect profile. The preferred medications and starting doses among the serotonergic antidepressants are given below. Nefazodone is also included in the list.

– paroxetine (Paxil)	10-20 mg AM
– sertraline (Zoloft)	25-50 mg AM

– fluoxetine (Prozac)	10-20 mg AM
– fluvoxamine (Luvox)	50-100 mg AM
– venlafaxine (Effexor)	12.5-25 mg BID-TID
– nefazodone (Serzone)	100-150 mg BID-TID

TCAs provide another option, but they are second to SSRIs in their safety and side effect criteria. In terms of antipanic effects, TCAs are as effective as SSRIs. For example, imipramine and desipramine are excellent antipanic medications, except for their TCA side effects. Examples of TCAs are as follows:

– imipramine (Tofranil)	25-150 mg HS or in divided doses
– desipramine (Norpramin)	25-100 mg HS or in divided doses
– nortriptyline (Pamelor)	25-50 mg HS or in divided doses
– amitriptyline (Elavil)	25-100 mg HS or in divided doses
– clomipramine (Anafranil)	25-100 mg HS or in divided doses

MAOIs are effective antipanic drugs but are second- or third-line drugs due to their side effects and diet/drug interaction problems. Two such examples follow:

– phenelzine (Nardil)	15-45 mg BID
– tranylcypromine (Parnate)	10-20 mg BID

Antidepressants for the treatment of Panic Disorder are usually started at very low doses and gradually increased to the maximum recommended dose as needed. They are not immediately effective, but are excellent for prophylaxis against panic attacks and anxiety. Since some patients with panic disorder are very sensitive to antidepressants during the drug treatment initiation period, it is prudent to start the patients on a low dose. However, the author's clinical experience suggests that most patients with panic disorder eventually need antidepressant doses in the higher dosage range.

Benzodiazepines are immediately effective and hence are excellent adjunctive medications for as-needed (PRN) use. Many psychiatrists advocate using benzodiazepines, particularly alprazolam (Xanax) and clonazepam (Klonopin), as primary first-line drugs of choice. This practice is not endorsed by the author because of significant risk of typical problems associated with sedatives in chronic use, such as cognitive impairment, memory impairment, tolerance, habituation, dependence, and depression. Patients with anxiety and panic disorder are not immune to these iatrogenic problems, despite some claims to the contrary. All potent benzodiazepines are equally effective in equivalent doses; however, alprazolam is most widely used for treatment of panic disorder, probably as a result of marketing focus. Some examples follow:

– alprazolam (Xanax)	0.5-2 mg TID-QID
– clonazepam (Klonopin)	0.5-1 mg BID-TID
– lorazepam (Ativan)	0.5-2 mg TID
– diazepam (Valium)	5-10 mg BID
– oxazepam (Serax)	15 mg TID

If, however, a benzodiazepine has to be used as the primary antipanic medication in the rare patient who cannot tolerate or who does not respond to antidepressants, the dosage required tends to be fairly high. For instance, alprazolam in the range of 1 to 3 mg TID is occasionally needed for control of panic attacks. Since alprazolam can cause marked interdose troughs in blood level leading to anxiety symptoms, TID-QID administration is necessary. Clonazepam, which is a potent benzodiazepine with a longer half-life, can be used on a BID schedule, and is preferred to alprazolam, to avoid interdose rebound anxiety.

Other medications that can be used adjunctively are beta-blockers, buspirone (Buspar), and clonidine (Catapres). The following are some examples:

– propranolol (Inderal)	10-40 mg BID-TID
– propranolol SR (Inderal LA)	60-120 mg per day
– buspirone (Buspar)	10 mg BID-TID
– clonidine (Catapres)	0.1-0.2 mg BID-TID

In the author's experience, bupropion (Wellbutrin) and trazodone (Desyrel) do not have impressive antipanic effects, though trazodone can be used at low doses adjunctively for augmentation purposes or as a sleep aid.

Panic disorder can occur with or without agoraphobia. The pharmacological treatment guidelines are similar to panic disorder in either condition. Patients with anticipatory anxiety or agoraphobia may benefit from adjunctive use of benzodiazepines, especially when situations that might generate anticipatory anxiety or agoraphobia can be determined.

Cognitive and behavioral therapeutic techniques are particularly beneficial and may help achieve complete resolution of the panic disorder when provided in conjunction with pharmacological treatment.

AGORAPHOBIA

The diagnostic criteria for agoraphobia, according to the *DSM-IV*, are as follows:*

A. Anxiety about being in places or situations from which escape might be difficult (or embarrassing) or in which help may not be available in the event of having an unexpected or situationally predisposed panic attack or panic-like symptoms. Agoraphobic fears typically involve characteristic clusters of situations that include being outside the home alone; being in a crowd or standing in a line; being on a bridge; and traveling in a bus, train, or automobile.

B. The situations are avoided (e.g., travel is restricted) or else are endured with marked distress or with anxiety about having a panic attack or panic-like symptoms, or require the presence of a companion.

C. The anxiety or phobic avoidance is not better accounted for by another mental disorder, such as social phobia (e.g., avoidance limited to social situations because of fear of embarrassment), specific phobia (e.g., avoidance limited to a single situation like elevators), obsessive-compulsive disorder (e.g., avoidance of dirt in someone with an obsession about contamination), post-traumatic stress disorder (e.g., avoidance of stimuli associated with a severe stressor), or separation anxiety disorder (e.g., avoidance of leaving home or relatives).

The treatment of agoraphobia is similar to that of panic disorder. Antidepressant medication and cognitive-behavioral therapy are the ideal treatments, with benzodiazepines, beta-blockers, buspirone, and clonidine used as possible adjunctive options.

One important clinical point is that if agoraphobia is chronic and severe, the patient should be carefully evaluated for the presence of underlying psychotic symptoms. Well-guarded psychosis can manifest itself as anxiety, panic attacks, agoraphobia, somatic preoccupation, depression, etc. If severe agoraphobia does not improve on antidepressants and/or benzodiazepines, a trial on low doses of antipsychotics should be considered in conjunction with antidepressants/benzodiazepines. In most of these cases, the low dose of antipsychotic medication can be withdrawn after several months, even when mild psychotic symptoms were initially present.

---

*Italicized text is reprinted with permission from the *Diagnostic and Statistical Manual of Mental Disorders*, Fourth Edition. Copyright 1994 American Psychiatric Association.

PHOBIA

DSM-IV diagnostic criteria for specific phobia are as follows:*

A. Marked and persistent fear that is excessive or unreasonable, cued by the presence or anticipation of a specific object or situation (e.g., flying, heights, animals, receiving an injection, seeing blood).

B. Exposure to the phobic stimulus almost invariably provokes an immediate anxiety response, which may take the form of a situationally bound or situationally predisposed panic attack. Note: In children, the anxiety may be expressed by crying, tantrums, freezing, or clinging.

C. The person recognizes that the fear is excessive or unreasonable. Note: In children, this feature may be absent.

D. The phobic situation(s) is avoided or else is endured with intense anxiety or distress.

E. The avoidance, anxious anticipation, or distress in the feared situation(s) interferes significantly with the person's normal routine, occupational (or academic) functioning, or social activities or relationships, or there is marked distress about having the phobia.

F. In individuals under age 18 years, the duration is at least six months.

G. The anxiety, panic attacks, or phobic avoidance associated with the specific object or situation are not better accounted for by another mental disorder such as obsessive-compulsive disorder (e.g., fear of dirt in someone with an obsession about contamination), post-traumatic stress disorder (e.g., avoidance of stimuli associated with a severe stressor), separation anxiety disorder (e.g., avoidance of school), social phobia (e.g., avoidance of social situations because of fear of embarrassment), panic disorder with agoraphobia, or agoraphobia without history of panic disorder.

Specify type:

- *Animal type*
- *Natural environment type (e.g., heights, storms, water)*
- *Blood-injection-injury type*
- *Situational type (e.g., airplanes, elevators, enclosed places)*
- *Other type (e.g., phobic avoidance of situations that may lead to choking, vomiting, or contracting an illness; in children, avoidance of loud sounds or costumed characters)*

The pharmacological treatment of phobias is similar to the treatment of panic disorder. Cognitive-behavioral therapy, including techniques such as progressive relaxation training, systematic desensitization, graded exposure, and flooding are particularly beneficial, along with medication management. Anticipatory anxiety is commonly associated with phobia, especially when a commonly encountered object or situation is the phobic stimulus.

As is the case with panic disorder, serotonergic antidepressants and clomipramine are the author's drugs of choice for treatment of phobic disorders, followed by TCAs and MAOIs, with PRN use of high-potency benzodiazepines such as alprazolam, clonazepam, and lorazepam.

SOCIAL PHOBIA

Diagnostic criteria for social phobia according to *DSM-IV* are as follows:*

A. A marked and persistent fear of one or more social or performance situations in which the person is exposed to unfamiliar people or to possible scrutiny by others. The individual fears that he or she will act in a way (or show anxiety symptoms) that will be humiliating or embarrassing. Note: In children, there must be evidence of the capacity for age-appropriate social relationships with familiar people and the anxiety must occur in peer settings, not just in interactions with adults.

B. Exposure to the feared social situation almost invariably provokes anxiety, which may take the form of a situationally bound or situationally predisposed panic attack. Note: In children, the anxiety may be expressed by crying, tantrums, freezing, or shrinking from social situations with unfamiliar people.

C. The person recognizes that the fear is excessive or unreasonable. Note: In children, this feature may be absent.

D. The feared social or performance situations are avoided or else are endured with intense anxiety or distress.

E. The avoidance, anxious anticipation, or distress in the feared social or performance situation(s) interferes significantly with the person's normal routine, occupational (or academic) functioning, or social activities or relationships, or there is marked distress about having the phobia.

---

*Italicized text is reprinted with permission from the *Diagnostic and Statistical Manual of Mental Disorders*, Fourth Edition. Copyright 1994 American Psychiatric Association.

F. In individuals under 18 years, the duration is at least six months.

G. The fear or avoidance is not due to the direct physiological effects of a substance (e.g., a drug of abuse, a medication) or general medical condition and is not better accounted for by another mental disorder (e.g., panic disorder with or without agoraphobia, separation anxiety disorder, body dysmorphic disorder, a pervasive developmental disorder, or schizoid personality disorder).

H. If a general medical condition or another mental disorder is present, the fear in criterion A is unrelated to it, e.g., the fear is not of stuttering, trembling in Parkinson's disease, or exhibiting abnormal eating behavior in anorexia nervosa or bulimia nervosa.

Specify if:

- ***Generalized:*** *if the fears include most social situations (also consider the additional diagnosis of avoidant personality disorder)*

If situations that give rise to symptoms of social phobia are not frequent, treatment using antidepressants is not necessary. Effective medications for performance anxiety, which should be administered one to two hours prior to the event, are as follows:

– propranolol (Inderal)	10-40 mg
– alprazolam (Xanax)	0.25-1 mg
– clonazepam (Klonopin)	0.5-1 mg
– lorazepam (Ativan)	0.5-1 mg
– oxazepam (Serax)	15-30 mg
– clonidine (Catapres)	0.1-0.2 mg

For moderate to severe social phobic symptoms, a combination of propranolol and a benzodiazepine may be used quite effectively. In cases that do not respond to these interventions, it may be necessary to place the patient on an antidepressant medication. In order of preference, the author's choices of antidepressants for treatment of social phobia are SSRIs, clomipramine, TCAs, and MAOIs.

As in other anxiety disorders, if symptoms and dysfunction are severe and if no improvement is seen with the medications mentioned above, consideration should be given to trial on low doses of antipsychotics for a short period of time. Extreme social phobia can be a severe form of "negative" symptomatology in a psychosis or could have a well-guarded paranoid basis.

OBSESSIVE-COMPULSIVE DISORDER

DSM-IV criteria for obsessive-compulsive disorder (OCD) are as follows:*

A. Either obsessions or compulsions: Obsessions as defined by 1, 2, 3, and 4:

1. *Recurrent and persistent thoughts, impulses, or images that are experienced, at some time during the disturbance, as intrusive and inappropriate and that cause marked anxiety or distress*
2. *The thoughts, impulses, or images are not simply excessive worries about real-life problems*
3. *The person attempts to ignore or suppress such thoughts, impulses, or images, or to neutralize them with some other thought or action*
4. *The person recognizes that the obsessional thoughts, impulses, or images are a product of his or her own mind (not imposed from without as in thought insertion)*

Compulsions as defined by 1 and 2:

1. *Repetitive behaviors (e.g., hand washing, ordering, checking) or mental acts (e.g., praying, counting, repeating words silently) that the person feels driven to perform in response to an obsession, or according to rules that must be applied rigidly*
2. *The behavior or mental acts are aimed at preventing or reducing distress or preventing some dreaded event or situation; however, these behaviors or mental acts either are not connected in a realistic way with what they are designed to neutralize or prevent or are clearly excessive*

B. At some point during the course of the disorder, the person has recognized that the obsessions or compulsions are excessive or unreasonable. Note: This does not apply to children.

C. The obsessions or compulsions cause marked distress, are time consuming (take more than one hour per day), or significantly interfere with the person's normal routine, occupational (or academic) functioning, or usual social activities or relationships.

---

*Italicized text is reprinted with permission from the *Diagnostic and Statistical Manual of Mental Disorders*, Fourth Edition. Copyright 1994 American Psychiatric Association.

D. If another Axis I disorder is present, the content of the obsessions or compulsions is not restricted to it (e.g., preoccupation with food in the presence of an eating disorder, hair pulling in the presence of trichotillomania, concern with appearance in the presence of body dysmorphic disorder, preoccupation with drugs in the presence of a substance use disorder, preoccupation with having a serious illness in the presence of hypochondriasis, preoccupation with sexual urges or fantasies in the presence of a paraphilia, or guilty ruminations in the presence of major depressive disorder).

E. The disturbance is not due to the direct physiological effects of a substance (e.g., a drug of abuse, a medication) or a general medical condition.

Specify if:

- ***With Poor Insight:** if, for most of the time during the current episode, the person does not recognize that the obsessions and compulsions are excessive or unreasonable*

Obsessive-compulsive disorder can present in innumerable variations, with the specific obsessions and compulsions differing in different people. Either obsessions or compulsions may be predominant in a particular patient. In some patients obsessions or compulsions may be seen exclusively. Any symptom that has an obsessional or compulsive trait has the potential to respond to treatment strategies described here.

SSRIs are the drugs of choice for OCD symptoms because of their effectiveness, safety in overdose, and favorable side-effect profile. Adequate treatment of OCD frequently requires doses higher than those usually employed for treatment of depression or anxiety. Examples:

— fluoxetine (Prozac)	60-80 mg per day
— fluvoxamine (Luvox)	200-300 mg per day
— paroxetine (Paxil)	40-60 mg per day
— sertraline (Zoloft)	150-200 mg per day
— venlafaxine (Effexor)	100-125 mg po TID

Although clomipramine is the most effective medication for OCD, it is generally used as a second-line medication because of its TCA side-effect liability, especially at high doses. In addition to typical TCA side effects, clomipramine at high doses lowers the seizure threshold significantly; hence, a total daily dose greater than 250 mg is not recommended. The author's practice is to prescribe anticonvulsants such as divalproex sodium (Depakote) or carbamazepine (Tegretol) if clomipramine dosage exceeds

225 mg per day. Clomipramine dosage above 150 mg should be given in divided doses. In treatment-resistant cases, in which monotherapy is not sufficient, clomipramine may be combined with SSRIs. In order to minimize the risk of seizure, the dose of clomipramine and the SSRI should not be high. When employing high doses, seizure prophylaxis should be instituted. Myoclonic jerks, which can be prodromal signs of seizure, should prompt decrease in dose or obtaining an EEG to rule out subclinical seizure activity.

Fluoxetine is approved by the FDA for treatment of OCD for which higher doses, such as 60 to 80 mg per day, may be needed. Though the manufacturer's recommendation for highest dose is 80 mg per day, several patients who needed 100 mg daily for adequate response tolerated the medication well without any side effects. Sertraline can also be used for the treatment of OCD. The dosage range is 50 to 200 mg daily. Patients have tolerated up to 300 mg daily without adverse effects.

Although sertraline is not approved by the FDA for treatment of OCD as of this writing, based on the author's experience, it is as effective as fluoxetine. Paroxetine is effective and FDA approved for treatment of OCD at the higher dose range of 45 to 80 mg per day, although the highest dose recommended by the manufacturer is 60 mg daily. The author has had excellent results using paroxetine for treatment of OCD.

Venlafaxine is yet another recently introduced antidepressant that is useful in the treatment of OCD. Its effective dosage range is from 150 to 375 mg daily in divided doses. Fluvoxamine is an FDA-approved antiobsessional drug in the SSRI group. Its dose range is 100 to 300 mg per day. It is as effective as any of the other SSRIs for the treatment of OCD. Its slightly sedating effect may be an advantage in anxious individuals and in patients who have insomnia. Nefazodone, trazodone, and bupropion have not been impressive as primary antiobsessional drugs in the author's experience. However, nefazodone and trazodone at low doses can be used as adjunctive medications to augment the antiobsessional effects of other primary medications. When used as an augmenter, nefazodone 50 mg TID and trazodone 50 mg TID are effective in some patients. See the clinical profiles of individual antidepressants in Chapter 4 for details.

High-potency benzodiazepines can be added to SSRIs or clomipramine. This intervention is effective in some cases. Some examples follow:

– clonazepam (Klonopin)	0.5-1 mg BID-TID
– alprazolam (Xanax)	0.5-1 mg TID-QID
– lorazepam (Ativan)	0.5-1 mg TID

Other adjunctive medication doses that are effective in an occasional patient are listed below:

– buspirone (Buspar)	10 mg BID-TID
– trazodone (Desyrel)	50-100 mg BID-TID
– nefazodone (Serzone)	50 mg BID-TID
– lithium carbonate	300 mg BID-TID
– clonidine (Catapres)	0.1 mg BID-TID
– guanfacine (Tenex)	1-2 mg HS
– risperidone (Risperdal)	0.5-1 mg HS or another antipsychotic at low doses
– olanzapine (Zyprexa)	2.5-5 mg HS

Severe OCD can be as debilitating as chronic psychosis and requires perseverance on the part of the physician. MAOIs can be tried if SSRIs and clomipramine are not effective; however, the success rate is not high. In severe refractory cases, the addition of low doses of an antipsychotic medication, preferably risperidone or olanzapine because of their relatively improved side effect profile, could be effective. Severely dysfunctional OCD patients who do not respond to the medication interventions listed above should be considered for a trial on clozapine prior to being considered for cingulotomy (although clozapine is not approved by the FDA for treatment of OCD).

There are numerous symptoms or disorders that have compulsive characteristics, sometimes known as obsessive-compulsive spectrum disorders. Patients exhibiting any behaviors that have compulsive or obsessive traits that are socially and culturally inappropriate or have negative consequences deserve to be considered for a trial of antiobsessional medications, especially if standard treatment for these conditions is unsatisfactory. These behaviors or conditions include sexual or any other perversions, fixation on any idea or issue, overinvolvement, concrete thinking, eating disorder, kleptomania, gambling, fanaticism, autistic behavior, stereotyped movements, tic disorders, elimination disorders, substance abuse, delusional disorders, somatoform disorders, paraphilias, and various impulse control disorders. Obviously, these disorders may not always be etiologically related to OCD, in which case antiobsessional medications may not work. For example, kleptomaniac behavior is always an antisocial act, but frequently (not always) also has an obsessive-compulsive etiology. Other etiologies, such as mania, psychosis, and antisocial personality disorder must be ruled out. Behaviors that have underlying obsessive-compulsive traits are so varied, and sometimes even esoteric, that the clinician should keep an obsessive-compulsive etiology in mind when evaluating such symptoms.

Since effective treatment is available for most obsessive-compulsive symptoms, especially using SSRIs and clomipramine, it is important not to miss an opportunity to help a patient eliminate the burden these disorders cause.

POST-TRAUMATIC STRESS DISORDER

Diagnostic criteria for post-traumatic stress disorder (PTSD) according to *DSM-IV* are listed below:*

A. The person has been exposed to a traumatic event in which both of the following were present:

1. *The person experienced, witnessed, or was confronted with an event or events that involved actual or threatened death or serious injury, or a threat to the physical integrity of self or others*
2. *The person's response involved intense fear, helplessness, or horror. Note: In children, this may be expressed by disorganized or agitated behavior*

B. The traumatic event is persistently reexperienced in one (or more) of the following ways:

1. *Recurrent and intrusive distressing recollections of the event, including images, thoughts, or perceptions. Note: In young children, repetitive play may occur in which themes or aspects of the trauma are expressed*
2. *Recurrent distressing dreams of the event. Note: In children, there may be frightening dreams without recognizable content*
3. *Acting or feeling as if the traumatic event were recurring (includes a sense of reliving the experience, illusions, hallucinations, and dissociative flashback episodes, including those that occur on awakening or when intoxicated)*
4. *Intense psychological distress at exposure to internal or external cues that symbolize or resemble an aspect of the traumatic event*

---

*Italicized text is reprinted with permission from the *Diagnostic and Statistical Manual of Mental Disorders*, Fourth Edition. Copyright 1994 American Psychiatric Association.

5. Physiological reactivity on exposure to internal or external cues that symbolize or resemble an aspect of the traumatic event

C. Persistent avoidance of stimuli associated with the trauma and numbing of general responsiveness (not present before the trauma), as indicated by three (or more) of the following:

1. Efforts to avoid thoughts, feelings, or conversations associated with the trauma
2. Efforts to avoid activities, places, or people that arouse recollections of the trauma
3. Inability to recall an important aspect of the trauma
4. Markedly diminished interest or participation in significant activities
5. Feeling of detachment or estrangement from others
6. Restricted range of affect (e.g., unable to have loving feelings)
7. Sense of a foreshortened future (e.g., does not expect to have a career, marriage, children, or a normal life span)

D. Persistent symptoms of increased arousal (not present before the trauma), as indicated by two (or more) of the following:

1. Difficulty falling or staying asleep
2. Irritability or outbursts of anger
3. Difficulty concentrating
4. Hypervigilance
5. Exaggerated startle response

E. Duration of the disturbance (symptoms in criteria B, C, and D) is more than one month.

F. The disturbance causes clinically significant distress or impairment in social, occupational, or other important areas of functioning.

Specify if:

- ***Acute:** if duration of symptoms is less than three months*
- ***Chronic:** if duration of symptoms is three months or more*
- ***With delayed onset:** if onset of symptoms is at least six months after the stressor*

PTSD can present with many different symptoms, such as anxiety, depression, paranoia, hallucinations, nightmares, insomnia, and irritability. Different symptoms predominate in different patients; hence, there is no standard medication treatment approach for PTSD. Antidepressants, anxiolytics, antipsychotics, mood stabilizers, buspirone, beta blockers, and clonidine have been used, depending on the symptoms. Common medications employed are combinations of serotonergic antidepressants, trazodone, antipsychotics, and anxiolytics, as well as buspirone. Various combinations of the above medications are beneficial in individual patients.

ACUTE STRESS DISORDER

The diagnostic criteria for acute stress disorder according to *DSM-IV* are as follows:*

A. The person has been exposed to a traumatic event in which both of the following were present:

1. *The person experienced, witnessed, or was confronted with an event or events that involved actual or threatened death or serious injury, or a threat to the physical integrity of self or others*
2. *The person's response involved intense fear, helplessness, or horror*

B. Either while experiencing or after experiencing the distressing event, the individual has three (or more) of the following dissociative symptoms:

1. *A subjective sense of numbing, detachment, or absence of emotional responsiveness*
2. *A reduction in awareness of his or her surroundings (e.g., "being in a daze")*
3. *Derealization*
4. *Depersonalization*
5. *Dissociative amnesia (i.e., inability to recall an important aspect of the trauma)*

C. The traumatic event is persistently reexperienced in at least one of the following ways: recurrent images, thoughts, dreams, illusions, flashback episodes, or a sense of reliving the experience; or distress on exposure to reminders of the traumatic event.

D. Marked avoidance of stimuli that arouse recollections of the trauma (e.g., thoughts, feelings, conversations, activities, places, people).

E. Marked symptoms of anxiety or increased arousal (e.g., difficulty sleeping, irritability, poor concentration, hypervigilance, exaggerated startle response, motor restlessness).

F. The disturbance causes clinically significant distress or impairment in social, occupational, or other important areas of functioning or impairs the individual's ability to pursue some necessary task, such as obtaining necessary assistance or mobilizing personal resources by telling family members about the traumatic experience.

G. The disturbance lasts for a minimum of two days and a maximum of four weeks and occurs within four weeks of the traumatic event.

H. The disturbance is not due to the direct physiological effects of a substance (e.g., a drug of abuse, a medication) or a general medical condition, is not better accounted for by brief psychotic disorder, and is not merely an exacerbation of a pre-existing Axis I or Axis II disorder.

Although, by definition, the symptoms of acute stress disorder last less than four weeks, the symptoms should still be treated since they are clinically significant and cause dysfunction. The choice of a medication or combination of medications is based on the nature and predominance of specific symptom complex seen in the individual patient, as in the case of PTSD. If symptoms last longer than four weeks, the diagnosis of PTSD must be considered.

ADJUSTMENT DISORDER WITH ANXIETY

Adjustment disorder with anxiety presents with symptoms such as anxiety, excessive worrying, increased tension, vague fears, nervousness, and, in children, separation anxiety. For classification as an adjustment disorder, the symptoms must develop within three months of onset of an identifiable psychosocial stressor. The symptoms should cause either marked distress or significant impairment in social or occupational functioning. The symptoms typically resolve within six months of the termination of the stressor unless the stressor or its consequences are enduring. If symptoms resolve within six months, the episode is considered "acute," and if symptoms last six months or longer, the adjustment disorder is described as "chronic." The treatment principles are similar to that of generalized anxiety disorder.

Chapter 8

Clinical Profiles of Antianxiety Medications: Advantages and Disadvantages

LORAZEPAM (ATIVAN)

Lorazepam is a benzodiazepine with a half-life of twelve hours. It is available in 0.5 mg, 1 mg, and 2 mg tablets, and in a parenteral form. Its peak activity after oral administration occurs in two hours. It has no active metabolites. Lorazepam is 85 percent bound to plasma proteins. It is contraindicated in patients with acute narrow-angle glaucoma. At low oral therapeutic doses, lorazepam has no significant effect on respiratory depression; however, when administered intravenously (IV) it can affect respiration in susceptible individuals.

Lorazepam is one of the best overall choices for antianxiety use for the following reasons: rapid onset of action; no active metabolites; intermediate half-life; reliable po, IM, and IV absorption; and generic availability. It has wide application as a hypnotic at 0.5 mg or 1 mg dose orally, as an effective IM medication at 1 to 2 mg dose for control of severe agitation in the emergency room or hospitalized patients (usually in conjunction with an IM neuroleptic), and as a short-term antianxiety medication given at 0.5 mg orally two to three times a day, once daily, or as needed. It can be given IV at 1 mg in 50 cc of normal saline administered over 30 minutes, or as 0.5 mg slow IV push over two minutes, repeated every four to six hours as needed in an inpatient setting if the patient cannot take oral medications or receive medication by the IM route. The advantage of IM administration over the oral route is that it is rapidly and reliably absorbed, with peak effect in about one hour. Obviously, sedation is the most common side effect. As mentioned previously, and as applicable to all benzodiazepines, lorazepam is usually administered as an adjunct to other medications, usually with an antidepressant or antipsychotic medication, and preferably for short-term use. Dosage in an outpatient practice generally should not exceed a total of 3 to 4 mg in divided doses. At higher doses, there is a significant risk of addiction.

Patients should be warned of the risk of dependence, tolerance, memory impairment, and of the risks of stopping the medication abruptly since sudden discontinuation can significantly lower the seizure threshold, in addition to causing withdrawal anxiety and insomnia. Generally, in the author's experience, if a patient needs more than 3 to 4 mg per day, it is because the patient has other diagnoses, such as depression, psychosis, or other specific anxiety disorders, such as obsessive-compulsive disorder, which have not been diagnosed and treated. Based on cases that have come to me from other physicians, in which patients have been kept on more than 3 to 4 mg of lorazepam per day (or the equivalent), various undiagnosed and untreated problems have been frequently uncovered. Usually these include mild psychosis, paranoia, obsessive or compulsive tendencies, irrational hostility, and other mild or vague disorders that are difficult to diagnose but that can present with massive anxiety and these are often misdiagnosed as generalized anxiety disorder.

Many problems occur when a patient is treated solely with benzodiazepines at fairly high doses over a long period of time. Most of these patients continue to experience breakthrough anxiety, depression (which can be a side effect of benzodiazepines), tolerance that necessitates the need for increasing the dose of the medication, dependence on the medication and on the physician (and resultant subconscious hostility), and cognitive impairment. Hence, the author's opinion, based on extensive clinical experience treating very complicated cases, is to avoid benzodiazepines as the primary medication at high doses over a long period of time even for GAD.

In many primary care practices and in some psychiatric practices, it is quite tempting to use benzodiazepines as the primary medication for a variety of emotional symptoms, probably because they are easy to use, immediately effective, and relatively free of initial serious side effects. Serotonergic antidepressants such as fluoxetine (Prozac), sertraline (Zoloft), paroxetine (Paxil), venlafaxine (Effexor), fluvoxamine (Luvox), and nefazodone (Serzone) should effectively control anxiety and should be used as the primary medication in an outpatient primary care or psychiatric practice, with use of benzodiazepines as the secondary medications in an adjunctive role. Lorazepam is the author's preferred benzodiazepine for short-term treatment of anxiety and insomnia, and for adjunctive use for treating psychotic agitation (usually in the IM form).

Summary of Advantages and Disadvantages of Lorazepam

Advantages

- No active metabolites; preferable in patients with hepatic disease
- Tablet and parenteral (IM or IV) forms
- Effective for treatment of anxiety
- Effective as a hypnotic for initial and middle insomnia
- Intermediate half-life
- Generic available at low cost

Disadvantages

- Fairly rapid onset of action increases abuse potential and dependence
- Abrupt discontinuation after long-term use can cause withdrawal symptoms

ALPRAZOLAM (XANAX)

Alprazolam tablets are available in 0.25 mg, 0.5 mg, 1 mg, and 2 mg doses. Peak plasma concentration occurs in 1.5 hours with a half-life of 11 hours. Although alprazolam has active metabolites, their potency and half-life are similar to the parent compound. Its protein binding is at approximately 80 percent. Alprazolam is primarily used for treatment of generalized anxiety disorder, panic disorder, and anxiety associated with depression. It has all the disadvantages associated with a potent, intermediate half life, fast-acting benzodiazepine, such as addiction potential and tolerance. Clinical experience suggests that the dependence potential has been underestimated. Despite FDA approval for generalized anxiety disorder and panic disorder and the marketing focus on these disorders, the author's clinical experience suggests that alprazolam is still a poor choice as a primary medication for these disorders, particularly for long-term use, as are all of the other benzodiazepines. Alprazolam is a good choice as an adjunctive medication, as are lorazepam (Ativan), oxazepam (Serax), clonazepam (Klonopin) and other benzodiazepines, for treatment of anxiety disorders. Alprazolam may be prescribed at 0.25 mg to 0.5 mg po TID for most anxieties for two- to four-week periods, and at 1 mg for severe anxieties for two to four weeks. Higher dosages for longer periods of time tend to lead to dependence. Physicians and psychiatrists have been encouraged to prescribe at much higher doses for treatment of panic disorder. This is not a prudent strategy in the long run. Panic attacks will be controlled at higher doses, but patients are at high risk for physiological dependence on the medication and resultant dependence on the prescribing physician.

Summary of Advantages and Disadvantages of Alprazolam

Advantages

- Effective for short-term treatment of acute anxiety
- Effective for initial and middle insomnia
- Intermediate half-life
- Available in generic form (since 1994) at low cost
- Rapid onset of action

Disadvantages

- Rapid onset of action, fairly short half-life, and high potency greatly increase potential for abuse and dependence
- No parenteral form
- Abrupt discontinuation after more than three to four weeks of regular use leads to withdrawal symptoms
- Active metabolites; half-life prolonged in patients with liver impairment and in the elderly
- Interdose breakthrough anxiety possible, needing TID-QID dosing

DIAZEPAM (VALIUM)

Diazepam is available in tablets of 2 mg, 5 mg, and 10 mg strength. Diazepam, along with its active metabolites, has a half-life of approximately 50 hours, and reaches peak plasma concentration in 1.5 hours after oral administration. Due to its long half-life, diazepam can be administered once a day, preferably at night. It can be used for adjunctive short-term treatment of anxiety and is also a muscle relaxant. It is an excellent choice for treating alcohol withdrawal or for treating withdrawal from sedatives that have short to intermediate half-lives, such as triazolam (Halcion), oxazepam (Serax), lorazepam (Ativan), temazepam (Restoril), and alprazolam (Xanax). Its long half-life provides a built-in taper, minimizing abrupt withdrawal effects.

Diazepam can be given via IM or IV route, though absorption by an IM route can be erratic. An IV route is generally employed for rapid control of seizure activity. Withdrawal symptoms do not appear until three to five days after abrupt discontinuation of diazepam and generally are less acute compared to sedatives with a short half-life. Since metabolites accumulate with repeated administration of diazepam, especially in the elderly, benzodiazepines with short to intermediate half-lives are preferred for the elderly and the medically ill.

Summary of Advantages and Disadvantages of Diazepam

Advantages

- Long half-life makes it suitable for treatment of sedative or alcohol withdrawal
- Once-a-day dosing possible
- Relatively easy to taper off when medication is to be discontinued
- Excellent oral and IV absorption
- Fairly safe with slow IV push at doses of 2 to 5 mg
- Effective for treatment of anxiety
- Low cost due to generic availability

Disadvantages

- Liver disease and old age prolongs half-life
- IM absorption is erratic
- Fairly rapid onset of action increases potential for abuse
- Long half-life and active metabolites lead to accumulation with repeated dosing

CLONAZEPAM (KLONOPIN)

Clonazepam is a high-potency benzodiazepine with a half-life of about 30 hours, rapid onset of action, and 85 percent protein binding. It is available in 0.5 mg, 1 mg, and 2 mg scored tablets. The peak plasma level is obtained in one and one-half hours after the oral dose. Clonazepam is FDA-approved for the treatment of seizures. It is also an effective short-term antianxiety medication at low doses such as 0.5 mg to 1 mg po BID. Clonazepam can be used for adjunctive treatment of mania, as an anxiolytic in panic disorder, and as a hypnotic, preferably for short-term intervention. It can be given twice a day, unlike alprazolam (Xanax) and lorazepam (Ativan), which are usually given three times a day. Clonazepam has addictive potential and, if used regularly for more than several months, tolerance develops. Hence, in the author's view, it should not be used as the primary medication either for anxiety disorders or for mania, but rather should be used as an adjunctive medication at low doses, preferably on a PRN schedule. If stopped abruptly after prolonged regular use at moderate or high doses, the risk of withdrawal seizure is significant.

Carbamazepine can decrease the plasma concentration of clonazepam. Common side effects at the low doses typically used for psychiatric application are sedation, fatigue, and mental dullness. Side effects are dose-related, as is true with most medications. At high doses, other side effects such as ataxia, confusion, slurred speech, agitation, motor incoordination, and respiratory depression can appear.

All benzodiazepines are relatively contraindicated in patients with a history of drug or alcohol abuse. Clonazepam, as well as other sedative medications, in long-term use at high doses, puts patients at risk for iatrogenic drug dependence.

Summary of Advantages and Disadvantages of Clonazepam

Advantages

- Effective for short-term treatment of anxiety, at low doses
- Effective as a hypnotic, at low doses
- Fairly long half-life provides stable interdose drug level, enabling twice-a-day dosing
- Fairly rapid onset of action
- May be used for mania
- Scored tablets convenient for flexible dosing
- Low cost due to generic availability

Disadvantages

- No parenteral form
- Abrupt discontinuation may cause withdrawal symptoms, particularly seizures
- Adverse side effects such as confusion and unsteadiness, somewhat more common than with lorazepam or alprazolam
- Half-life prolonged in elderly and in patients with hepatic impairment

CHLORDIAZEPOXIDE (LIBRIUM)

Chlordiazepoxide is a benzodiazepine agonist with active metabolites and a combined half-life of approximately 70 hours with repeated dosing, making it a drug of choice in alcohol detoxification in patients without significant liver disease. Its oral and IV absorption are excellent, but IM absorption is erratic. The onset of action is fairly slow, compared to diazepam (Valium), clorazepate (Tranxene), and alprazolam (Xanax).

It can be used as an antianxiety medication in doses of 10 to 50 mg in divided doses or at bedtime, for short periods of time. However, as discussed in the introduction, the author's preference is to use antidepressants as the primary medication for treatment of anxiety.

For individuals without evidence of liver disease, chlordiazepoxide is a drug of choice for treatment of alcohol withdrawal, though any benzodiazepine or sedative can be used. Average oral dose for treatment of alcohol withdrawal ranges from 25 to 150 mg, depending on the severity of alcohol dependence, tapered off over a period of three to five days. Chlordiazepoxide can be given as a slow IV push over one to two minutes at doses of 25 to 100 mg in divided doses if oral administration is not possible or for severe alcohol withdrawal symptoms, with a switch to an oral dose whenever possible.

Summary of Advantages and Disadvantages of Chlordiazepoxide

Advantages

- Long half-life convenient for alcohol detoxification
  Low potency and fairly slow onset of action makes it relatively less attractive as a drug of abuse
- Relatively easy to taper off when medication is to be discontinued
- Excellent po and IV absorption
- Fairly safe with slow IV push at doses of 10 to 25 mg
- Low cost due to generic availability

Disadvantages

- Relatively less effective for treatment of acute anxiety attacks
- Liver disease prolongs half-life
- Active metabolites can accumulate with repeated administration
- IM absorption is erratic

CLORAZEPATE (TRANXENE)

Clorazepate is a rapidly acting benzodiazepine with active metabolites and an effective half-life of approximately 60 hours. It can be used for short-term treatment of anxiety, and for treatment of alcohol withdrawal symptoms. For anxiety, the usual dosage range is between 7.5 to 30 mg in divided doses or at bedtime. It is available in 3.75 mg, 7.5 mg, and 15 mg strengths. It is converted to the active metabolite desmethyldiazepam in the stomach and absorbed as such. It is also available in 11.25 mg and 22.5 mg slow release preparation as Tranxene-SD. A slow-release preparation may be convenient for use in partial seizures, which is one of the indications for clorazepate.

The dosages used for treatment of alcohol withdrawal is between 15 mg and 60 mg in divided doses, depending on the severity of alcohol dependence, tapered off in three to five days.

Any of the long half-life benzodiazepines can be used for treating withdrawal from a sedative with a shorter half-life. The dose of the treating drug and the length of taper depend on individual circumstances.

Summary of Advantages and Disadvantages of Clorazepate

Advantages

- Once-a-day dosing possible
- Indicated for adjunctive treatment of partial seizures
- May be used for alcohol/sedative withdrawal symptoms
- Easier to discontinue because of long half-life
- Low cost due to generic availability

Disadvantages

- No IM or IV form available
- Long half-life causes accumulation with repeated administration
- Rapid onset of action increases abuse potential

PRAZEPAM (CENTRAX)

Prazepam is a long half-life benzodiazepine with active metabolites, available for oral dosing in 5, 10, and 20 mg capsules and tablets. Its half-life is about 70 hours. Its onset of action is slow, compared to other benzodiazepines. It can be used for short-term treatment of anxiety, alcohol withdrawal, and sedative withdrawal.

Summary of Advantages and Disadvantages of Prazepam

Advantages

- Once-a-day dosing possible, due to long half-life
- May be used for alcohol/sedative withdrawal
- Easier to discontinue because of long half-life

Disadvantages

- No IM or IV form available
- Long half-life with active metabolites leads to accumulation with repeated dosing
- Liver disease prolongs half-life
- Product not widely available, since manufacturing stopped several years ago

OXAZEPAM (SERAX)

Oxazepam is a relatively slow-acting benzodiazepine with no active metabolites, available in 10, 15, and 30 mg capsules, and 15 mg tablets. Its half-life is approximately 12 hours. It can be used for the short-term treatment of anxiety in doses ranging from 30 to 90 mg in three divided doses, as well as for the treatment of alcohol withdrawal. Due to its relatively short half-life, if used for treatment of alcohol or sedative withdrawal symptoms, the dosage should be gradually decreased over a period of seven to eight days. Since oxazepam has no active metabolites, it is fairly safe for use in patients with liver disease, which is common among severe alcoholics.

A patient with liver disease who is dependent on two to three six-packs of beer daily may be treated on the following oxazepam dosage schedule, more or less:

- Day 1–Oxazepam 30 mg po QID
- Day 2–Oxazepam 30 mg po TID
- Day 3–Oxazepam 15 mg po TID
- Day 4–Oxazepam 15 mg po TID

- Day 5–Oxazepam 10 mg po TID
- Day 6–Oxazepam 10 mg po BID
- Day 7–Oxazepam 10 mg po HS, then discontinue

Summary of Advantages and Disadvantages of Oxazepam

Advantages

- No active metabolites; preferable for patients with hepatic dysfunction
- Relatively slow onset of action decreases abuse potential compared to medications with rapid onset
- May be used for treating middle and terminal insomnia
- Generic available at low cost

Disadvantages

- No IM or IV form
- Relatively short half-life requires multiple dosing
- Discontinuation of medication requires gradual taper

QUAZEPAM (DORAL)

Quazepam is a fairly rapid-acting benzodiazepine with active metabolites, approved by the FDA for short-term treatment of insomnia. The approximate half-life of the parent compound and its metabolites is 50 hours. It can cause daytime drowsiness due to its long duration of action. It is available in 7.5 mg and 15 mg tablets, and is comparable to flurazepam (Dalmane) 15 mg and 30 mg strengths, respectively.

Summary of Advantages and Disadvantages of Quazepam

Advantages

- Improves initial, middle, and terminal insomnia
- Less rebound anxiety (as sometimes seen with ultra-short-acting hypnotics, such as triazolam or zolpidem)

Disadvantages

- Possible daytime drowsiness
- Liver disease prolongs half-life
- Generic not available, making it fairly expensive

TEMAZEPAM (RESTORIL)

Temazepam is a relatively rapid-acting benzodiazepine with no active metabolites, available in 15 and 30 mg capsules, and the recently introduced 7.5 mg capsule. It has a half-life of approximately 12 hours. It is marketed and FDA-approved as a hypnotic, but has a pharmacokinetic profile similar to oxazepam (Serax). Its clearance is not significantly affected by liver disease. Temazepam is effective for short-term treatment of initial and middle insomnia, as well as for early morning awakening. Many patients do well on the recently introduced 7.5 mg strength without significant daytime drowsiness.

Summary of Advantages and Disadvantages of Temazepam

Advantages

- No active metabolites; clearance not significantly affected by liver dysfunction or old age
- Effective for initial insomnia, middle insomnia, and early morning awakening
- Available in 7.5, 15, and 30 mg strengths
- Low cost due to generic availability

Disadvantage

- No IM or IV form

TRIAZOLAM (HALCION)

Triazolam is a rapid-onset, ultra short-acting benzodiazepine available in 0.125 and 0.25 mg dose tablets. Its half-life is approximately three hours. Triazolam is particularly effective for treatment of initial insomnia. No significant adverse effects were noted in the author's experience in using triazolam for short-term treatment in patients with insomnia. However, recent news reports of amnesia, anterograde amnesia, hyperexcitability, delirium, and hallucinations associated with use of triazolam have surfaced, leading to a decrease in the number of prescriptions for triazolam. Its short half-life could cause rebound anxiety in some patients.

Summary of Advantages and Disadvantages of Triazolam

Advantages

- Rapid-acting; effective for initial insomnia
- Short-acting; lack of daytime drowsiness

Disadvantages

- Reports of anterograde amnesia, delirium, and hallucinations (rare adverse reactions of all short-acting sedatives)
- No IM form
- May cause rebound anxiety in some patients, due to ultra-short half-life
- Generic not available; fairly expensive

FLURAZEPAM (DALMANE)

Flurazepam is a long half-life benzodiazepine with a fairly rapid onset, which is marketed for treatment of insomnia. It is effective for short-term treatment of initial insomnia, middle insomnia, and early morning awakening. It has active metabolites that have a half-life of approximately 90 hours, resulting in drug accumulation with repeated dosing. Flurazepam is available in 15 and 30 mg capsules. Hepatic dysfunction and old age can prolong its hepatic clearance. Its long half-life makes it a good choice for patients who have insomnia as well as daytime anxiety. Other long-acting benzodiazepines such as diazepam, clorazepate, and quazepam have similar pharmacokinetic profiles and hence can be used for insomnia just as well as flurazepam, which is marketed specifically as a hypnotic.

Summary of Advantages and Disadvantages of Flurazepam

Advantages

- Effective for insomnia
- No rebound anxiety
- Generic available at low cost

Disadvantages

- Long half-life can cause daytime sedation
- Liver disease and old age prolong half-life
- No IM form

ESTAZOLAM (PROSOM)

Estazolam is a fairly fast-acting benzodiazepine with active metabolites and an average half-life of 16 hours. It is available as 1 and 2 mg tablets. Estazolam is marketed for treatment of insomnia. It is comparable to temazepam in terms of uses, pharmacokinetics, and side effects. It may be used for short-term treatment of initial and middle insomnia, and for early morning awakening.

Side effects at therapeutic doses include ataxia, sedation, dizziness, and fatigue. The potential for dependence, tolerance, and withdrawal is to be expected, as with all sedative-hypnotics.

Summary of Advantages and Disadvantages of Estazolam

Advantages

- Minimal daytime drowsiness
- Effective for short-term treatment of initial, middle, and terminal insomnia

Disadvantages

- Generic form not available, making it fairly expensive
- Liver disease prolongs half-life
- No parenteral form

ZOLPIDEM (AMBIEN)

Zolpidem is a rapid onset hypnotic with a half-life of two and one-half hours, available in 5 and 10 mg tablets. It has no significant antianxiety effects. It is claimed that zolpidem neither decreases sleep stages three and four, nor has appreciable effects on REM sleep. Its potential for dependency, tolerance, and abuse is similar to other short-acting hypnotics, as clinical experience has shown. Hence, abrupt discontinuation of high doses after long-term use can lead to sedative withdrawal symptoms. If prescribed and used within the FDA-approved guidelines, such adverse effects are rare. Zolpidem is particularly beneficial for patients with initial and middle insomnia. The maximum recommended daily dose is 10 mg. Patients should be initially tried on 5 mg and the dose increased to 10 mg if 5 mg is not effective.

Summary of Advantages and Disadvantages of Zolpidem

Advantages

- No daytime sedation
- Effective for initial insomnia
- Normal sleep architecture apparently not significantly affected

Disadvantages

- No IM form
- No generic form, making it fairly expensive
- Potential for tolerance, dependence, and abuse similar to short-acting sedatives
- Can cause anterograde amnesia

BUSPIRONE (BUSPAR)

Buspirone is a nonbenzodiazepine antianxiety drug with a half-life of two and one-half hours. It is available in unscored 5 and 10 mg and scored 15 mg tablets. Buspirone does not cause physiological dependence or addiction. It does not treat sedative or alcohol withdrawal symptoms. Buspirone has no muscle relaxant, anticonvulsant, or sedative properties. Its antianxiety effects take more than ten days to manifest, and are moderate at best. In clinical practice, it is used predominantly as an adjunctive medication with benzodiazepines and antidepressants. Buspirone is a logical choice for treatment of anxiety disorder in patients with addictive history or potential, or in patients in whom sedation is undesirable, such as in patients with breathing difficulties or in patients with sleep apnea. It does not potentiate the sedative effects of antidepressants, alcohol, and benzodiazepines.

Buspirone can be tried as an adjunctive medication for patients with a variety of psychiatric conditions such as depression, anxiety, phobia, obsessive-compulsive disorder, and post-traumatic stress disorder.

The usual dose range is 20 to 45 mg per day in two or three divided doses. Since any antianxiety effects may not be evidenced for one to two weeks, a low dose of benzodiazepines may have to be prescribed during the first ten days. The recent introduction of scored 15 mg tablets provides the convenience of a BID dosing schedule that will improve compliance.

Buspirone has no acute antianxiety effects and hence has no use as a PRN medication. It cannot treat a panic attack. Its effectiveness in treating acute anxiety is much less compared to benzodiazepines.

Buspirone may cause transient nausea, diarrhea, headache, dizziness, and nervousness. It is contraindicated with MAOIs.

Summary of Advantages and Disadvantages of Buspirone

Advantages

- Lack of potential for addiction, dependence, or abuse
- Lack of sedative effects
- Appropriate for use in patients with substance abuse potential
- Adjunctive use for a variety of conditions, including depression, anxiety, phobia, obsessive-compulsive disorder, and post-traumatic stress disorder
- Mild to moderate antianxiety effect with prolonged regular use

Disadvantages

- Antianxiety effect takes one to two weeks to manifest
- Neither useful as a PRN medication, nor for acute anxiety
- No cross-tolerance with sedatives or alcohol
- No generic availability, making it expensive

CHLORAL HYDRATE (NOCTEC)

Chloral hydrate is a hypnotic medication with a half-life of eight hours. The usual adult dose is 500 to 1,000 mg at bedtime. It can be used in children at a dose of 50 mg/kg. The maximum recommended dose for adults and children is 2 grams and 1 gram, respectively. It is available in 250 and 500 mg capsules, in liquid concentrate, and in 500 mg rectal suppositories. Chloral hydrate is particularly effective for treatment of initial insomnia. Since it is a gastric irritant, oral administration along with a snack or plenty of fluid is preferable. Since it has low lethal to therapeutic ratio, it is relatively contraindicated in patients with suicidal risk. Since the advent of benzodiazepines, the popularity of chloral hydrate has justifiably decreased markedly. It is hardly ever used as an antianxiety agent.

Rapid tolerance develops to the hypnotic effects of chloral hydrate; hence, it is best used for less than two weeks or on an as-needed schedule. In patients who have liver disease or who are on oral anticoagulants, benzodiazepines such as lorazepam, temazepam, and oxazepam are preferred.

Summary of Advantages and Disadvantages of Chloral Hydrate

Advantages

- Effective for initial and middle insomnia
- Established safety in children (at appropriate doses)
- Available in capsule, liquid, and rectal suppository forms
- Safety and reliability established over a century of use (within dosage range)
- Fairly short half-life minimizes daytime sedation
- Generic available at low cost

Disadvantages

- Low toxic-to-therapeutic ratio
- Gastric irritant
- No IM form
- Can cause displacement of oral anticoagulants from protein-binding sites causing potentiation of effects
- Relatively contraindicated in patients with hepatic disease, gastritis, or renal disease

HYDROXYZINE (ATARAX, VISTARIL)

Hydroxyzine, available in 10, 25, 50, and 100 mg tablets; 25, 50, and 100 mg capsules; in liquid concentrate form; and in IM form, has sedating and antipruritic properties. It can be used for treatment of anxiety at doses of 25 to 50 mg po TID, and for insomnia at doses of 50 to 100 mg as one bedtime dose. A 25 to 50 mg IM dose will produce a rapid effect. The main side effects are sedation and dry mouth. Tolerance develops to the sedative and hypnotic effects with long-term use. It has the advantage of having fairly low potential for dependence and abuse, making it preferable for use in patients with addiction risk. It is contraindicated in the first trimester of pregnancy, due to teratogenic potential.

Summary of Advantages and Disadvantages of Hydroxyzine

Advantages

- Low risk of abuse or dependence
- Preferred in patients with addiction potential
- IM form available
- Fairly effective for initial insomnia and middle insomnia
- Generic form available at low cost

Disadvantages

- Causes dry mouth
- Less effective when compared to hypnotics
- Tolerance develops in two to four weeks

DIPHENHYDRAMINE (BENADRYL)

Diphenhydramine is an antihistamine that can be used for sedation and for anticholinergic effects. It is available over-the-counter in 25 mg strength, and by prescription in 50 mg strength capsules, as well as in liquid form and parenteral form for IM and IV use. Its duration of action is four to six hours. Besides use as a hypnotic, it can be used for treatment of acute dystonia and other extrapyramidal symptoms caused by antipsychotics. As a hypnotic, the dosage is 50 mg at bedtime. For acute dystonic reaction it can be used at 25 to 50 mg IM or IV. For extrapyramidal symptoms, the dosage range is 25 to 50 mg TID. Side effects are sedation, dry mouth, gastrointestinal distress, and other anticholinergic side effects. Tolerance to the sedative and hypnotic effects develops with continued use. Diphenhydramine is a good choice for use as a hypnotic in patients who are at risk for addiction.

Summary of Advantages and Disadvantages of Diphenhydramine

Advantages

- Low risk of abuse/dependence
- May be used in patients with addiction potential
- Capsule, liquid, IM, and IV form
- Fairly effective for initial insomnia
- Generic and over-the-counter forms (25 mg) available at low cost

Disadvantages

- Anticholinergic side effects
- Less effective for anxiety, compared to benzodiazepines
- Tolerance develops in two to three weeks

PHENOBARBITAL (LUMINAL)

Phenobarbital is a long-acting barbiturate sedative with a half-life of four days. The primary use in psychiatry is to treat sedative withdrawal symptoms. Its long half-life makes withdrawal safer and smoother in a detoxification regimen. It is an excellent choice for treatment of withdrawal from nonbarbiturate sedatives, barbiturate sedatives, and alcohol. It is available in 15, 30, 60, and 100 mg tablets, liquid form, and parenteral form for IM and IV administration. It has been successfully used to withdraw patients from very high doses of alprazolam, lorazepam, and clonazepam (such as 6 to 8 mg per day or more).

Its major side effects are sedation and cognitive impairment. When used for detoxification purposes, its hepatic enzyme induction effect is not a major concern since the use is usually limited to seven to ten days at the most.

Phenobarbital can be combined with carbamazepine or valproate for control of sedative withdrawal symptoms, particularly if the target sedative was being taken in very high doses and/or if severe withdrawal symptoms are expected or manifested. Although phenobarbital has antianxiety and hypnotic properties, it is a poor choice for these purposes, especially with the availability of benzodiazepines, which are safer and have less potential for abuse. The usual adult dosage range for sedative withdrawal treatment is 150 to 400 mg per day in three divided doses with 15 to 20 percent reduction daily, completed over five to seven days. Slower taper may be necessary for severe dependence, especially if the offending sedative has a fairly long half-life. The maximum recommended dose as a detoxification agent is 600 mg per day. Since phenobarbital is well-absorbed after an oral dose, the IM route is used only in the unusual case when oral intake is not possible. The IM dose is approximately two-thirds of the oral dose.

Summary of Advantages and Disadvantages of Phenobarbital

Advantages

- Excellent choice for treatment of sedative or alcohol withdrawal
- Tablet, liquid, IM, and IV form available

- Benign side effect profile
- Once-a-day administration (doses less than 200 mg) possible, usually given at bedtime
- Low cost due to generic availability

Disadvantage (as a detoxification agent)

- Contraindicated in patients with acute intermittent porphyria

OTHER ANTIANXIETY AGENTS, SEDATIVES, AND HYPNOTICS

Medications that are still available but only rarely used in modern psychiatric practice include meprobamate (Equanil, Miltown), glutethimide, ethchlorvynol (Placidyl), secobarbital (Seconal), pentobarbital (Nembutal), and amobarbital (Amytal). Since the introduction of various benzodiazepines that have several advantages over the above-mentioned medications, their use has declined. Rarely, one still sees a patient who has been taking one of the above medications for many years and is doing well; hence, one may be obliged to continue prescribing the same medication.

Chapter 9

Bipolar Disorder

The main forms of bipolar disorder are bipolar I disorder and bipolar II disorder. Bipolar I disorder is characterized by the occurrence of one or more manic episodes or mixed episodes, with or without a history of a major depressive episode. Bipolar II disorder is characterized by the presence or a history of one or more major depressive episodes and at least one hypomanic episode, but no manic or mixed episodes.

MANIC EPISODE

Criteria for a manic episode according to *DSM-IV* are given below:*

A. A distinct period of abnormally and persistently elevated, expansive, or irritable mood, lasting at least one week (or any duration if hospitalization is necessary).

B. During the period of mood disturbance, three (or more) of the following symptoms have persisted (four if the mood is only irritable) and have been present to a significant degree:

1. *Inflated self-esteem or grandiosity*
2. *Decreased need for sleep (e.g., feels rested after only three hours of sleep)*
3. *More talkative than usual or pressure to keep talking*
4. *Flight of ideas or subjective experience that thoughts are racing*
5. *Distractibility (i.e., attention too easily drawn to unimportant or irrelevant external stimuli)*
6. *Increase in goal-directed activity (either socially, at work or school, or sexually) or psychomotor agitation*

---

7. *Excessive involvement in pleasurable activities that have a high potential for painful consequences (e.g., engaging in unrestrained buying sprees, sexual indiscretions, or foolish business investments)*

C. The symptoms do not meet criteria for a mixed episode.

D. The mood disturbance is sufficiently severe to cause marked impairment in occupational functioning or in usual social activities or relationships with others, or to necessitate hospitalization to prevent harm to self or others, or there are psychotic features.

E. The symptoms are not due to the direct physiological effects of a substance (e.g., a drug of abuse, a medication, or other treatment) or a general medical condition (e.g., hyperthyroidism).

Note: Manic-like episodes that are clearly caused by somatic antidepressant treatment (e.g., medication, electroconvulsive therapy, light therapy) should not count toward a diagnosis of bipolar I disorder.

HYPOMANIC EPISODE

A less severe form of manic episode with less marked impairment in social or occupational functioning is known as a hypomanic episode. The criteria for a hypomanic episode according to *DSM-IV* are as follows:*

A. A distinct period of persistently elevated, expansive, or irritable mood, lasting throughout at least four days, that is clearly different from the usual nondepressed mood.

B. During the period of mood disturbance, three (or more) of the following symptoms have persisted (four if the mood is only irritable) and have been present to a significant degree:

1. *Inflated self-esteem or grandiosity*
2. *Decreased need for sleep (e.g., feels rested after only three hours of sleep)*
3. *More talkative than usual or pressure to keep talking*
4. *Flight of ideas or subjective experience that thoughts are racing*
5. *Distractibility (i.e., attention too easily drawn to unimportant or irrelevant external stimuli)*

---

*Italicized text is reprinted with permission from the *Diagnostic and Statistical Manual of Mental Disorders*, Fourth Edition. Copyright 1994 American Psychiatric Association.

6. Increase in goal-directed activity (either socially, at work or school, or sexually) or psychomotor agitation
7. Excessive involvement in pleasurable activities that have a high potential for painful consequences (e.g., the person engages in unrestrained buying sprees, sexual indiscretions, or foolish business investments)

C. The episode is associated with an unequivocal change in functioning that is uncharacteristic of the person when not symptomatic.

D. The disturbance in mood and the change in functioning are observable by others.

E. The episode is not severe enough to cause marked impairment in social or occupational functioning, or to necessitate hospitalization, and there are no psychotic features.

F. The symptoms are not due to the direct physiological effects of a substance (e.g., a drug of abuse, a medication, or other treatment) or a general medical condition (e.g., hyperthyroidism).

Note: Hypomanic-like episodes that are clearly caused by somatic antidepressant treatment (e.g., medication, electroconvulsive therapy, light therapy) should not count toward a diagnosis of bipolar II disorder.

MIXED EPISODE

Mixed episodes are characterized by full manic episodes and full depressive episodes rapidly alternating almost daily. It is sometimes difficult to distinguish a mixed episode from a depressive or manic episode with predominant agitation, irritability, anxiety, and anger. The criteria for a mixed episode according to *DSM-IV* are as follows:*

A. The criteria are met both for a manic episode and for a major depressive episode (except for duration) nearly every day during at least a one-week period.

B. The mood disturbance is sufficiently severe to cause marked impairment in occupational functioning or in usual social activities or relationships with others, or to necessitate hospitalization to prevent harm to self or others, or there are psychotic features.

C. The symptoms are not due to the direct physiological effects of a substance (e.g., a drug of abuse, a medication, or other treatment) or a general medical condition (e.g., hyperthyroidism).

---

*Italicized text is reprinted with permission from the *Diagnostic and Statistical Manual of Mental Disorders*, Fourth Edition. Copyright 1994 American Psychiatric Association.

Note: Mixed-like episodes that are clearly caused by somatic antidepressant treatment (e.g., medication, electroconvulsive therapy, light therapy) should not count toward a diagnosis of bipolar I disorder.

SEVERITY/PSYCHOTIC/REMISSION SPECIFIERS FOR MANIC EPISODE

There are several subcategories of mania, based on the severity level, presence or absence of psychotic symptoms, and degree of remission. The specific *DSM-IV* criteria for each of these specifiers are listed below:*

- ***Mild:*** *minimum symptom criteria are met for a manic episode*
- ***Moderate:*** *extreme increase in activity or impairment in judgment*
- ***Severe Without Psychotic Features:*** *almost continual supervision required to prevent physical harm to self or others*
- ***Severe With Psychotic Features:*** *delusions or hallucinations (If possible, specify whether the psychotic features are mood-congruent or mood-incongruent)*
  - ***Mood-Congruent Psychotic Features:*** *delusions or hallucinations whose content is entirely consistent with the typical manic themes of inflated worth, power, knowledge, identity, or special relationship to a deity or famous person*
  - ***Mood-Incongruent Psychotic Features:*** *delusions or hallucinations whose content do not involve typical manic themes of inflated worth, power, knowledge, identity, or special relationship to a deity or famous person. Included are symptoms such as persecutory delusions (not directly related to grandiose ideas or themes), thought insertion, and delusions of being controlled*
- ***In Partial Remission:*** *symptoms of a manic episode are present but full criteria are not met, or there is a period without any significant symptoms of a manic episode lasting less than two months following the end of the manic episode*
- ***In Full Remission:*** *during the past two months no significant signs or symptoms of the disturbance were present*
- ***Unspecified***

---

*Italicized text is reprinted with permission from the *Diagnostic and Statistical Manual of Mental Disorders*, Fourth Edition. Copyright 1994 American Psychiatric Association.

These criteria are similar for mixed episode except that both manic and depressive episodes are considered in arriving at the proper classifications. Therefore, a mixture of specific criteria for both major depressive episode and manic episode is employed.

Bipolar I disorder and bipolar II disorder can present with rapid cycling features characterized by the occurrence of four or more mood episodes in one year. Criteria for a rapid-cycling specifier according to *DSM-IV* are as follows:*

***With Rapid Cycling** (can be applied to bipolar I disorder or bipolar II disorder): At least four episodes of a mood disturbance in the previous 12 months that meet criteria for a major depressive, manic, mixed, or hypomanic episode.*

Note: Episodes are demarcated either by partial or full remission for at least two months or a switch to an episode of opposite polarity (e.g., major depressive episode to manic episode).

Bipolar I disorder can occur with mixed features, psychotic features, and rapid cycling features. Bipolar II disorder can occur with psychotic features and rapid-cycling features, but not mixed features.

Moodiness and mood irritability are not necessarily indicative of bipolar disorder or of responsiveness to mood stabilizers. If a patient reports mood swings, it is important to obtain more details: Does it mean that the patient gets episodically depressed and then feels euthymic or is it episodic depression alternating with mania? What are the behavioral and subjective symptoms during the various episodes? Obtain descriptions of actual behavior and thoughts during these different phases of moods. In clinical experience, most patients who report mood swings, mood irritability, and moodiness do not have bipolar disorder and hence do not need mood stabilizers. Many patients who have dysthymia, major depression, and anxiety present with complaints of mood swings, which are usually described as episodes of dysphoria or anxiety alternating with feeling euthymic or happy, but not manic. Another easily confusing symptom is the patient's complaint of racing thoughts. Again, in most cases, detailed inquiry will reveal that racing thoughts are manifestations of anxiety, obsessional preoccupation, or excessive worrying, rather than mania. In the case of mania, racing thoughts are accompanied by behavior consistent with mania. Compulsive shopping is a common example of pseudomanic behavior that is frequently confusing to

---

*Italicized text is reprinted with permission from the *Diagnostic and Statistical Manual of Mental Disorders*, Fourth Edition. Copyright 1994 American Psychiatric Association.

clinicians because it is easily interpreted to suggest manic behavior whereas further evaluation, taking into consideration the context and compulsive nature of the behavior, could reveal an obsessive-compulsive basis. Table 9.1 gives a list of characteristics differentiating mania and pseudomania.

Most pseudomanic behavior reflects obsessive-compulsive disorder, histrionic features, cyclothymia, or atypical depression. If there is no evidence of manic behavior, either related to racing thoughts or mood irritability, the primary treatment should not, in most cases, be with antimanic medications. In these cases, antidepressants and adjunctive antianxiety medications should be considered. The author has seen a number of patients who were placed on antimanic medications, particularly lithium, based on the patient's report of mood irritability or mood swings, when in fact careful history revealed dysthymia or major depression. These disorders are responsive to antidepressants, which are particularly effective for treatment of symptoms such as irritability, anger outbursts, reactive mood changes, mood swings, and obsessional worrying.

Bipolar disorder with mixed features is also known as dysphoric mania. Carbamazepine, gabapentin, lamotrigine, and valproic acid are preferentially effective for bipolar disorder with mixed features and rapid-cycling features, whereas lithium is the drug of choice for typical manic episodes. This should be considered a generalization, since the author has had good results with lithium for bipolar patients with mixed and rapid cycling features. Similarly, carbamazepine and valproic acid can be effective for treating manic episodes.

As is emphasized throughout this text, medication selection is based on symptoms, not diagnosis. A patient with a diagnosis of bipolar disorder is typically treated using a mood stabilizer. In addition, that patient might also be placed on an antidepressant and on a variety of medications from other classes of psychotropic drugs, depending on the specific assortment of symptoms.

Dysphoric mania and rapid-cycling bipolar disorder may require treatment using more than one mood stabilizer. Some common combinations are the following:

- Lithium and carbamazepine
- Lithium and gabapentin
- Lithium and lamotrigine
- Lithium and valproic acid

Carbamazepine and valproic acid may be given concurrently with closer monitoring of liver function tests, complete blood count (CBC), and serum levels of both drugs. Most hospitalized bipolar patients require multiple

TABLE 9.1. Characteristics Distinguishing Mania from Pseudomania

Mania/Hypomania	Pseudomania
Severity:	
Significant dysfunction in almost all spheres of functioning is common	Dysfunction primarily limited to interpersonal functioning or to one aspect of behavior
Duration:	
Behaviors and thoughts persist, lasting days or weeks	Behaviors and thoughts are episodic, lasting hours, not days or weeks
Progression:	
Behaviors and thoughts tend to worsen if untreated	Behaviors and thoughts return to baseline within hours
Thought Content:	
Grandiosity, inflated self-esteem, or extreme hostility are persistent	Gradiosity and increased self-confidence are usually absent; the degree of hostility is less intense, and reactive, and usually directed at close family or co-workers
Rationality:	
Irrational thinking is usually present	Irrational thinking is absent
Mood:	
Mood may be elevated or irritable, but lability of affect is almost always present	Mood may be irritable, but is not elevated; affect lability is usually absent
Insight:	
Usually impaired	Usually preserved
Activity Level:	
Reckless, usually unrestrained, repetitive, unremorseful, escalating, and not limited to one type of behavior	Can be excessive, but has a compulsive episodic character, usually limited to one type of behavior, accompanied by guilt, remorse, and distress

medications for effective and rapid resolution of symptoms. Recently introduced anticonvulsants such as gabapentin and lamotrigine have also been found to be effective in the treatment of bipolar disorder. A brief clinical profile of each of these new drugs is presented later in this chapter.

Although ECT, paradoxically, is effective for mania, its actual use for treatment of mania is extremely rare. Prudent use of available medications as described in this text should control virtually all acute manic episodes. ECT is perhaps more beneficial in severe dysphoric mania, which occasionally does not respond to aggressive medication management.

Bipolar disorder with mixed features and bipolar II disorder frequently require antidepressant medication along with a mood stabilizer. All antidepressants are effective, although the author tends to prefer serotonergic antidepressants and bupropion over TCAs and MAOIs because of advantages in side effect profiles.

Thyroid supplementation may decrease cycling in rapid cyclers and improve mood stability in a mixed bipolar disorder. However, in the author's experience, the success rate of thyroid augmentation in euthyroid patients is fairly low when used for decreasing mood swings. Levothyroxine (Synthroid) at a dose of 0.025 to 0.075 mg per day may be tried for euthyroid individuals. The starting dose should be low, with a slow dosage increase, accompanied by clinical monitoring of symptoms of thyrotoxicosis and laboratory monitoring of the thyroid profile, including the thyroid-stimulating hormone (TSH). The thyroid dose should not be high enough to suppress TSH. Since lithium has antithyroid effects, thyroid supplementation may be necessary for some patients on long-term maintenance on lithium.

Some of the very severe manias, mixed manias, and rapid-cycling bipolar disorder, which do not respond to management using standard medications, may respond to clozapine. Although the FDA-approved use of clozapine is currently for treatment-resistant schizophrenia, other uses may be clinically justified and effective, especially in severe treatment-resistant cases.

PRACTICAL MANAGEMENT OF MANIA

Mania is a psychiatric emergency, and in almost all cases, requires immediate hospitalization. Negative vocational, financial, interpersonal, and social consequences, as well as suicidal and homicidal risks, are high. Since insight and judgment are extremely impaired in virtually all severely manic patients, involuntary hospitalization and treatment are usually necessary. Mood stabilizers such as lithium, carbamazepine, valproic acid, and verapamil do not work rapidly and are not sufficient during the first several days of acute mania. All manic episodes are accompanied by psychotic symptoms such as grandiose delusions, disorganized thoughts, irrational beliefs, extreme lability of affect, racing thoughts, flight of ideation, hostility if frustrated, and extreme irritability, in varying degrees of intensity. Unlike chronic psychotic disorders, such as schizophrenia and paranoid disorder, the acute psychotic symptoms in mania in most cases subside within a short period of time with appropriate treatment.

The immediate treatment approach is to medicate the patient with fast-acting medications. Parenteral antipsychotics along with parenteral benzodiazepines should be the medications of choice to control acute agitation and floridly psychotic symptoms during the first 24 to 48 hours of treatment. Examples of effective combinations are the following:

One of the Following Antipsychotics	+	One of the Following Benzodiazepines
haloperidol 5 mg IM		lorazepam 0.5 to 1 mg IM
fluphenazine HCL 5 mg IM		diazepam 5 mg IM
trufluoperazine 5 mg IM		chlordiazepoxide 25 mg IM
perphenazine 10 mg IM		
thiothixene 10 mg IM		
loxapine 25 mg IM		

An example of an effective initial medication order for an acutely manic patient might be as follows:

- Haloperidol 5 mg po or IM every hour as needed for agitation–maximum 30 mg per 24 hours
- Lorazepam 1 mg po or IM every hour as needed for agitation–maximum 6 mg per 24 hours
- Haloperidol and Lorazepam may be given concurrently
- If the patient refuses medication orally, give IM
- If given orally, check for "cheeking" (i.e., holding the pill in the cheek, with the intent to spit it out), or substitute liquid form if available
- Lithium carbonate 300 mg po QID
- Lorazepam 1 mg po PRN insomnia

Several days later, when the patient is cooperative, the order may be as follows:

- Risperidone 1 mg po TID or olanzapine 10 mg HS*
- Lorazepam 0.5 mg po BID
- Lithium carbonate 600 mg po BID or valproate 250 mg TID

*Olanzapine can induce or worsen hypomania in some patients.

Generally, low-potency antipsychotics are to be avoided because of increased risk of hypotension with parenteral use. If the patient is willing to take the medications voluntarily, oral concentrate, if available, is preferred for two reasons: (1) it assures that the medication has been taken and not "cheeked," and (2) it is absorbed more rapidly. Manic patients, while acutely ill, are manipulative, clever, and sneaky; hence, even if an agitated patient appears cooperative, the clinician must be extra vigilant to be sure the patient actually ingests the medication.

Of all the benzodiazepines, lorazepam is the author's preferred medication choice for emergency use. It is well-absorbed by the IM route, has an intermediate half-life (giving better control of dosing), and is well-tolerated by most patients. Several of the common benzodiazepines such as alprazolam, clonazepam, oxazepam, and clorazepate are not available in the United States for IM use. Since diazepam and chlordiazepoxide are absorbed erratically after IM administration and have long half-lives, they should be used as second-line benzodiazepines, if lorazepam is not tolerated by, or is ineffective for, a particular patient.

The combination of antipsychotic and benzodiazepine may be repeated every one to two hours until the patient's agitation is controlled and the patient accepts medication orally. After the first one to three doses, the majority of patients respond. Some may require up to six IM doses, but this is rare. For the elderly and children, the dose should be half of the dose listed.

As soon as the patient is willing to accept medications orally, all medications–including medications for control of acute symptoms (antipsychotics and benzodiazepines) and mood stabilizers–may be given by mouth. Mood stabilizers should be started concurrently. Since they are not available in parenteral form in the United States, the patient's cooperation is necessary to administer them (valproic acid may become available in parenteral form in the United States in the future).

Mood stabilizers should be started at fairly low doses with gradual increase in dose to give time to develop tolerance to gastrointestinal and neurological side effects. Although giving large doses of lithium, valproic acid, or carbamazepine in a "loading dose" (a high initial dose) format is effective and theoretically appealing, it is clinically not prudent. Since gastrointestinal side effects such as nausea, gastric irritation, heartburn, and diarrhea are common even with enteric-coated and sustained-release forms when initially introduced, giving high initial doses orally runs the risk of acute gastrointestinal side effects. Such side effects may lead to the patient's refusal to take these highly effective medications. When parenteral forms that bypass the gastrointestinal tract become available, "loading dose" will probably make clinical sense. Valproic acid is expected to be available for IV administration in the future under the trade name Depacon. A loading dose should then have greatly improved tolerability and patient acceptance since the GI tract is bypassed, sparing many common initial side effects. Furthermore, the IV form could produce rapid clinical effects. Consult the package insert for dosing guidelines and other details.

Since it is a benzodiazepine, clonazepam is a poor long-term prophylactic mood stabilizer because of typical long-term problems associated with benzodiazepines. It is highly effective, as are all of the potent benzodiazepines such as lorazepam, alprazolam, oxazepam, and diazepam for short-term control of severe anxiety and agitation including those associated with mania and psychosis.

After the patient's acute symptoms such as agitation, extreme lability, hostility, and resistance to treatment are controlled, the dose of the antipsychotic can be reduced and eventually tapered off completely. Approximately 50 percent of manic patients will benefit from and need a longer maintenance period on neuroleptics. The maintenance period may last anywhere from one week to several months. Most manic patients need antipsychotics for the first several days for efficient and effective control of symptoms. Some may need low doses of antipsychotics as an adjunctive medication for more than six months, depending on the extent of the severity and chronicity of psychotic symptoms. Theoretically, a manic patient can possibly be treated using mood stabilizers alone. However, monotherapy using only a mood stabilizer will lengthen the time to achieve the desired result of stability. With the recent focus on cost-effectiveness, short-term hospitalization, and outpatient treatment–which should always be the goal–patients currently do not have the luxury of staying in psychiatric hospitals for a month or longer (which was the case some years ago). In fact, patients are now fortunate if they are able to stay in the hospital for several weeks. Regardless of the availability of inpatient days, the physician has a responsibility to treat the patient as rapidly and efficiently as possible, and to return the patient to the community as soon as possible. Immediate treatment using a combination of an antipsychotic and a sedative along with concurrent initiation of a mood stabilizer will frequently result in rapid stabilization of the patient and avoidance of prolonged inpatient confinement. Reliance on a mood stabilizer alone, though eventually effective, usually takes longer for achieving stabilization, thus lengthening the period of hospitalization.

Risperidone and olanzapine are antipsychotics with improved side effect profiles as compared to traditional antipsychotics. They may be used for maintenance when the patient is ready to accept medication by mouth.

Risperidone and olanzapine are not yet available parenterally. Risperidone is available in liquid form.

Since acutely manic patients tend to process lithium more efficiently, resulting in a lower blood level compared to the euthymic state, the initial lithium dose for acute manic patients is 900 mg to 1,200 mg per day in divided doses. The dose may need to be increased to achieve a blood level of 1.0 to 1.3 mEq/L for control of acute mania. It takes about five days for lithium to reach a steady state. Serum level should be obtained five days after lithium initiation or dosage adjustment, unless toxicity is suspected or unless more frequent monitoring is medically necessary. All blood drug-level monitoring should be based on the pharmacokinetic profile of the individual drug, and should be obtained only if and when medically necessary to manage the patient. Routine blood-level monitoring on fixed days (such as every Monday, for example) without regard to individual patient needs and individual drug pharmacokinetics should be discouraged.

Once the mania begins to subside, the serum level of lithium tends to increase while on the same daily dose. Therefore, lithium levels should be checked several times a week if the patient is on fairly high doses of lithium, especially if the previous lithium level was at or above 1.2 mEq/L. As the patient improves, the dose of lithium may need to be decreased to prevent toxicity. Once the patient is euthymic, the dose should be monitored to give a lithium level of 0.5 to 0.8 mEq/L. The phenomenon of differential utilization of a drug by the body as seen with lithium, based on acuity of the illness, is not seen with other mood stabilizers such as carbamazepine or valproic acid, although small decreases in the dose of the above medications during euthymia may be desirable and possible without losing therapeutic benefits.

The correlation between lithium dose and serum level is fairly linear, except when patients are stabilizing after a manic episode. For example, if a lithium dose of 1,200 mg per day yields a steady-state serum level of 0.6 mEq/L, it can be calculated that every 200 mg of lithium contributes to 0.1 mEq/L of serum level. Since a lithium level in the range of 1.0 to 1.3 mEq/L is the generally desired serum level for effective treatment of acute mania, based on application of the dose-to-level ratio for this patient, it is calculated that a lithium dose of approximately 2,100 mg per day is required to raise the serum level to 1.1 mEq/L. Due to increased gastrointestinal and neurological side effects associated with rapid and large dosage increments, the dose should be increased from 1,200 mg per day to 2,100 mg per day over a period of two to three days. The lithium level is likely to remain the same if the patient's clinical condition does not change. However, when the mania begins to subside, the level is likely to rise on the same dose, requiring a decrease in the dose to prevent toxic levels. It is conceivable that the patient who had a serum level of 1.1 mEq/L on lithium 2,100 mg per day could yield a level of 1.6 mEq/L or higher on the same dose in a euthymic state; this patient may have a lithium level of 1.1 mEq/L on 1,500 mg per day of lithium when not acutely manic. Since maintenance lithium level for prophylactic purposes during euthymia is between 0.5 and 0.8 mEq/L for most patients, the corresponding lithium dose is also lower, usually in the range of 600 to 1,200 mg per day. During maintenance phase, the linear relationship between lithium dose and serum level is more valid. A slightly lower steady-state lithium level is obtained on sustained-release preparation compared to the same dose of regular preparation.

Acutely manic patients frequently have symptoms such as hostility, lability of affect, impatience, narcissism, ambivalence, intrusiveness, manipulative and demanding behavior, idealizing and devaluing attitudes, and behavior that can lead to staff splitting and disruption of the inpatient unit homeostasis. It is tempting for the staff to attribute these symptoms to a personality disorder, most commonly to borderline, narcissistic, or histrionic personality disorders, thereby justifying their hostile countertransference. It is important for clinicians not to assume that a patient's symptoms while acutely ill are due to a personality disorder, however disagreeable the symptoms may be. The author has seen many cases of the so-called personality disorders fading with appropriate treatment. In most cases, these patients had atypical bipolar disorders, schizoaffective disorders, depression, cyclothymia, ADD, PTSD or substance abuse problems. The effective and practical pharmacotherapy of personality disorders is discussed in detail in the author's text *Personality Disorders: New Symptom-Focused Drug Therapy, With 50 Clinical Cases* (The Haworth Press, 1997).

Once a patient is branded as having a personality disorder, there emerges a sense of futility and negative countertransference that is subconsciously communicated to the patient and can interfere with the patient-clinician rapport, patient compliance, and successful treatment outcome.

PRACTICAL MAINTENANCE TREATMENT OF BIPOLAR DISORDER

Patients with bipolar disorders are likely to have periodic relapses. Lithium, carbamazepine, and valproic acid are the mainstays of maintenance and prophylaxis. Gabapentin and lamotrigine can also be used for maintenance treatment. One of the mood stabilizers is continued beyond the acute phase of the illness for two major reasons:

1. To maintain improvement and stability
2. To act as a prophylactic against manic episodes

The length of time a patient is maintained on mood stabilizers depends on the severity of the current episode, the severity and number of previous episodes, the duration of intensive treatment required for control of current or previous episodes, and the level of dysfunction associated with episodes. The more pronounced any one or more of these factors are, the longer the duration of prophylactic medication maintenance recommended. Occurrence of manic episodes without any clear precipitants and the presence of strong family history of bipolar disorder also favor the need for maintenance treatment for long periods of time. After the first episode of mania, treatment should be continued for about one year prior to attempting a very slow taper over a period of three months. If prodromal symptoms such as insomnia, irritability, increased energy, grandiosity, intrusiveness, increased daydreaming, preoccupation, and increased sociability occur, a higher dose can be easily reinstated. The greater the number of exacerbations, the higher the chance of bipolar disorder developing rapid-cycling characteristics, causing what is generally considered a more severe form of bipolar disorder. For patients who have had several relapses, long-term prophylaxis is the rule. Some of the severe cases may need life-long maintenance on a mood stabilizer. Patients should be advised of the serious consequences associated with relapse, and of the benefit-to-risk ratio that strongly favors being maintained on medication on a long-term basis.

Many hypomanic and manic patients enjoy the feeling of having racing and grandiose thoughts and are resistant to treatment. They are more energetic and possess a belief that they accomplish more and are more creative while in a hypomanic mood. It is important for the clinician to identify this phenomenon in a particular patient, to acknowledge the reality of these feelings, and to convince the patient of the need to accept the treatment. Using the following example of a speeding vehicle illustrates this point to the patient in a manner that can easily be understood. Although driving at 100 miles an hour is very efficient and exciting, it is also extremely dangerous because it decreases control and increases the likelihood of accidents. On the other hand, driving at 60 miles per hour provides a reasonable balance between efficiency and safety. Figuratively speaking, the purpose of treating hypomanic patients is to bring them to a "safe speed." Patients recovering from a manic episode or patients who are in a hypomanic state are capable of fair insight, when the reasoning is presented in a manner with which they can identify. Floridly manic patients are not amenable to logical thinking and hence any insight-oriented discussions should await their recovery from the acute phase of their illness.

Most symptoms exist in a continuum from mild to severe, and so do psychotic symptoms. Many primarily bipolar patients manifest mild psychotic symptoms which are not controlled by mood stabilizers. In clinical practice, it is the rare bipolar patient who does well on a mood stabilizer alone. Adjunctive treatment using low doses of an antipsychotic is often necessary for optimal treatment of a patient with bipolar disorder. An excellent first-line choice of an antipsychotic is risperidone at 0.5 to 2 mg po AM or HS or olanzapine 5 to 10 mg HS. Higher doses are not usually necessary for patients who have predominantly affective symptoms as in the case of bipolar disorders.

There is overlap between the symptoms of bipolar disorder and those of attention deficit hyperactivity disorder, which in some cases can coexist. If both bipolar disorder and ADHD are present, both conditions should be treated using mood stabilizers and stimulants, respectively. Similarly, other conditions can coexist with bipolar disorder. In these cases, each distinct symptom complex should be separately evaluated and treated.

In individuals predisposed to mania who present with depression, antidepressants or ECT can cause a switch to mania. If this occurs, antidepressant dosage should be lowered or discontinued and mania should be treated. These patients will most often need a combination of a mood stabilizer and an antidepressant for optimal results because if the antidepressant is discontinued, depression usually recurs.

CYCLOTHYMIA

Cyclothymia is characterized by chronic mood swings, involving periods of hypomanic and depressive symptoms. Diagnostic criteria according to *DSM-IV* are given below:*

A. For at least two years, the presence of numerous periods with hypomanic symptoms and numerous periods with depressive symptoms that do not meet criteria for a major depressive episode. Note: In children and adolescents, the duration must be at least one year.

B. During the above two-year period (one year in children and adolescents), the person has not been without the symptoms in criterion A for more than two months at a time.

---

*Italicized text is reprinted with permission from the *Diagnostic and Statistical Manual of Mental Disorders*, Fourth Edition. Copyright 1994 American Psychiatric Association.

C. No major depressive episode, manic episode, or mixed episode has been present during the first two years of the disturbance.

Note: After the initial two years (one year in children and adolescents) of cyclothymic disorder, there may be superimposed manic or mixed episodes (in which case both bipolar I disorder and cyclothymic disorder may be diagnosed) or major depressive episodes (in which case both bipolar II disorder and cyclothymic disorder may be diagnosed).

D. The symptoms in Criterion A are not better accounted for by schizoaffective disorder and are not superimposed on schizophrenia, schizophreniform disorder, delusional disorder, or psychotic disorder not otherwise specified.

E. The symptoms are not due to the direct physiological effects of a substance (e.g., a drug of abuse, a medication) or a general medical condition (e.g., hyperthyroidism).

F. The symptoms cause clinically significant distress or impairment in social, occupational, or other important areas of functioning.

Cyclothymia, for practical clinical purposes, should be seen as a mild form of bipolar disorder and should be managed accordingly, using mood stabilizers and antidepressants, as indicated. For example, if hypomanic symptoms are prominent with clinically insignificant depressive symptoms, one of the mood stabilizers should be sufficient. However, if depressive symptoms predominate, with negligible hypomanic symptoms, an antidepressant alone may be all that is needed. Low doses of antipsychotics may be desirable initially for rapid control of hypomanic symptoms.

MOOD STABILIZERS

Lithium Salts

Lithium is an effective medication for treatment of manic episodes and for maintenance treatment of bipolar disorders. It is the drug of choice for the treatment of mania. It also has some antidepressant properties but is not effective by itself as an antidepressant. Lithium can be used for adjunctive treatment of refractory depression in combination with antidepressants, including MAOIs. Other uses include treatment of impulsivity and aggressive behavior. For rapid-cycling bipolar conditions, dysphoric mania, bipolar disorder NOS, it appears that valproate (Depakene, Depakote), gabapentin (Neurontin), carbamazepine (Tegretol), and lamotrigine (Lamictal) may be slightly more effective. Since lithium has excellent mood-stabilizing properties, it is an overall good choice to try for a patient with extreme mood swings, regardless of whether the patient fits the description of classical bipolar disorder, rapid-cycling bipolar disorder, or dysphoric mania. Lithium can be combined with antidepressants, antipsychotics, and antianxiety medications, although the combination can result in more pronounced central nervous system side effects. It can also be used with valproate, carbamazepine, gabapentin, lamotrigine, and verapamil, with the same caution. Since lithium has a narrow therapeutic range and can be lethal in serious overdoses, its use in suicidal patients should be supervised carefully.

Lithium is available as lithium carbonate 300 mg tablets and as lithium citrate syrup for oral administration. Two slow-release forms are Eskalith CR 450 mg and Lithobid 300 mg. The slow-release form tends to cause significantly less gastrointestinal irritation, and hence is the preferred form. Since Eskalith CR is available in 450 mg strength, this may be less expensive because of the higher dose per pill. Eskalith CR 450 mg is a scored tablet and can be broken for ease of dosage titration, and for multiple dosing.

Lithium, when used as an adjunctive to antipsychotics, can increase central nervous system side effects. Since lithium has a narrow therapeutic range, close blood-level monitoring is required, especially in the initial period of treatment and at the high end of the therapeutic range. The serum level necessary for effective treatment of acute mania is between 1.0 and 1.3 mEq/L, and for maintenance or prophylactic use, the serum level is between 0.5 and 0.8 mEq/L. Patients in an acute manic state tend to need very high doses of lithium to reach the effective serum level; whereas as mania subsides, the blood level rises on the same dose that was required initially. Hence, to prevent toxicity and to keep the serum level within the safe range appropriate for the acuity of the illness, the dosage will need to be decreased as the patient improves. Acutely manic patients respond on a dose of 1,500 to 2,400 mg per day, and most hypomanic or maintenance patients need a dose of 600 to 1,200 mg per day. Both clinical monitoring and serum level monitoring are important. The author has had the experience of treating several patients in severe manic states who needed a dose of 3,000 mg per day to yield a serum level of 1.3 mEq/L, while the same patients, when euthymic, needed only a dose of 1,200 mg per day to obtain a serum level of 0.8 mEq/L. Thus, the relationship between dosage and serum level is not linear during the acute and recovery phases, when serum levels are variably responsive to dosages; however, during maintenance periods, the dose-serum level relationship seems to be fairly linear. Hence, lithium levels should be obtained at least once a week until the patient's acute symptoms are controlled. Since most manic patients need inpatient treatment, close serum-level monitoring is not a consideration for the outpatient office practice that treats hypomanic and bipolar patients who are in fair control. Since serum levels are dosage-dependent in a fairly linear fashion in patients who are neither acutely manic nor in the recovery phase, and since the serum levels aimed for in an office setting are in the maintenance range of 0.5 to 0.8 mEq/L, the need for close serum-level monitoring is not as stringent. The usual starting dose in an outpatient office is 600 to 900 mg per day. However, in an inpatient unit, the usual starting dose is 900 to 1,200 mg per day, with further dosage titration based on serum level obtained after a steady state is reached (usually five days after lithium is initiated). Since the half-life of lithium is 24 hours, one needs to wait about five days to get a valid serum level after starting lithium or after a dosage adjustment, unless blood level is obtained to monitor toxicity or for other medical reasons. The blood sample should be drawn approximately 12 hours after the previous dose, and is usually obtained in the morning, before the first dose of lithium is given.

Eskalith CR 450 mg 1/2 po AM and 1 po with supper is a convenient and well-tolerated regimen for starting lithium in an outpatient. Another option is the slow-release Lithobid 300 mg po BID. The slow-release formula gives fairly even blood levels. Since lithium side effects can become evident even at low serum levels, it is best to start an outpatient at low doses and then titrate the dose upward over several weeks so the patient has time to become tolerant of the side effects. An oral loading dose is likely to result in severe side effects, such as nausea, diarrhea, and vomiting, thereby causing the patient to develop an aversion to lithium. Besides, lithium usually takes five to seven days to begin to work; hence, there is no advantage in risking acute side effects by giving a high dose to start, even for an out-of-control, floridly manic patient. Acutely manic patients should be managed using other adjunctive medications during the first several days of treatment. Side effects tend to rise as the dosage is increased. Children and the elderly are more susceptible to side effects at relatively lower serum levels; hence, starting dose and dosage increments should be low.

The most common side effects of lithium are nausea, diarrhea, fine hand tremors, increased thirst, polydypsia, polyuria, fatigue, polyphagia, and weight gain. Other side effects include dermatological reactions such as rash and worsening of psoriasis, flattening or inversion of the T-wave in the EKG, sinus bradycardia, hypothyroidism, renal effects, leukocytosis, ataxia, joint swelling, and memory impairment. Lithium should not be given to patients with sick sinus syndrome, or if it causes bradycardia, which can predispose to ventricular arrhythmias, congestive heart failure, and syncope.

Angiotensin converting enzyme inhibitors, NSAIDs, thiazide diuretics, and metronidazole (Flagyl) can increase lithium level by 30 to 40 percent. If any of these medications are added to lithium, decrease the lithium dose by at least 40 percent while the patient is on one of the above medications and recheck the serum level within three days. For example, if a patient is on lithium 900 mg per day, the total daily dosage should be reduced to 450 mg per day if the patient is on one of the above medications, and to 300 to 450 mg per day if the patient is on two or more of the above medications. Theophylline (Theodur), phenothiazines, and excessive caffeine can decrease lithium levels. Since lithium is not bound to plasma proteins, it is not likely to be affected by other medications that are highly protein-bound.

The lithium dose should be decreased in patients with renal functioning abnormalities, fever, dehydration, and diarrhea. Patients should be instructed to maintain their normal salt intake and to increase fluid intake to 2 to 2.5 liters a day to ensure efficient renal functioning. Thyroid supplementation may be necessary if hypothyroidism develops. Lithium given as a one-time dose preferably with supper is thought to cause less polyuria and to decrease the risk of renal impairment. However, single dosing can cause more gastrointestinal irritation and is not practical if the patient needs greater than 900 mg per day. Lithium can cause nephrogenic diabetes insipidus, probably requiring its discontinuation in most instances. It is relatively contraindicated in patients with cardiac or renal problems and if given, should be monitored by EKG and frequent serum levels. Loop diuretics such as furosemide (Lasix), bumetanide (Bumex), and ethacrynic acid (Edecrin) tend to affect the lithium level relatively less.

As with all medications, lithium use in pregnancy should be weighed against the risks. Lithium in rare instances has been implicated in causing heart defects (such as Ebstein's anomaly) in the first trimester. The author has successfully used verapamil for several bipolar, manic patients who became pregnant. Lithium use after the first trimester of pregnancy is considered less risky. If possible, lithium should be tapered off one week prior to delivery to avoid lithium side effects in the neonate. Increase in salt intake should be considered in patients likely to lose electrolytes such as in excessive sweating, diarrhea, or vomiting.

Prior to starting lithium, the recommended baseline laboratory studies are urinalysis, electrolytes, blood urea nitrogen, creatinine, thyroid profile (with TSH), CBC, and EKG. Since lithium is relatively contraindicated in the first trimester of pregnancy, a pregnancy test is also appropriate in females of child-bearing age.

Nephrogenic diabetes insipidus secondary to lithium can be controlled at times, paradoxically by using hydrochlorothiazide (Hydrodiuril) 50 mg po daily, or amiloride (Midamor) 5 to 10 mg daily. A 40 to 50 percent lithium dosage reduction, frequent monitoring of lithium level, and monitoring of electrolytes are necessary if any of the above medications are to be added to lithium. In the author's opinion, such an intervention is recommended only if absolutely necessary in cases where alternate mood stabilizers such as divalproex sodium (Depakote), carbamazepine (Tegretol), lamotrigine (Lamictal), gabapentin (Neurontin), or verapamil (Calan SR) are either ineffective or poorly tolerated by the patient, necessitating the use of lithium. These situations arise only rarely in clinical practice, and when they do, internal medicine or nephrology consultation is advisable.

Hypothyroidism leading to goiter–induced by the antithyroid action of lithium–can be treated using levothyroxine 50 to 100 mcg daily, monitoring TSH, creatinine, and lithium levels every three to four months for maintenance treatment. Since coadministration with carbamazepine and neuroleptics can increase central nervous system side effects, the dosage of both drugs should be lowered slightly.

Maintenance Treatment

How long should patients be maintained on lithium? The length of lithium maintenance depends on the chronicity of the illness, the severity of manic episodes, presence of side effects, relapses, and whether or not other medications are used. If the patient has a chronic illness with several relapses in the past when taken off lithium or has relapsed while on lithium, the author recommends keeping these patients on lithium indefinitely. Even though patients can have breakthrough manic episodes while on lithium, these episodes are likely to be less frequent and less severe, thus easier to control. A patient with hypomanic episodes may be able to be slowly tapered off of lithium after six months to one year. People with cyclothymia, which by definition is a chronic condition, may need maintenance doses for several years prior to an attempt at discontinuation. It is the author's opinion that if a patient has had a severe manic episode that required prolonged hospitalization and multiple medications for control, it is safer to recommend that the patient stay on lithium prophylactically for four to five years, even if this was the first manic episode. Any discontinuation of lithium in general should be done very gradually over a period of three to four months under close clinical supervision, with office visits every three to four weeks. Patients and significant others should be thoroughly educated to identify prodromal symptoms of a relapse, such as insomnia, increased anxiety, grandiose thoughts, or irritability and instructed to call the physician when these appear. (*Note:* The importance of including significant others is related to the fact that patients, as stated previously, enjoy the hypomanic feeling and may resist returning to treatment.) The author has found it helpful to prescribe #10 each of haloperidol 5 mg and lorazepam 1 mg pills for emergency use. A combination of haloperidol 5 mg and lorazepam 1 mg orally for several nights will control most of the manic episodes if identified early, probably preventing hospitalization, especially if patients are already on maintenance lithium. Immediate availability of the suggested medications or substitutes will enable patients to control their emerging symptoms, thereby giving them a sense of control over their illness and an incentive to monitor their symptoms. This leads to better compliance with the treatment protocol and acceptance of the illness. In addition, these medications help to keep patients under control until the increased dose of lithium or another mood stabilizer becomes effective.

Valproate

Valproic acid (Depakene capsules), sodium valproate (Depakene syrup), and divalproex sodium (Depakote), which contain both sodium valproate and valproic acid, are primarily indicated for seizures. Recently, valproate received FDA approval for treatment of mania. Sodium valproate is converted to valproic acid, which is the primary form in the blood. The pharmacokinetics of the various forms are similar. Valproic acid (Depakene) is available in 250 mg strength capsules in both brand name and in less-expensive generic forms. It tends to cause slightly more gastrointestinal irritation and nausea, compared to other formulations. Divalproex sodium (Depakote) is available in enteric coated 125 mg, 250 mg, and 500 mg tablets. Since gastrointestinal side effects are fairly common with the generic form valproate, especially during the first several weeks of treatment, the author recommends Depakote although it is more costly. Patients should be warned of these side effects and instructed to tolerate side effects if possible since they will subside after one to two weeks of continued use in most cases. For those who have preexisting dyspepsia, ulcer, or gastrointestinal reflux, an even more tolerable form is available as Depakote Sprinkle capsule 125 mg strength. This formulation is designed for children and is to be taken mixed with food. The capsule can be opened and the coated granules sprinkled over food and then ingested. For those who can swallow the capsule, there is no need to open it and sprinkle it. This formulation causes the least gastrointestinal side effects and is recommended for anyone with GI problems or in those who have a low threshold for tolerating GI side effects. Taking the pills with food further reduces the GI side effects. Valproic acid is expected to be available for IV administration in the near future under the trade name Depacon. Starting oral dosages in healthy adults are as follows:

- Depakote (divalproex sodium): 250 mg po BID and HS with meals
- Depakote sprinkle capsules (divalproex sodium): 250 mg po TID
- Depakene capsules (valproic acid): 250 mg po BID and HS with meals

Valproate can cause liver function abnormalities. Weekly monitoring of these laboratory studies is recommended for the first two weeks, and should be followed by monthly intervals for two months, bimonthly intervals for four months, then once every four to six months for as long as the patient is on valproate.

The therapeutic blood level range is between 50 and 100 mcg/ml for management of seizures. Generally, this blood level range is recommended for psychiatric purposes, but the author has seen satisfactory improvements in symptoms at lower than this blood level range and has decided to keep patients at the corresponding dosage. Ultimately, more important than blood level range is symptom monitoring, with blood level monitoring primarily for assuring that there is no toxicity. Valproate is particularly effective for the treatment of rapid-cycling bipolar disorder and mixed mania.

Side effects include sedation, tremor, fluid retention, increased appetite and consequent weight gain, elevation in liver function tests, and increase in ammonia level that is usually benign and transient. Rare hepatotoxicity has occurred in children. Symptoms of hepatotoxicity are anorexia, severe nausea, vomiting, weakness, and jaundice. Infrequent side effects include thrombocytopenia and pancreatitis.

The half-life of valproate is 14 hours. It reaches steady-state plasma level in three to four days. Valproate is usually started at 250 mg twice a day for three to four days, then increased to three times a day or one in the morning and two tablets with the evening meal. Given its pronounced gastrointestinal side effects, an oral "loading dose" should be avoided. Loading dose by the IV route (when an IV formulation becomes available) should be convenient, tolerable, and rapidly effective. The IV dosing guidelines for the treatment of a manic episode were not available at the time of this writing.

Valproate can be combined with lithium, antipsychotics, and antidepressants. The dosage of an antidepressant should be reduced since valproate can increase antidepressant blood levels.

Carbamazepine (Tegretol)

Carbamazepine, approved for the treatment of temporal lobe epilepsy and trigeminal neuralgia, is an effective agent for treatment of impulse control problems, rapid-cycling bipolar disorder, mixed mania, and atypical bipolar disorder. Carbamazepine tends to be somewhat more effective than lithium for this subgroup of patients. It can be used for control of manic episodes. Given the concern with hematological abnormalities such as leukopenia, thrombocytopenia, rare aplastic anemia, and agranulocytosis, as well as hepatitis, the author prefers valproate for first-line treatment of rapid cyclers and for mixed mania. Agranulocytosis or aplastic anemia is estimated to occur in 1 in 20,000 patients. Carbamazepine may have some antidepressant properties, but it is not considered an effective antidepressant on its own.

The starting dose in a healthy adult patient is 100 mg TID, increased to 200 mg BID in the first week, with the therapeutic serum concentration for seizure control being between 6 and 12 mcg/ml. For psychiatric use, a serum level in the same therapeutic range is recommended. Since carbamazepine induces its own metabolism, higher doses may be needed after two to four weeks to maintain the therapeutic serum level. Blood level monitoring, CBC, and liver function tests are obtained weekly for the first several weeks, then monthly for several months, and every two to three months thereafter. Other side effects include rash, sedation, nausea, dizziness, hyponatremia, headache, diarrhea, and diplopia. Dermatological reactions, including rash, may require discontinuation. Patients taking carbamazepine should be instructed to contact the physician if they develop signs of illness, such as pallor, fever, weakness, sore throat, or easy bruising. Fluoxetine and verapamil can increase the carbamazepine level. Carbamazepine can reduce the effectiveness of antipsychotics and TCAs to some extent.

There are additional concerns for women taking carbamazepine. Blood levels of oral contraceptives may be decreased while taking carbamazepine, probably by increasing the metabolism of estrogen. Female patients should be cautioned about this possibility. One gram of ascorbic acid (Vitamin C) daily has the potential to increase estrogen level and may be considered for patients who need to be on carbamazepine while taking oral contraceptives. As another option, the patient could be advised to contact her gynecologist or family physician to consider prescribing an oral contraceptive with a higher estrogen content or consider using a supplemental form of contraception for greater protection while the patient is on carbamazepine. Carbamazepine can be combined with lithium if necessary, but there is an increased risk of central nervous system toxicity. Carbamazepine has a half-life of 15 hours, and reaches steady state in four days. It is 75 percent protein-bound.

Concurrent use of MAOIs with carbamazepine is not generally recommended because carbamazepine is chemically related to tricyclic compounds. However, the author has used combinations of carbamazepine and phenelzine (Nardil) without complications. Carbamazepine is available in generic form as chewable tablets of 100 mg; tablets of 200 mg; extended-release (XR) tablets of 100, 200, and 400 mg, for BID dosing; and as an oral suspension of 100mg/5 mL (teaspoon).

Gabapentin (Neurontin)

Gabapentin is an anticonvulsant that may be effective as a mood stabilizer in patients with bipolar disorder. It is supplied as 100, 300, and 400 mg capsules. The recommended dosage range is 300 to 600 mg TID for its FDA-approved indication, which is as an adjunctive agent in the treatment of partial seizures. It has low protein-binding. It is eliminated by the kidneys, without significant metabolism by the liver. Although the dosage range for psychiatric application is considered the same as recommended for partial seizures, in practice, a lower dosage range of 300 to 400 mg TID has been effective in patients with bipolar disorder. Titration to an effective dose can be achieved starting with 300 mg at bedtime on day one, 300 mg BID on day two, and 300 mg TID on day three. Further dosage increments can be instituted at a rate of 300 mg every six to seven days up to the maximum total daily dose of 1,800 mg. The dose may be given on a BID schedule for psychiatric applications. Gabapentin does not significantly interact with lithium, valproate, carbamazepine, lamotrigine, or common psychiatric drugs. The total dose should be reduced by half in patients with compromised renal function.

The most commonly observed side effects related to gabapentin were somnolence, dizziness, ataxia, fatigue, mystagmus, and tremor. Gabapentin is well tolerated by patients. Since it has no bone marrow suppressing effects, it may be administered as a seizure prophylactic in patients placed on high doses of clozapine. Appetite stimulation is not a common side effect of gabapentin. Routine laboratory monitoring is not necessary.

Lamotrigine (Lamictal)

Lamotrigine is a recently introduced anticonvulsant drug approved by the FDA for adjunctive therapy in the treatment of partial seizures in adults. The proposed mechanism of action is enhanced stabilization of neuronal membranes, thereby inhibiting presynaptic release of excitatory neurotransmitters such as glutamate and aspartate. It is not highly protein bound. Lamotrigine is available as scored 25, 100, 150, and 200 mg tablets. It is metabolized by the liver and excreted primarily through the kidneys.

Lamotrigine is well tolerated and is effective as a mood stabilizer in patients with bipolar disorder. If necessary, it can be administered with lithium. For psychiatric indications, it should be avoided in patients taking valproic acid due to increased incidence of serious rash and drug interaction, resulting in significantly increased plasma concentration of lamotrigine.

The most commonly reported side effects were dizziness, headache, diplopia, ataxia, nausea, blurred vision, somnolence, rash, and vomiting. A worsening rash, particularly associated with fever, lymphadenopathy, facial swelling, and hematologic and hepatologic abnormalities, is an indication for immediate discontinuation of lamotrigine and appropriate medical intervention. The incidence of rash is greater when (1) coadministered with valproate and carbamazepine, (2) higher than recommended initial dose is given, and (3) dosage escalation is instituted rapidly. Most of the side effects tend to subside gradually over a period of several weeks.

The recommended starting dose and dosage escalation schedule for the management of partial seizures is 50 mg for two weeks, followed by 50 mg BID during weeks three and four. Thereafter, the dose is increased by 100 mg every week until a maintenance dose of 300 to 500 mg per day in divided doses is reached. The maximum recommended dose is 700 mg per day in divided doses. This dosage recommendation is followed in the application of lamotrigine for the treatment of bipolar disorders, except that clinical outcome should primarily determine the decision to increase the dose. As is observed with other anticonvulsants used for the treatment of bipolar disorder, such as valproate, carbamazepine, and gabapentin, considerable variability in the effective dosage range is possible with lamotrigine. For example, if a patient achieves mood stability on lamotrigine 50 mg BID, there is no clinical necessity to increase the dose further, unlike in seizure-control applications where maintenance on an established therapeutic dosage range might be desirable.

Routine blood level or laboratory monitoring is not necessary unless other enzyme-inducing antiepileptic drugs such as carbamazepine, phenytoin, phenobarbital, or valproate are coadministered, or toxicity is suspected. If lamotrigine is discontinued, a gradual decrease over a week is preferred over abrupt discontinuation, as is true regarding the strategy for discontinuing all anticonvulsants, unless safety concerns require a more rapid or abrupt withdrawal.

Verapamil (Calan)

Verapamil is a calcium-channel blocker, indicated primarily for treatment of hypertension. It can also be used for treatment of manic episodes at doses of 40 to 80 mg po TID or as a slow-release preparation (Calan SR) 120, 180, or 240 mg po once daily. Verapamil is employed in clinical practice only when other, more effective mood stabilizers such as lithium, valproate, carbamazepine, lamotrigine, and gabapentin fail or are not tolerated by the patient. Verapamil interacts with carbamazepine, causing increased central nervous system side effects. Therefore, if a combination is used, the dosage of both drugs should be lowered to minimize the risk of side effects. Verapamil can cause constipation, hypotension, bradycardia, nausea, headache, anxiety, malaise, AV (atrioventricular) block, and edema. It should not be used with other cardiac medications without close medical supervision. Blood pressure and pulse rate should be monitored when the patient is initiated on verapamil.

Verapamil is occasionally effective for control of impulsivity and aggression. The author has successfully used verapamil to control manic and hypomanic symptoms in several pregnant patients. Theoretically, other calcium-channel blockers also should have an antimanic effect, but the author has no experience in using them for treatment of mania.

Clonazepam (Klonopin)

See section on benzodiazepines.

Combinations of Mood Stabilizers

In many cases, monotherapy may not be sufficient to control symptoms, necessitating the addition of a second mood stabilizer as an adjunctive medication. This is particularly applicable in complicated mania and in patients who have chronic dysfunctional symptoms that do not readily respond to simple treatment strategies. Effective combinations are lithium plus valproate, lithium plus gabapentin, lithium plus lamotrigine, lithium plus carbamazepine, or lithium plus a low dose of clonazepam. Combination treatment increases the risk of side effects. The patient should be given a full trial on the first medication and be kept on a stable dose before the second medication is added. The first medication is discontinued if there is no improvement at all. However, if at least moderate improvement is obtained on a medication, that medication is continued, while a second medication is added to achieve an improved response. Once the patient is on the second medication, and if there is significant improvement, the first medication is gradually tapered off unless the patient deteriorates, in which case the patient is kept on both medications. When combination treatment is attempted, the blood levels of medications having a narrow therapeutic range should be monitored frequently to detect changes in blood levels due to hepatic enzyme induction, inhibition, increased free drug in the serum due to substrate competition, protein-binding competition, or a combination of these.

Atypical Antipsychotics as Mood Stabilizers

Atypical antipsychotics that are currently available such as clozapine, risperidone, and olanzapine have mood-stabilizing effects. They are typically used in an adjunctive or augmenting role, in combination with one or more of the primary mood stabilizers such as lithium, valproate, carbamazepine, gabapentin, and lamotrigine.

Among the atypical antipsychotics, clozapine has the most pronounced mood-stabilizing effects. In complicated bipolar disorders that do not respond satisfactorily to the primary mood stabilizers, a trial of clozapine should be considered, though it must be pointed out that clozapine is not approved by the FDA for this purpose. In the author's experience, several severe treatment-resistant cases of bipolar disorder have had excellent stabilization of mood on clozapine alone. A clozapine dosage range of 150 to 250 mg is usually sufficient for mood-stabilizing effects. Refer to Chapter 11 for a detailed discussion of the clinical profile of clozapine.

Risperidone and olanzapine also have some mood-stabilizing properties, but are not effective as primary mood stabilizers. However, they are typically employed as adjunctive medications along with a primary mood stabilizer. Both risperidone and olanzapine, on rare occasions, can induce hypomanic or manic behavior. The switch to mania has not been observed with clozapine. For adjunctive mood-stabilizing effects, a risperidone dosage range of 1 to 3 mg daily, and olanzapine dosage range of 2.5 to 7.5 mg HS is optimal in the author's experience. Refer to Chapter 11 for clinical profiles of risperidone and olanzapine.

Chapter 10

Psychotic Disorders

GENERAL CLINICAL CONCEPTS

Psychotic symptoms are prominent in the following disorders:

- Schizophrenia
- Schizophreniform disorder
- Schizoaffective disorder
- Delusional disorder
- Brief psychotic disorder
- Shared psychotic disorder
- Psychotic disorder due to a medical condition
- Substance-induced psychotic disorder
- Psychotic disorder not otherwise specified
- Treatment refractory severe depression with psychotic features

Antipsychotic medications are the mainstay of treatment of psychotic disorders. Adjunctive medications are commonly used for treating nonpsychotic symptoms and for treating the side effects of the primary medication. Like most symptoms in psychiatry, psychotic symptoms exist in a continuum, from mild to severe as illustrated in Figure 10.1, and from transient to chronic. There is considerable overlap between contiguous states of mind. It follows that patients with mild psychotic symptoms may only need low doses of antipsychotics and patients with moderate to severe psychotic symptoms will need higher doses.

Psychotic symptoms are the most predominant and clinically significant in psychotic disorders, whereas mild psychotic symptoms that do not meet the criteria for one of the psychotic disorders can occur independently or in association with nonpsychotic disorders. Psychotic disorders of moderate or severe intensity can usually be diagnosed fairly easily. However, it is clinically challenging to detect mild psychotic symptoms, to persuade the patient to accept treatment, and then to manage the treatment.

FIGURE 10.1. Normalcy-Psychosis Continuum

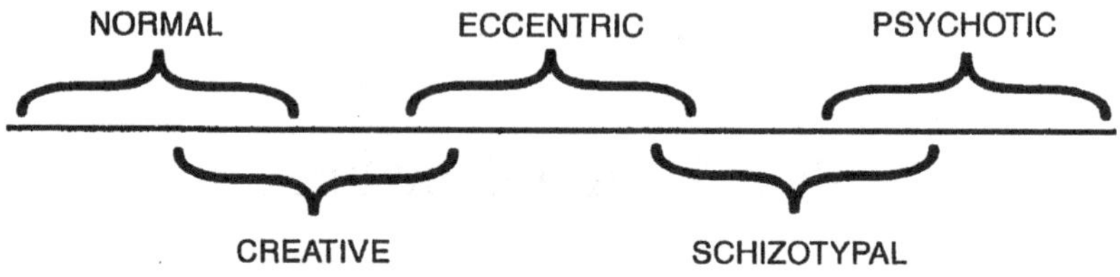

Since treatment of chronic psychoses such as schizophrenia, schizoaffective disorder, and delusional disorders represent a substantial percentage of psychiatric practice, detailed clinical profiles of various anti-psychotic drugs are included in this text. Schizophrenia is the most common disorder among chronic psychotic disorders.

SCHIZOPHRENIA

There are five types of schizophrenia:

- Paranoid type
- Disorganized type
- Catatonic type
- Undifferentiated type
- Residual type

Diagnostic criteria for schizophrenia, according to *DSM-IV* are as follows:*

A. Characteristic Symptoms: Two (or more) or the following, each present for a significant portion of time during a one-month period (or less if successfully treated):

1. Delusions
2. Hallucinations
3. Disorganized speech (e.g., frequent derailment or incoherence)

*Italicized text is reprinted with permission from the *Diagnostic and Statistical Manual of Mental Disorders*, Fourth Edition. Copyright 1994 American Psychiatric Association.

4. *Grossly disorganized or catatonic behavior*
5. *Negative symptoms (i.e., affective flattening, alogia, or avolition)*

Note: Only one criterion A symptom is required if delusions are bizarre or hallucinations consist of a voice keeping up a running commentary on the person's behavior or thoughts, or two or more voices conversing with each other.

B. Social/Occupational Dysfunction: For a significant portion of the time since the onset of the disturbance, one or more major areas of functioning such as work, interpersonal relations, or self-care are markedly below the level achieved prior to the onset (or when the onset is in childhood or adolescence, failure to achieve expected level of interpersonal, academic, or occupational achievement).

C. Duration: Continuous signs of the disturbance persist for at least six months. This six-month period must include at least one month of symptoms (or less if successfully treated) that meet criterion A (i.e., active-phase symptoms) and may include periods of prodromal or residual symptoms. During these prodromal or residual periods, the signs of the disturbance may be manifested by only negative symptoms or two or more symptoms listed in criterion A present in an attenuated form (e.g., odd beliefs unusual perceptual experiences).

D. Schizoaffective and Mood Disorder Exclusion: Schizoaffective disorder and mood disorder with psychotic features have been ruled out because either (1) no major depressive, manic, or mixed episodes have occurred concurrently with the active-phase symptoms; or (2) if mood episodes have occurred during active-phase symptoms, their total duration has been brief relative to the duration of the active and residual periods.

E. Substance/General Medical Condition Exclusion: The disturbance is not due to the direct physiological effects of a substance (e.g., a drug of abuse, a medication) or a general medical condition.

F. Relationship to a Pervasive Developmental Disorder: If there is a history of autistic disorder or another pervasive developmental disorder, the additional diagnosis of schizophrenia is made only if prominent delusions or hallucinations are also present for at least a month (or less if successfully treated).

Classification of longitudinal course (can be applied only after at least one year has elapsed since the initial onset of active-phase symptoms):

- *Episodic with interepisode residual symptoms (episodes are defined by the reemergence of prominent psychotic symptoms); also specify if: with prominent negative symptoms*

- *Episodic with no interepisode residual symptoms*
- *Continuous (prominent psychotic symptoms are present throughout the period of observation); also specify if: with prominent negative symptoms*
- *Single episode in partial remission; also specify if: with prominent negative symptoms*
- *Single episode in full remission*
- *Other or unspecified pattern*

Antipsychotic medications are the primary drugs used for the treatment of schizophrenia. Treatment of catatonic stupor may respond to a combination of an antipsychotic and a benzodiazepine, or ECT if medication intervention fails. Antipsychotic medications can be broadly categorized as traditional and atypical. Currently used traditional antipsychotics and atypical antipsychotics are listed below.

Traditional Antipsychotics

- chlorpromazine (Thorazine)
- thioridazine (Mellaril)
- mesoridazine (Serentil)
- perphenazine (Trilafon)
- trifluoperazine (Stelazine)
- fluphenazine (Prolixin)
- fluphenazine Enanthate (IM Depot use only)
- fluphenazine Decanoate (IM Depot use only)
- haloperidol (Haldol)
- haloperidol Decanoate (IM Depot use only)
- molindone (Moban)
- thiothixene (Navane)
- chlorprothixene (Taractan)
- loxapine (Loxitane)

Atypical Antipsychotics

- risperidone (Risperdal)
- clozapine (Clozaril)
- olanzapine (Zyprexa)
- sertindole (Serlect); expected to be introduced in 1997
- Others are expected to be introduced in the future

Individual profiles of antipsychotic medications are given in Chapter 11. Traditional antipsychotics have major drawbacks in long-term use. Since schizophrenia by definition is a chronic disorder needing long-term medication treatment, these drawbacks are significant. The major and unique disadvantages of traditional antipsychotics are:

- Tardive dyskinesia/tardive dystonia
- Limited efficacy for negative symptoms
- High incidences of intolerable EPS

Although there are many side effects and deficiencies associated with antipsychotics in general, the most distinguishing and the most clinically relevant differences between traditional and atypical antipsychotics are based on the factors listed above. For short-term treatment of psychotic symptoms, the above disadvantages are not a major consideration. For example, brief psychotic disorder may be effectively treated using traditional antipsychotics.

Three currently available atypical antipsychotic medications are clozapine, risperidone, and olanzapine. Of these, clozapine is not generally associated with tardive dyskinesia and is extremely effective for both positive and negative symptoms. Because of a 1 percent incidence of agranulocytosis, weekly WBC monitoring is required to detect early stages of neutropenia that may be due to bone marrow suppression so that clozapine can be stopped prior to development of a serious medical complication. Hence, clozapine is currently approved for use in treatment of refractory schizophrenics who have failed to respond to traditional antipsychotics. Clozapine also lowers the seizure threshold.

Risperidone is very effective for treatment of positive symptoms, as are clozapine and traditional antipsychotics, and is fairly effective for treatment of negative symptoms. Traditional antipsychotics do not significantly improve negative symptoms. Risperidone can cause tardive dyskinesia but less frequently when compared to traditional antipsychotics. Risperidone does not cause agranulocytosis and does not lower the seizure threshold any more than traditional antipsychotics.

Olanzapine is another atypical antipsychotic that is effective for both positive and negative symptoms. Its potential for causing tardive dyskinesia and EPS is estimated to be significantly less than that of traditional antipsychotics and slightly less compared to risperidone. Olanzapine does not cause agranulocytosis. Refer to Chapter 11 for detailed descriptions of the clinical profiles of all antipsychotics.

In terms of overall clinical efficacy alone, clozapine is clearly superior to all antipsychotics currently available in the United States, with the efficacy of risperidone and olanzapine probably between that of clozapine and traditional antipsychotics. Yet, since risperidone and olanzapine are moderately effective for negative symptoms, have less potential to cause tardive dyskinesia compared to traditional antipsychotics, and have better side effect profiles compared to clozapine and traditional antipsychotics, risperidone and olanzapine may be used as the first-line general purpose antipsychotics for most patients if cost is not a major consideration. The author's considerable experience in treating patients by using traditional antipsychotics, risperidone, olanzapine, and clozapine has shown that clozapine's efficacy in treating negative, positive, dysphoric, manic, and anxiety symptoms is generally better than any other antipsychotic medication currently available. Fatality from agranulocytosis can be significantly reduced by weekly WBC monitoring and education of patients to watch for and to report signs and symptoms of infection. The risk of seizures is a concern when the dosage exceeds 500 mg per day. If this dose is exceeded, the patient may be started on an anticonvulsant for seizure prophylaxis.

Given the superior efficacy of clozapine and virtual lack of tardive dyskinesia compared to other antipsychotics, it is the author's clinical opinion that it is in the best interest of patients with a confirmed diagnosis of schizophrenia to start clozapine as the first-line medication. Weekly CBC monitoring will detect in excess of 98 percent of cases of agranulocytosis in time to initiate discontinuation of clozapine and medical treatment, providing significant protection from fatalities that can occur from agranulocytosis. Prophylactic anticonvulsant treatment can protect the patient from seizures.

The rankings of various groups of antipsychotic medication based on important target effects and side effects are given in Table 10.1. Table 10.2 gives a rank order of choice of antipsychotics based on diagnosis and presenting symptoms.

It is clear from the author's experience that clozapine offers the best treatment for schizophrenia, severe forms of schizoaffective disorders, and other functional disorders characterized by severe chronic psychotic symptoms. The earlier clozapine is started, the better the recovery in functioning, and the fewer the functional deficit. Irreversible tardive dyskinesia is a substantial and foreseeable risk associated with chronic antipsychotic treatment using traditional antipsychotics. Chronic psychosis typically requires lifelong antipsychotic therapy. The risk of suicide among chronically psychotic patients is significantly greater than 1 percent even when maintained on traditional antipsychotics. Why wait for TD to emerge when it could be irreversible, and why let the chronically psychotic patient subsist with an unacceptably high suicide risk when clozapine therapy can prevent TD and

TABLE 10.1. Rarkings of Antipsychotics Based on Target Effects and Side Effects

	Efficacy for positive symptoms	Efficacy for negative symptoms	Tardive dyskinesia	Seizure	Bone marrow suppression	Neuroleptic malignant syndrome	Extra-pyramidal symptoms	Hypotension	Cost
Most Desirable	all antipsychotics	clozapine olanzapine sertindole risperidone	clozapine sertindole olanzapine	high-potency antipsychotics risperidone olanzapine sertindole	risperidone high-potency antipsychotics olanzapine sertindole	clozapine sertindole olanzapine risperidone	clozapine sertindole olanzapine	high-potency antipsychotics risperidone olanzapine	traditional antipsychotics
Moderately Desirable			risperidone	low-potency antipsychotics	low-potency antipsychotics	risperidone low-potency antipsychotics	low-potency antipsychotics risperidone	sertindole	
Least Desirable		traditional antipsychotics	traditional antipsychotics	clozapine	clozapine	high-potency antipsychotics	high-potency antipsychotics	low-potency antipsychotics clozapine	risperidone clozapine sertindole? olanzapine

TABLE 10.2. Practical Choice of Antipsychotics Based on Diagnosis and Symptoms

	Schizophrenia	Schizoaffective	Delusional disorder (low dose)	Brief psychotic disorder	Schizophreniform	Psychotic features	Severe bipolar with chronic psychosis	Mild psychotic symptoms (low dose)	Acute extreme hostility and agitation	Chronic hostility and prominent chronic negative symptoms
Most Desirable	clozapine risperidone olanzapine sertindole	clozapine risperidone olanzapine sertindole	risperidone olanzapine sertindole	risperidone traditional antipsychotics olanzapine	risperidone traditional antipsychotics olanzapine sertindole	risperidone olanzapine sertindole	clozapine olanzapine sertindole risperidone	risperidone traditional antipsychotics olanzapine sertindole	risperidone traditional antipsychotics olanzapine	clozapine risperidone olanzapine sertindole
Moderately Desirable	traditional antipsychotics	traditional antipsychotics	traditional antipsychotics	sertindole		traditional antipsychotics	traditional antipsychotics		sertindole	
Least Desirable			clozapine	clozapine	clozapine	clozapine		clozapine	clozapine	traditional antipsychotics

substantially reduce the suicide risk? Given these observations, it seems cost-effective to offer clozapine as the first-line antipsychotic medication in chronic, severe psychotic patients. Limiting clozapine for use only for the refractory and "burned out" schizophrenic is not clinically in the best interest of the patient. Such restrictions are reasonable and warranted if weekly WBC monitoring is not obtained. The physician's responsibility to the patient is to offer the best treatment in terms of efficacy and safety. The goal should be to arrest or to prevent the functional deterioration by treating with clozapine early. Weekly WBC monitoring during the first six months of treatment when there is a 1 percent risk of agranulocytosis, and the availability of highly effective filgrastim (Neupogen) therapy for agranulocytosis should improve clozapine's risk-benefit index to a tolerable level that is sufficient to position it as a serious contender as a first-line antipsychotic for selected patients, in the author's opinion.

In general, risperidone and olanzapine are clearly superior to traditional antipsychotics on all criteria, as outlined in Tables 10.1 and 10.2. They should be the first-line antipsychotics for the treatment of most functional psychotic symptoms. At low doses, they are excellent adjunctive medications, and are well-tolerated by patients. Psychotic features associated with various emotional disorders and mild psychotic symptoms respond nicely to risperidone at dosages as low as 0.5 mg to 2 mg per day and to olanzapine 2.5 to 5 mg HS. The author has effectively and successfully used doses as low as 0.25 mg per day of risperidone and 1.25 to 2.5 mg per day of olanzapine in some patients.

Given the long-term advantages of clozapine, olanzapine, and risperidone, regarding efficacy for positive and negative symptoms and decreased risk of tardive dyskinesia, it makes clinical sense to switch patients who are on traditional antipsychotics to risperidone, olanzapine, or clozapine, depending on the clinical considerations described. Effectiveness for negative symptoms and decreased risk of tardive dyskinesia should be sufficient clinical criteria to consider such a switch, especially when the long-term benefits to the patient outweigh the temporary disadvantages, inconvenience, effort, and expense associated with the switch.

SWITCHING TO RISPERIDONE

The switch from traditional antipsychotics to risperidone can be fairly easily done as an outpatient, with complete tapering off of the old antipsychotic over a span of five to seven days. Risperidone should be initiated at low doses on the first one or two days and gradually increased over a period of four to five days to a therapeutic dose. Since risperidone has an effective dosage range of 2 to 10 mg with 6 mg per day as the optimal dose, a linear conversion from the old antipsychotic to risperidone may not be applicable. However, there are some guidelines that have worked well in clinical practice. A potency ratio of 2:1 between haloperidol and risperidone is reasonable for doses up to haloperidol 10 mg per day. Above haloperidol 10 mg per day, risperidone dosage should be maintained at 6 mg per day in divided doses for several weeks, and increased by 2 mg increments every one to two weeks until satisfactory results are obtained. If there is no significant improvement at a dose of 16 mg per day, it is unlikely that the patient will respond at higher doses. Most patients respond satisfactorily on doses between 2 to 6 mg, in the author's experience. A patient taking haloperidol 15 mg per day is switched over in the following manner:

Day 1:	haloperidol 10 mg	risperidone 1 mg BID
Day 2:	haloperidol 5 mg	risperidone 1 mg BID
Day 3:	haloperidol 5 mg	risperidone 1 mg TID
Day 4:	haloperidol 2.5 mg	risperidone 2 mg BID
Day 5:	discontinue haloperidol	risperidone 2 mg TID

A patient on haloperidol 5 mg per day may be switched over as follows:

Day 1:	haloperidol 2.5 mg	risperidone 1 mg BID
Day 2:	haloperidol 1 mg	risperidone 1 mg BID
Day 3:	discontinue haloperidol	risperidone 1 mg TID

If the patient has been on an antiparkinsonian medication, this should be continued during the switchover period. After the patient is stabilized on risperidone, the antiparkinsonian medication may be gradually withdrawn over a period of 10 to 14 days. Although the incidence and severity of extrapyramidal symptoms (EPS) is less on risperidone compared to traditional high-potency antipsychotics, there are some patients on risperidone who experience acute dystonia and other EPS, which may benefit from concurrent treatment using antiparkinsonian agents.

SWITCHING TO OLANZAPINE

Patients taking traditional antipsychotics can be rapidly switched to olanzapine over a period of four to five days. Traditional high-potency antipsychotics can be discontinued more rapidly than low potency antipsychotics. Refer to the section on olanzapine in Chapter 11 for further details and examples of switching schedules.

SWITCHING TO CLOZAPINE

In most instances, switching to or starting on clozapine should ideally be done in an inpatient facility where careful dosage titration, and close medical and psychiatric monitoring, which are necessary, can be instituted. When switching from the old antipsychotic to clozapine, an overlapping period of four to six days is reasonable. During the first four to six days of clozapine initiation, the clozapine dose may not be sufficient to control psychotic symptoms. Escalating the clozapine dosage too rapidly, even if to control severe psychosis, is medically risky due to the potential for hypotension and rare cardiorespiratory collapse. Therefore, it is important to follow the manufacturer's recommendation as to the starting dose and the increment rate. If psychotic symptoms are out of control during the first week of clozapine therapy, which is possible, it may be necessary to use a traditional high-potency antipsychotic or risperidone on a PRN basis or on a regular tapering schedule during the first seven to ten days of clozapine treatment. The author's practice is to use a non-phenothiazine, high-potency antipsychotic such as haloperidol, thiothixene, or risperidone to avoid the nearly negligible risk of bone marrow suppression associated with phenothiazines. Such adjunctive treatment–using a second antipsychotic–is usually necessary because of the slow and gradual dosage titration required for clozapine therapy. When other antipsychotics are used as the primary antipsychotic, dosage can be more rapidly increased, obviating the need for a second antipsychotic.

A switching protocol for a patient on haloperidol 15 mg per day may involve a decrease in the dosage of haloperidol by 2 mg daily until the patient is off haloperidol, and a simultaneous increase in the dose of clozapine according to the manufacturer's guidelines, with the first dose being 12.5 mg starting on the same day that haloperidol dose is decreased. Low-potency antipsychotics such as chlorpromazine or thioridazine should be stopped prior to starting clozapine in order to minimize the synergistic hypotensive effects. If such a patient becomes floridly psychotic, high-potency antipsychotics can be used adjunctively while clozapine dosage is being slowly increased. If switching is attempted after completely stopping the existing antipsychotic, there is great risk of acute psychotic deterioration, which clozapine would not be able to control on the low starting doses and which would necessitate the temporary use of concurrent traditional antipsychotics. Refer to the clozapine clinical profile in Chapter 11 for further practical information.

All of the various types of schizophrenia are sufficiently chronic and disabling in nature that all of them deserve long-term treatment. Although from an academic standpoint, paranoid, catatonic, and residual types may have a better prognosis, the pharmacological approach to treatment and medications is similar. Since negative symptoms tend to worsen over time and since they are resistant to treatment using traditional antipsychotics, it is all the more important to consider starting clozapine or risperidone or olanzapine as the first-line medication in patients presenting with chronic psychotic disorders.

It is extremely important to diagnose prodromal symptoms of schizophrenia and start antipsychotic treatment as early as possible in order to preserve as much cognitive abilities as possible and prevent deterioration. Psychiatrists are frequently reluctant to diagnose schizophrenia in patients in their early teens when the clinical presentation can be with mild prodromal symptoms such as social withdrawal, mild dysphoria, anhedonia, tendency to isolate oneself, irritability, increased anger, anergia, excessive preoccupation or daydreaming, excessive interest in abstract topics, lack of interest in daily routines, and blunting of the affect, all of which can readily be misinterpreted as manifestations of depression or phase of life problems. Perhaps consciously or subconsciously, the clinician may not wish to "stigmatize" the young teenager or the family with a diagnosis that requires treatment using an antipsychotic. It is much easier for the clinician and easily acceptable to the family to start the patient on a course of psychotherapy or on an antidepressant medication. There is even a risk that the parents may not return to the clinician if told that their 15-year-old child has prodromal symptoms of schizophrenia and that antipsychotic treatment should be started as soon as possible. However, early diagnosis and treatment of even mild prodromal symptoms of schizophrenia are essential in ensuring normal cognitive, perceptual, and emotional development, despite the risk of possible stigma and parental ambivalence or denial. With the availability of superior atypical antipsychotics such as olanzapine and risperidone (sertindole may be introduced in the near future) the treatment of psychoses should be nearly as effective as that of the treatment of depression. Again, the key is accurate and early diagnosis.

SCHIZOPHRENIFORM DISORDER

The *DSM-IV* diagnostic criteria for schizophreniform disorder are as follows:*

A. Criteria A, D, and E of schizophrenia are met.

B. An episode of the disorder (including prodromal, active, and residual phases) lasts at least one month but less than six months. (When the

---

diagnosis must be made without waiting for recovery, it should be qualified as "Provisional.")

Specify if:

- ***Without Good Prognostic Features***
- ***With Good Prognostic Features:*** *as evidenced by two (or more) of the following:*
  1. *Onset of prominent psychotic symptoms within four weeks of the first noticeable change in usual behavior or functioning*
  2. *Confusion or perplexity at the height of the psychotic episode*
  3. *Good premorbid and social and occupational functioning*
  4. *Absence of blunted or flat affect*

Schizophreniform disorder is similar to schizophrenia except that the duration of schizophreniform disorder is less than six months. Since most patients initially diagnosed with schizophreniform disorder eventually are classified as having schizophrenia or schizoaffective disorder, the treatment considerations for schizophrenia are also applicable to schizophreniform disorder, except that clozapine would not ordinarily be considered for the treatment of schizophreniform disorder.

BRIEF PSYCHOTIC DISORDER

DSM-IV diagnostic criteria for brief psychotic disorder are as follows:*

A. Presence of one (or more) of the following symptoms:

1. *Delusions*
2. *Hallucinations*
3. *Disorganized speech (e.g., frequent derailment or incoherence)*
4. *Grossly disorganized or catatonic behavior*

Note: Do not include a symptom if it is a culturally sanctioned response pattern.

B. Duration of an episode of the disturbance is at least one day but less than one month, with eventual full return to premorbid level of functioning.

---

*Italicized text is reprinted with permission from the *Diagnostic and Statistical Manual of Mental Disorders*, Fourth Edition. Copyright 1994 American Psychiatric Association.

C. The disturbance is not better accounted for by a mood disorder with psychotic features, schizoaffective disorder, or schizophrenia and is not due to the direct physiological effects of a substance (e.g., a drug of abuse, a medication) or a general medical condition.

Specify if:

- ***With Marked Stressor(s)** (brief reactive psychosis): if symptoms occur shortly after and apparently in response to events that, singly or together, would be markedly stressful to almost anyone in similar circumstances in the person's culture*
- ***Without Marked Stressor(s):** if psychotic symptoms do not occur shortly after, or are not apparently in response to events that, singly or together, would be markedly stressful to almost anyone in similar circumstances in the person's culture*
- ***With Postpartum Onset:** if onset within four weeks postpartum*

Since brief psychotic disorder by definition is of brief duration (of less than one month), short-term treatment using traditional antipsychotics, olanzapine, or risperidone is sufficient. If psychotic symptoms persist beyond one month, the diagnosis is changed to schizophreniform disorder or to another diagnosis, depending on specific symptom characteristics. The treatment is also revised accordingly.

SCHIZOAFFECTIVE DISORDER

Schizoaffective disorder may occur as bipolar type or as depressive type. *DSM-IV* diagnostic criteria are given below:*

A. An uninterrupted period of illness during which, at some time, there is either a major depressive episode, a manic episode, or a mixed episode concurrent with symptoms that meet criterion A for schizophrenia.

Note: The major depressive episode must include criterion A1: depressed mood.

B. During the same period of illness, there have been delusions or hallucinations for at least two weeks in the absence of prominent mood symptoms.

---

*Italicized text is reprinted with permission from the *Diagnostic and Statistical Manual of Mental Disorders*, Fourth Edition. Copyright 1994 American Psychiatric Association.

C. Symptoms that meet the criteria for a mood episode are present for a substantial portion of the total duration of the active and residual periods of the illness.

D. The disturbance is not due to the direct physiological effects of a substance (e.g., a drug of abuse, a medication) or a general medical condition.

Specify type:

- ***Bipolar Type:*** *if the disturbance includes a manic or mixed episode (or a manic or a mixed episode and major depressive episodes)*
- ***Depressive Type:*** *if the disturbance only includes major depressive episodes*

Although the prognosis for schizoaffective disorder is considered better than that of schizophrenia, it still represents a chronic disorder with psychotic features that tend to occur fairly frequently. Hence, medication treatment for the psychotic component of the illness is similar to that of schizophrenia. Since schizoaffective disorder, by definition, has components of depression or mania, or features of mixed bipolar disorder, patients with this diagnosis will need either an antidepressant or mood stabilizer or both, in addition to an antipsychotic. As always, the choice of medication is based on the presence of specific symptoms. In schizoaffective disorder, the presence of psychotic and affective symptoms requires combination treatment in virtually all cases. Additionally, ECT is an option for patients not responding well to aggressive medication management. Clozapine is recommended by the author for severe chronic cases of schizoaffective disorder if psychotic symptoms are prominent and chronic.

DELUSIONAL DISORDER

Delusional disorders are classified into six different types as follows:

- Grandiose type
- Erotomanic type
- Jealous type
- Persecutory type
- Somatic type
- Mixed type

DSM-IV criteria are given below:*

A. Nonbizarre delusions (i.e., involving situations that occur in real life, such as being followed, poisoned, infected, loved at a distance, or deceived by spouse or lover, or having a disease) of at least one month's duration.

B. Criterion A for schizophrenia has never been met.

Note: Tactile and olfactory hallucinations may be present in delusional disorder if they are related to the delusional theme.

C. Apart from the impact of the delusion(s) or its ramifications, functioning is not markedly impaired and behavior is not obviously odd or bizarre.

D. If mood episodes have occurred concurrently with delusions, their total duration has been brief relative to the duration of the delusional periods.

E. The disturbance is not due to the direct physiological effects of a substance (e.g., a drug of abuse, a medication) or a general medical condition.

Specify type (the following types are assigned based upon the predominant delusional theme):

- ***Erotomanic Type:*** *delusions that another person, usually of higher status, is in love with the individual*
- ***Grandiose Type:*** *delusions of inflated worth, power, knowledge, identity, or special relationship to a deity or famous person*
- ***Jealous Type:*** *delusions that the individual's sexual partner is unfaithful*
- ***Persecutory Type:*** *delusions that the person (or someone to whom the person is close) is being malevolently treated in some way*
- ***Somatic Type:*** *delusions that the person has some physical defect or general medical condition*
- ***Mixed Type:*** *delusions characteristic of more than one of the above types but no one theme predominates*
- ***Unspecified Type***

Patients with delusional disorders typically do not seek treatment voluntarily. They reluctantly come to the clinician's office because of pressure and persuasion from relatives, work supervisor, or legal authorities.

---

*Italicized text is reprinted with permission from the *Diagnostic and Statistical Manual of Mental Disorders*, Fourth Edition. Copyright 1994 American Psychiatric Association.

Even when they come, it is usually to appease others rather than to accept the diagnosis and treatment. In the author's experience, delusional disorders are characterized by obsessive features and psychotic features. Consistent with the author's thesis that medication selection is based on symptoms, and given the obsessive quality associated with their psychotic beliefs, the effective treatment for most patients with delusional disorder is a combination of low doses of antiobsessional medication and low doses of antipsychotics. A particularly effective and well-tolerated combination that has been successfully used by the author in several cases of delusional disorder is SSRIs at low doses or clomipramine 25 to 100 mg po HS and risperidone 0.5 mg to 2 mg po HS. The clinician should be careful to start at very low doses such as paroxetine 10 mg or clomipramine 25 mg and risperidone 0.5 mg po HS and increase the dose very slowly as needed. Another excellent antipsychotic drug option is the recently introduced olanzapine at a starting dose of 1.25 to 2.5 mg HS. Since patients with delusional disorder are very sensitive to any side effects, low initial doses and minimization of the initial side effects are more important in the first several weeks of treatment than symptom resolution. Once the patient is comfortable with the medication and establishes some rapport with the clinician–even if this is achieved due to external pressure–the chances of eventual development of some insight and cooperation are increased. All antiobsessional medications should be effective. The key clinical strategy is using very low starting doses. Some examples follow:

– Fluoxetine 10 mg		Olanzapine 1.25 to 2.5 mg
– Sertraline 25 mg		Risperidone 0.5 mg
– Clomipramine 25 mg	+	Haloperidol 0.5 mg
– Paroxetine 10 mg		or equivalent
– Fluvoxamine 25 mg		antipsychotic

Antipsychotic medication alone is unlikely to be sufficient for a patient with delusional disorder because the presence of obsessional features requires concurrent treatment of this symptom. Yet, antipsychotic medication is necessary. Antiobsessional medication in the absence of antipsychotics in delusional disorders can make the patient even more psychotic, just as antidepressants when given alone improve the dysphoric and negative symptoms in schizophrenics, but tend to make the psychosis worse. For severely delusional patients who are treatment-refractory and chronically dysfunctional, clozapine may be considered.

Chapter 11

Antipsychotic Medications: Advantages and Disadvantages

GENERAL CLINICAL CONCEPTS

Antipsychotic medications are primarily indicated for the treatment of psychotic symptoms that can be associated with various disorders. Typically, psychotic disorders include schizophrenia, brief psychotic disorder, schizophreniform disorder, delusional disorder, schizoaffective disorder, shared psychotic disorder, psychotic disorder due to a medical condition, and substance-induced psychotic disorder. In addition, psychotic symptoms can be associated with other disorders, such as depression, bipolar disorders, and personality disorders. Regardless of the diagnosis, treatment using antipsychotic medications is to be considered if psychotic symptoms are present. To some extent, the severity of symptoms determines the dosage. Generally, patients with severe psychotic symptoms tend to require higher doses compared to patients with milder psychotic symptoms who may do well on low doses.

Many patients present with mild psychotic symptoms, which are often missed by clinicians. In most of these cases, the presenting complaints are depression, anxiety, poor concentration, insomnia, anergia, anxiety attacks, vague somatic complaints, etc. Primary psychotic disorders, as listed in the first paragraph, when presented with textbook features are easily diagnosed by mental health professionals. Most severe depression and severe mania present with varying degrees of psychotic symptoms that should be recognized and treated for efficient resolution of the illness. In many of these situations, the adjunctive use of antipsychotics can be short-term. Once the acute phase of the illness is resolved, the antipsychotic may be gradually withdrawn and the patient may be maintained on an antidepressant or mood stabilizer.

A thorough working knowledge of the clinical uses and subtle clinical techniques of the application of all antipsychotic medications is necessary for every practicing psychiatrist, and for primary care physicians treating patients with psychotic symptoms. Given the expectation of managed care companies and HMOs, primary care physicians are likely to be pressured to take responsibility for the maintenance of patients on antipsychotics once they have been stabilized on medications by the psychiatrist.

Psychotic symptoms can be classified into positive and negative symptoms. Positive symptoms include delusions, hallucinations, illogical thinking, ideas of reference, hostility, and agitation. Negative symptoms include apathy, anergia, social withdrawal, demoralization, lack of spontaneity, and constricted or blunted affect.

A wide variety of antipsychotics are currently available for treatment. The three most recently introduced antipsychotics, risperidone (Risperdal), olanzapine (Zyprexa), and clozapine (Clozaril), offer significant advantages over the older antipsychotics such as the phenothiazines, haloperidol, thiothixene, molindone, and loxapine. One of the major advantages of atypical antipsychotics such as clozapine, risperidone, olanzapine, and the soon-to-be-introduced sertindole is that they improve negative symptoms. A recent report (Bodkin et al., 1996) suggested that selegiline (Eldepryl) 5 mg BID may be effective in further improving negative symptoms when given in combination with antipsychotics. Selegiline selectively inhibits monoamine oxidase B at a dosage of 15 mg or less per day, with no pharmacologically significant effect on norepinephrine or serotonin metabolism, thus sparing the need for strict adherence to dietary and medication interaction precautions (related to medications containing pharmacologically active amines), and theoretically eliminating the chances of hypertensive or hyperthermic crises. Since negative symptoms are very disabling from a quality-of-life standpoint, they need aggressive intervention. Selegiline 5 mg BID may be administered with traditional and atypical antipsychotics including clozapine.

Antipsychotics are useful in the treatment of psychotic symptoms of various etiologies. Depending on the presenting etiology, the usage can range from one dose to chronic use for many years. An example of the former is the use of a one-time dose of haloperidol 2 to 5 mg IM or IV for a patient with delirium, seen in the so-called "ICU Psychosis," in which no further administration of haloperidol is necessary once the delirium has cleared. However, antipsychotics are the mainstay in the treatment of schizophrenia, and a patient may need to be maintained on the medication for many years, if not for life. Antipsychotics are also used temporarily for control of discrete symptoms such as extreme hostility, anger, and agitation (for which other interventions are not effective) and when rapid control is necessary.

RISPERIDONE (RISPERDAL)

Risperidone is a serotonin-dopamine receptor antagonist, approved for the treatment of psychotic disorders. It is metabolized by the cytochrome P-450 enzyme system and has an active metabolite. Its half-life is 20 hours, and plasma-protein binding is 90 percent. Its metabolism can be inhibited by drugs that inhibit cytochrome P-450 II D6, such as fluoxetine, paroxetine, sertraline, and quinidine. It can interfere with, or its metabolism can be interfered by, other drugs that are metabolized by the cytochrome P-450 II D6 enzyme. Examples of such drugs include nortriptyline, desipramine, fluoxetine, paroxetine, beta-blockers, and various antipsychotics. A slight dosage reduction of risperidone should be considered if any of the above medications are coadministered. As with almost all medications, the dosage should be decreased in elderly patients and in patients who have liver disease or renal impairment. Its alpha-adrenergic blocking effect can cause orthostatic hypotension, tachycardia, dizziness, and syncope in patients susceptible to hypotension and in patients with cardiovascular disease. Lower initial dosage and slower increments are recommended in these patients.

The significant advantage of risperidone compared to traditional antipsychotics is that it has a low incidence of EPS in the optimal therapeutic dosage range of 2 to 6 mg daily and is believed to have a decreased risk of inducing tardive dyskinesia, although many more years of clinical experience will be necessary to obtain any conclusive information regarding the tardive dyskinesia risk. Risk of acute dystonia and neuroleptic malignant syndrome (NMS) is present but may be lower in comparison to traditional high-potency antipsychotics. The risk of EPS rises in a dose-dependent manner above a dose of 4 to 6 mg daily. Clinical experience so far has confirmed the expectation of lower EPS. The possibility (and probability) of decreased risk of tardive dyskinesia should make risperidone attractive to psychiatrists and other physicians treating patients on an antipsychotic. The other antipsychotics currently available in the United States with decreased risk of tardive dyskinesia, low EPS, and effectiveness for negative and positive symptoms are clozapine (Clozaril) and olanzapine (Zyprexa). However, clozapine has a 1 percent risk of agranulocytosis (and a 3 to 5 percent risk of seizures in therapeutic doses), requiring mandatory weekly WBC for as long as the patient is on the medication. Risperidone has no such risks, avoiding the need for laboratory monitoring. Although clozapine is superior to risperidone in terms of a fairly balanced effectiveness for positive and negative symptoms, clozapine's potential for serious side effects and consequent need for weekly WBC monitoring make it a complicated medication. Hence, clozapine's FDA-approved use is reserved for treatment of refractory cases of schizophrenia in current clinical practice. Risperidone is effective in treating positive symptoms such as hallucinations, delusions, agitation, hostility, anxiety, ideas of reference, thought disorders, and pressured speech, and fairly effective for improving negative or "deficit" symptoms such as apathy, social withdrawal, ambivalence, dysphoria, anergia, demoralization, lack of spontaneity, poor initiative, constricted or blunted affect, and concrete thinking.

For treatment of psychotic symptoms that are less acute or those that are likely to be fairly transient, the risperidone dosage range can be from 0.5 mg to 2 mg per day. Many patients with mild psychotic symptoms do well on a dose of risperidone 0.5 mg daily. For the previous indications, the length of treatment is usually weeks to several months, after which the dose is gradually tapered off over a period of several weeks.

Risperidone can cause insomnia in some patients. In these cases, AM administration is preferred. Most patients are able to tolerate it at bedtime. The most common side effects include extrapyramidal symptoms, insomnia, fatigue, anxiety, somnolence, hyperprolactinemia, and galactorrhea. Acute extrapyramidal symptoms such as acute dystonia and parkinsonism can be treated using anticholinergic medications as described in Chapter 12.

For patients with acute and chronic psychotic conditions, the starting dose recommended by the author is 0.5 mg po QID for two days. The dose should be increased by 1 mg increments every two days until 4 mg per day is reached. The 4 mg dose should be maintained for one week before further dosage increase is considered because clinical experience suggests that most patients respond well to 4 mg or less per day. For the elderly, debilitated, hypotensive, and renally or hepatically impaired patients, the initial dose should be 0.5 mg per day or 0.5 mg BID, with a dosage increase of 0.5 mg per day every two to three days until 2 mg per day is reached. These patients should be kept on 2 mg per day in divided doses for a week prior to considering dosage adjustment.

Risperidone may be combined with antidepressants, anticholinergics, anxiolytics, and mood stabilizers. Occasionally it is combined with clozapine, chlorpromazine, and thioridazine for optimal clinical response including sedation.

Risperidone is available in tablet form for oral use in doses of 1, 2, 3, and 4 mg strengths and in liquid form. The tablet can be easily broken into smaller doses. The liquid form makes it convenient to dispense intermediate doses as well as makes it difficult for uncooperative and manipulative patients to "cheek" the medication. Given the high cost of risperidone, it makes sense to obtain the higher dose tablet and divide it. For example, if a patient is on 1 mg per day, there may be some savings by purchasing seven 4 mg tablets and dividing each pill into four parts, yielding a four week supply (see Table 11.1). Once the patient is stabilized on a dose, minor variations in dose that may occur when a pill is divided into smaller pieces is not likely to be clinically significant, particularly since risperidone has a half-life of 20 hours. Rarely, risperidone can induce hypomania/mania.

Summary of Advantages and Disadvantages of Risperidone

Advantages

- Superior effectiveness for positive symptoms of psychosis
- Moderate effectiveness for negative symptoms
- Fairly low incidence of EPS and NMS, compared to traditional high-potency antipsychotics (dose-dependent)
- Mild antianxiety and antidepressant effects at low doses
- Well-tolerated by most patients
- First-line general purpose antipsychotic for a broad range of psychotic conditions and for all severity levels; effective for first-episode psychosis and some treatment-resistant schizophrenias
- Possible decreased risk of tardive dyskinesia, compared to traditional antipsychotics (many more years of experience will be necessary to obtain actual estimates)
- Availability of liquid form
- Improved efficacy and tolerability decrease relapses and rehospitalizations
- Potential significant long-term cost savings due to decreased illness-related direct and indirect costs

Disadvantages

- Risk of tardive dyskinesia, although considered less frequent than that of traditional antipsychotics
- Can cause EPS and NMS, though less frequently, compared to traditional high-potency antipsychotics; incidence of EPS higher at the 6 to 18 mg dosage range
- High cost of medication (average cost of $2,100 per year for a patient on a dose of 2 mg BID)
- Parenteral form not available, as of this writing
- Increases prolactin level, as do all of the traditional antipsychotics

CLOZAPINE (CLOZARIL)

In terms of overall efficacy for improvement in both positive and negative symptoms, clozapine is superior to all antipsychotics currently avail-

TABLE 11.1. Cost of Risperidone

Daily Risperidone Dose	Quantity	Cost per Month	Cost per Pill	Cost per 1 mg Unit
1 mg	30	$ 60.00	$2.00	$2.00
2 mg	30	$ 95.00	$3.16	$1.58
3 mg	30	$120.00	$4.00	$1.33
4 mg	30	$158.00	$5.26	$1.31

able in the United States, including risperidone and olanzapine. Clozapine has a half-life of 12 hours and is 95 percent bound to plasma protein. It is available in 25 mg and 100 mg scored tablets. Clozapine is approved by the FDA for use in patients with treatment-resistant schizophrenia who fail to respond satisfactorily to at least two standard antipsychotic medications. Weekly monitoring of the WBC is required for the duration of treatment and for four weeks after it is discontinued. Because of the rare incidence of syncope and respiratory depression and respiratory collapse, the starting dose should be 12.5 mg once or twice the first day. It is preferable to administer the starting dose after safely discontinuing benzodiazepines, which tend to increase the chances of respiratory depression, a concern primarily in the elderly. If the patient tolerates the first day's dose well, the dosage may be increased by 25 to 50 mg daily, up to 450 mg over a period of two weeks. If further dosage increase is necessary, it is implemented by maximum increments of 100 mg per week up to a maximum dose of 900 mg per day. Clinical experience indicates that most patients respond satisfactorily to between 200 and 500 mg per day in divided doses. The initial clozapine dosage titration schedule recommended by Sandoz Pharmaceuticals is listed in Table 11.2. Some elderly patients may require a lower starting dose of 6.25 mg and slower titration.

Since clozapine is highly protein-bound, it can displace other highly protein-bound drugs and increase their levels. This is of concern primarily for drugs that have a relatively narrow therapeutic range, for example warfarin or digoxin. However, the possible increase in the free-drug level in plasma of these latter medications is considered temporary because of compensatory hepatic clearance.

Clozapine has been used successfully in the treatment of schizoaffective disorder when the patient is not responding well to a combination of traditional antipsychotics, antidepressants, and/or mood stabilizers. It has

TABLE 11.2. Sandoz-Recommended Initial Clozapine Dosage Titration Schedule

Week 1	AM (mg)	HS (mg)	Total (mg)
Day 1	12.5	12.5*	12.5 - 25.0
Day 2	25	---	25
Day 3	25	25	50
Day 4	25	50	75
Day 5	50	50	100
Day 6	50	75	125
Day 7	50	100	150
Week 1	**AM (mg)**	**HS (mg)**	**Total (mg)**
Day 8	50	100	150
Day 9	100	100	200
Day 10	100	100	200
Day 11	50	200	250
Day 12	50	200	250
Day 13	100	200	300
Day 14	100	200	300

*Optional

also been successful in the treatment of complicated and chronic rapid-cycling bipolar disorder, which is unresponsive to standard combination treatment, particularly if antipsychotics in moderate to high doses are required to control the symptoms and to maintain stability. In any psychotic disorder of a chronic nature requiring at least moderate doses of antipsychotics, clozapine could be considered as an option, particularly if traditional antipsychotics are not optimally effective. As is true with all antipsychotics, clozapine has antimanic properties. Moreover, it seems to have mood-stabilizing properties, unlike traditional antipsychotics. Given its risk of agranulocytosis and seizures, clozapine should not be used as a first-line drug for bipolar disorders. However, for treatment-resistant and chronic bipolar patients who do not respond well to antidepressants, traditional antipsychotics, mood stabilizers, ECT, or combinations of some of these treatments, clozapine should be considered. For chronic conditions that carry a high risk of suicide, such as severe depression with psychotic features, severe dysphoric mania, severe rapid-cycling bipolar disorder, or severe borderline personality disorder with regressive and dissociative features, or any other severe chronic conditions with regressive or psychotic features, a trial of clozapine with its 1 percent risk of agranulocytosis and 3 to 5 percent risk of seizures is a risk worth taking for the patient if other antipsychotics have given suboptimal results, since clozapine leads to significant clinical improvement. Similarly, if a patient has extreme homicidal hostility that is chronic and unresponsive to all other medications, a clozapine trial should be considered. Severe chronic obsessive-compulsive disorder characterized by regressive features, psychotic features, and significant functional deterioration, and intractable to aggressive standard treatment attempts, is another example in which there may be clinical justification for a clozapine trial prior to considering cingulotomy. In all of these cases, the benefit-to-risk ratio related to the use of clozapine is favorable, in the author's opinion.

Clozapine may be considered for treatment of various chronic and severe treatment-refractory and dysfunctional conditions that would benefit from long-term maintenance on an antipsychotic, as listed below. It must be emphasized that for most of the conditions listed here and elsewhere, there have been no controlled studies evaluating the efficacy of clozapine. Its use for these indications is not endorsed by the FDA or the drug manufacturer, and essentially represents my clinical opinion. Justification for off-label uses should be discussed in detail with the patient and family, and consent documented with particular reference to clozapine's unique risk-benefit considerations.

- Treatment refractory schizophrenia (currenly the only FDA-approved indication)
- All schizophrenias
- Schizoaffective disorders
- Treatment refractory delusional disorders with severe dysfunction
- All chronic psychotic disorders
- Treatment refractory severe bipolar disorders with predominant manic and/or psychotic features
- Treatment refractory severe obsessive compulsive disorder, with regressive and psychotic features and significant functional deficits prior to considering cingulotomy (neuroleptics can occasionally worsen OCD)
- Treatment refractory severe borderline personality disorder, with psychotic and dissociative features
- Treatment refractory severe depression with psychotic features
- Treatment refractory severe impulse control disorders
- Treatment refractory severe dissociative disorders
- Treatment emergent tardive dyskinesia/tardive dystonia
- Psychotic patients with idiopathic parkinsonism who poorly tolerate other antipsychotics
- Psychosis induced by dopaminergic antiparkinsonian medication

Schizophrenia by definition is a chronic condition. If the diagnosis of schizophrenia can be confirmed, especially if the subtype is that of the disorganized or undifferentiated type with young age at onset in which the course is expected to be very chronic and where the prognosis is poor, it is the author's opinion that clozapine should be offered to the patient as a first-line maintenance medication. This eliminates the likelihood that the patient and family will go through the agony of multiple antipsychotic medication failures. Although risperidone and olanzapine are significant improvements over the traditional antipsychotics, clozapine is clearly more effective for negative symptoms compared to risperidone and olanzapine, and hence has overall superiority in the treatment of poor prognosis types of schizophrenia. Additionally, it has been the author's experience that insight, judgment, compliance, and acceptance of the chronic nature of the illness and recognition of the need for continuing the medication are improved once the patient achieves stabilization on clozapine. As a result, a great majority of patients comply with weekly monitoring of the WBC. This is somewhat surprising as many of these patients have a history of noncompliance with traditional antipsychotics, and the required weekly needle sticks are not a pleasant experience.

The combination of clozapine with other medications such as valproate, lithium, antidepressants, stimulants, benzodiazepines, and low doses of high-potency neuroleptics including risperidone has been successfully used by the author.

At a clozapine dosage in the range of 400 mg to 600 mg per day, the incidence of seizures is estimated at 5 percent, a substantial risk. Therefore, the author routinely prescribes prophylactic valproate if clozapine dosage exceeds 500 mg per day. When this combination is used, liver function tests should be monitored to detect any additive liver toxicity. Gabapentin (Neurontin) and lamotrigine (Lamictal) are options if valproate is not tolerated or is ineffective.

Clozapine can be combined with lithium, but must be monitored closely for increased central nervous system side effects. Many patients on clozapine will benefit from adjunctive treatment using serotonergic antidepressants, which have the potential to further improve negative symptoms, especially dysphoria, obsessive worrying, anxiety, demoralization, apathy, and anergia. Fluoxetine and paroxetine can increase clozapine level slightly by inhibition of cytochrome P-450 II D6. Venlafaxine, sertraline, fluvoxamine, and nefazodone do not affect clozapine metabolism significantly. Liver enzyme inhibition should ordinarily be a clinical consideration only if the patient is already on a high dose of clozapine, or if the dose of the antidepressant is at or near the maximum dosage limit.

Clozapine can be successfully employed in the treatment of patients with parkinsonism accompanied by psychotic symptoms. The dosage in this population is usually on the low side, for example between 25 mg and 100 mg per day.

Unlike traditional antipsychotics and risperidone, clozapine does not affect libido or sexual functioning significantly. Since clozapine has sedative properties, no additional sleep medication is necessary in most cases.

If clinical improvement is noted below the dose of 600 mg per day, there is probably no need for a clozapine blood level. Levels are recommended (1) if toxicity is suspected, (2) to monitor compliance if there is a question regarding this, (3) to guide dosage at the higher dosage range with its increased risks of side effects, (4) if other medications that inhibit or induce clozapine's hepatic metabolism are concurrently used, and (5) to guide dosage adjustment in nonresponders. It is not necessary to obtain clozapine blood levels routinely. A plasma clozapine concentration above 350 ng/ml, or a total plasma concentration of clozapine plus the active metabolite norclozapine above 450 ng/ml is correlated with a high probability of response. The upper therapeutic range of plasma clozapine levels and toxic levels have not been determined. The author has patients who responded satisfactorily at a blood level of less than 200 ng/ml, and at a blood level above 900 ng/ml (without toxic effects).

Clozapine is contraindicated in patients with myeloproliferative disorders. If patients with a low seizure threshold need clozapine, prophylactic treatment with an anticonvulsant should be considered even at low doses of clozapine. Seizure disorder is not a contraindication to the use of clozapine if the seizure is well-controlled on an antiseizure medication and if clozapine is initiated slowly and cautiously with close monitoring of seizure status. Carbamazepine should be avoided in a patient on clozapine because of carbamazepine's potential effects on bone marrow. Cigarette smoking and phenytoin (Dilantin) can decrease clozapine blood levels, and cimetidine (Tagamet) can increase blood levels. Hence, smoking should be discouraged, and the clozapine dose may need adjustment if these medications are started or stopped in a patient on clozapine.

Since the greatest risk of agranulocytosis is within the first six months of starting clozapine, it is reasonable to decrease the frequency of CBC monitoring to biweekly or monthly intervals after the first six months to one year. However, weekly monitoring of the WBC is required currently for as long as the patient is on clozapine, and for four weeks after stopping clozapine. Patients should be instructed to call the physician if any signs of infection are noted, such as fever, sore throat, pallor, tonsillitis, flu, pneumonia, lethargy, or urinary symptoms. Such precautions could alert the patient to any precipitous decline in WBC that can occur rarely. If any of these symptoms occur, vital signs and a CBC should be obtained immediately. WBC-related adverse events and suggested actions are summarized in Table 11.3.

Most patients who do well on clozapine end up remaining on the medication long-term for maintaining clinical improvement. This is because clozapine does not cure psychosis; similar to the use of insulin in diabetes, clozapine only controls psychosis. Another important clinical observation is that some patients become more floridly psychotic when taken off clozapine, even after they are switched to another antipsychotic, including risperidone and olanzapine. When risperidone was introduced in early 1994, it was felt that risperidone would give antipsychotic efficacy similar to clozapine, without the risk of agranulocytosis and seizure and without the need for weekly CBCs. Thus, it was reasonable to consider switching patients from clozapine to risperidone. The author, following this line of reasoning, attempted to switch several patients from clozapine to risperidone with disastrous results. It is as if patients go through a period of rebound psychosis in which their psychotic symptoms, such as delusions, hallucinations, and agitation, are much worse than prior to starting clozapine. Hence, if clozapine is discontinued, gradual tapering along with close clinical supervision and monitoring are recommended. Refer to Table 11.5 for clozapine discontinuation schedule. Clozapine tends to improve tardive dyskinesia and tardive dystonia caused by traditional neuroleptics in some patients.

Clozapine is typically used for maintenance treatment on a long-term basis. Patients with chronic schizophrenia need to stay on maintenance medication indefinitely since the risk of relapse and subsequent disruption and deterioration of functioning is great if medication is discontinued. Hence, from a clinical standpoint, the physician has to recommend that patients stay on the medication indefinitely, perhaps for life, depending on the individual case. It is perhaps a legal necessity that the drug manufacturer publications recommend that efforts should be made periodically to decrease the dose of clozapine and to discontinue the medication if possible. Conversely, clinical reasoning would indicate that the physician and the patient are taking considerable risks if clozapine is discontinued when the patient is doing well on it. In many cases, psychosis may not recur immediately after stopping the medication. A symptom-free period of weeks to months is the norm, but in the majority of cases, symptoms are bound to return within one year of stopping the medication. Clinical experience suggests that the more frequent the episodes of psychotic exacerbation, the more difficult it is to treat subsequent episodes, and the worse the

TABLE 11.3. White Blood Cell Count/Granulocyte-Related Events and Suggested Actions

	WBC Count/Granulocyte	Actions
Screening	Before treatment: WBC<3,500/mcl	Treatment not initiated Other contraindications: Myeloproliferate disorders Previous Clozaril-induced agranulocytosis or severe granulocytopenia Simultaneous use with other agents having a well-known potential to suppress bone marrow function
	WBC>3,500/mcl No previous agranulocytosis	Initiate treatment
Normal WBC results	After Clozaril treatment initiated: WBC>3,500/mcl No substantial drop from baseline	Continue treatment with weekly WBC testing/drug dispensing
Mild Leukopenia	WBC<3,500/mcl or substantial drop in baseline, even if WBC>3,500/mcl or immature forms present	1. Repeat WBC and do differential count; Continue twice-weekly WBC and differential until WBC exceeds 3,500/mcl
Moderate Leukopenia	After action 1: Total WBC<3,000/mcl or granulocyte (bands plus polys) count is <1,500/mcl	2. Interrupt clozapine therapy; Institute daily WBC and differential counts; Monitor patient for flu-like symptoms or other symptoms of infection
	If after action 2: No symptoms of infection develop	3A. Resume Clozaril therapy*
	Total WBC returns to levels >3,000/mcl Granuloctyes return to levels >1,500/mcl	Continue twice-weekly WBC and differential counts until total WBC counts return to levels >3,500/mcl

	WBC Count/Granulocyte	Actions
Severe Leukopenia or Agranulocytosis	WBC falls to <2,000/mcl or granulocytes fall to <1,000/mcl	Discontinue clozapine at once. Consider bone marrow aspiration to ascertain granulopoietic status
	Granulocytes fall to <500/mcl	If granulopoiesis is deficient, protective isolation may be indicated
		Consider treatment using granulocyte colony stimulating factor such as filgrastim (Neupogen)
		If evidence of infection develops, take appropriate cultures and start patient on appropriate antibiotic regimen
		Do not rechallenge with Clozaril
		Continue WBC counts for four consecutive weeks after discontinuation of Clozaril

Notes: Granulocyte defined as bands plus polys (absolute neutrophil count)
*When patients have been off Clozaril for two days or longer and are restarted, it is recommended that treatment be initated with one-half of a 25 mg tablet (12.5 mg)
Source: Table modified from Sandoz Pharmaceuticals, *Clozaril—Management of Adverse Effects*, 1993. Used with permission.

prognosis. Any psychosocial gains the patient had achieved through maintainance medication are probably wiped out by each acute exacerbation, not to mention the loss of confidence, increase in frustration, expense, and disruption of daily functioning associated with each episode of relapse. However, the patient's and family's requests to stop the medication are understandable and should be acknowledged. The physician has the responsibility to explain the advantages and disadvantages in simple terms and to strongly recommend that maintenance medication be continued. The disruption caused by a relapse can potentially lead to loss of job, prolonged disability, divorce, financial problems, loss of self-esteem, psychosocial deterioration, increased suicide risk, and more.

Given the morbidity associated with psychosis and given the superiority of clozapine in the control of psychotic symptoms, consideration should be given to clozapine as a first-line medication for patients who are likely to have a poor prognosis suggested by the following features:

- Early onset of symptoms (adolescent vs. adult)
- Family history of schizophrenia
- Preexisting personality disorder among cluster A (schizoid, schizotypal, and paranoid)
- Absence of precipitating stressors
- Preponderance of negative or deficit symptoms
- Insidious onset
- Prodromal symptoms
- Violent acting-out tendencies
- Apathy or blunted affect
- Features of disorganized type or undifferentiated type
- Poor social support
- Disorganized delusions
- Chronic hostility and agitation

Effective Combinations Involving Clozapine

Clozapine plus a low dose of risperidone or other high-potency nonphenothiazine antipsychotics are at times clinically necessary and effective. The possible clinical contexts in which such a combination can be successfully used include the following:

- When initiating clozapine therapy, it is frequently necessary to treat the patient using a high-potency antipsychotic during the first four to seven days or until a reasonable clozapine dose is reached, usually above 150 to 200 mg per day. Among the high potency antipsychotics, risperidone, haloperidol and thiothixene are preferred. Phenothiazines should be avoided because of their rare effects on bone marrow.
- If a patient derives partial and unique benefits from clozapine at a particular dose, but a further needed dosage increase leads to intolerable side effects, the dose of clozapine may be kept at a tolerable dose and a high-potency antipsychotic may be added to obtain optimal benefit.
- If seizure is a particular concern and if the patient is unable to tolerate anticonvulsants, the dose of clozapine may be reduced to a statistically safe range at which seizure risk is low (less than 400 mg per

day), and a high-potency antipsychotic may be added for best results.

- In rare instances, the clozapine dose yielding a therapeutic plasma clozapine level still may not optimally control psychotic symptoms. Addition of a high-potency antipsychotic, including risperidone, may be considered in this context.

A benzodiazepine may be added to clozapine for treatment of insomnia or anxiety. Low doses of trazodone or nefazodone also can be added for treatment of insomnia. If depression is identified, an antidepressant (preferably one of the SSRIs) may be added. Clomipramine, bupropion, TCAs, and MAOIs are preferably avoided with clozapine, if possible, to minimize various side-effect synergism. Valproate, lamotrigine, and gabapentin are preferred for seizure prophylaxis. Clozapine can be used with lithium and valproate for treatment of manic symptoms not controlled on clozapine. Mirtazapine should not be given with clozapine due to increased risk of neutropenia.

The author's general approach is first to introduce clozapine and to get the dose to a fair therapeutic range of 200 to 500 mg daily. If there are still residual symptoms that need treatment, various adjunctive medications as have been described are then added sequentially, depending on the specific needs of an individual patient. It has been a frequent clinical observation that many patients whose symptoms have barely been controlled on a combination of multiple psychotropic medications, when switched to clozapine, are able to function well on clozapine alone. Hence, the chances are that clozapine's superior and broad therapeutic effects will supersede the need for various adjunctive medications. However, treatment using clozapine alone is not sufficient for some patients; thus, combinations involving clozapine and other medications are necessary for optimal outcome. Useful combinations are listed in Table 11.4.

Weekly CBC monitoring is expected to identify the 1 percent of patients at risk for agranulocytosis. By strictly following a weekly CBC during the first year, more than 98 percent of the occurrences of bone marrow suppression can be diagnosed promptly and immediate treatment initiated, thereby considerably decreasing the chances of mortality. Furthermore, patients are routinely advised to report any signs of infection and to get an immediate CBC at the first sign or suspicion of infection. When both precautions are adhered to, the author's opinion is that mortality due to agranulocytosis can be decreased significantly.

Data on file at Sandoz Pharmaceutical Corporation revealed that there were 13 deaths due to agranulocytosis in a five-year period from February 1990 through June 1995, when 109,550 patients had taken clozapine, sug-

TABLE 11.4. Medications That May Be Combined with Clozapine for Optimal Outcome

Residual Symptoms	Medications to Add to Clozapine
Depression	Antidepressants; SSRIs preferred
Anxiety	Benzodiazepines*, buspirone
"Positive" symptoms of psychosis	High-potency antipsychotics; risperidone preferred (low dose of depot haloperidol decanoate may improve noncompliance and residual "positive" symptoms)
Extreme mood instability	Lithium, valproic acid, lamotrigine, gabapentin
Marked anergia	Stimulants, caffeine
Obsessive-compulsive symptoms	Antiobsessional medications, SSRIs preferred
Substance abuse, including alcoholism	Naltrexone
Compulsive self-mutilation	SSRIs, naltrexone, buspirone
Persistent negative symptoms	SSRIs, bupropion, stimulants, selegiline 5mg BID, caffeine

*Watch for respiratory depression or excessive sedation when a benzodiazepine and clozapine are given concurrently during the first week of initiation of clozapine, in the elderly. After the first week, coadministration of a benzodiazepine has been well tolerated, in the author's experience.

gesting a mortality rate* of one death due to agranulocytosis per 8,426 patients treated with clozapine. Given the substantial risk of suicide (estimated at approximately 10 percent) among the poorly treated severely mentally ill patients, the mortality rate if not treated with clozapine is

*"Mortality rate" has a specific statistical meaning that is different from its meaning in this context where it is used nontechnically and descriptively to denote a general index of risk or probability of death.

expected to be much higher than the mortality rate due to agranulocytosis, making clozapine treatment of the severely ill safer than not treating with clozapine. Assuming a 10 percent mortality rate due to suicide among the poorly treated chronically psychotic patient population, it can be estimated that there would be 10,950 suicides (10 percent of 109,550 patients) if all 109,550 patients had treatment-refractory illness and if clozapine was not made available to these patients. This can be compared to 13 deaths attributed directly to clozapine among 109,550 patients on clozapine therapy. Although there are other confounding variables including availability of risperidone and prolonged inpatient hospitalization as options that can alter the analysis described above, it is clear that clozapine still has a favorable benefit-to-risk ratio despite the risk of fatality as a result of agranulocytosis.

Given the probability that most patients with schizophrenia and schizoaffective disorder eventually develop treatment resistance when treated long enough on traditional antipsychotic agents, "treatment resistance" may be considered one of the characteristics of schizophrenia or one of the inherent long-term consequences of treatment using traditional antipsychotic agents. This supports the clinical wisdom of considering the use of clozapine as a first-line treatment option for selected patients expected to need long-term antipsychotic therapy.

Traditional antipsychotics cause numerous side effects such as extrapyramidal symptoms and increased risk of tardive dyskinesia. In addition, they do not satisfactorily treat negative symptoms; hence, compliance is a perennial problem. Although risperidone and olanzapine are superior to traditional antipsychotics in this regard and therefore should be preferred over traditional antipsychotics, the author's experience indicates that clozapine is superior to even risperidone and olanzapine, and much superior to traditional antipsychotics. Hence, if a patient presents with several of the poor prognosticators, there are many clinical reasons, as outlined–notwithstanding cost considerations–to consider clozapine as the first-line antipsychotic for long-term maintenance if the diagnosis is schizophrenia or schizoaffective disorder.

A cost analysis indicates that to maintain a patient on haloperidol 5 mg daily (which is a reasonable maintenance dose), the monthly cost is expected to average $8.00. Even when an adjunctive anticholinergic such as benzotropine mesylate 1 mg BID is needed, the total cost for a month's supply of medications is likely to be approximately $18.00. This can be compared to the cost of $175 per month for risperidone 2 mg BID, and $220 per month for olanzapine 10 ms HS, which are reasonable maintenance doses. The cost of maintaining a patient on clozapine 300 mg daily (which should be a reasonable maintenance dose in clinical practice), including the cost of weekly CBCs at $15 per CBC, should be approximately $370 per month. Although the cost savings with the use of haloperidol are considerable compared to olanzapine, risperidone, and clozapine, any significant overall clinical advantage to the patient suffering from such a debilitating illness should be worth the additional cost, both from a humane perspective and from a long-term economic impact perspective. An illness or symptom that is not so debilitating probably deserves more attention to cost considerations. For example, temazepam (Restoril) 15 mg costs $7 per month, whereas zolpidem (Ambien) 10 mg costs $50 for a one-month supply. Both of these medications can be used for short-term treatment of insomnia. In this example, even though zolpidem is superior to temazepam for initial insomnia, the cost difference in excess of $40 per month is significant, given the clinical observation that both treat insomnia fairly well. Hence, the clinically and economically prudent strategy is to prescribe the least expensive medication for the treatment of fairly inconsequential symptoms. It follows, then, that it is equally prudent to prescribe the most superior medication obtainable for one of the most debilitating of medical conditions, schizophrenia, despite the high cost.

Discontinuation of Clozapine

It is generally not prudent to discontinue clozapine if it is effective. However, clozapine may have to be discontinued in the following contexts:

- Clozapine is not effective.
- Clozapine side effects prevent continued treatment.
- Maintenance on clozapine is difficult due to economic or other reasons.
- The patient decides to discontinue clozapine for whatever reason.

In ideal conditions clozapine should be gradually tapered off at a rate of 10 to 15 percent decrease daily, over a span of 10 to 20 days while the patient is being introduced to the new antipsychotic. Prior to the conclusion of the clozapine taper, the new antipsychotic should be at the optimal therapeutic dose to prevent relapse of psychosis. Rapid discontinuation of clozapine can lead to a "rebound psychosis," characterized by confusion, agitation, mania, paranoia, hyperactivity, insomnia, auditory and visual hallucinations, loose associations, and even disorientation, necessitating immediate hospitalization. The rebound psychosis may require treatment using sedating medications, including low-potency antipsychotics and benzodiazepines. Clinical experience indicates that patients who had a superior response to clozapine and who were on doses higher than 300 mg daily tend to develop rebound psychosis more frequently compared to those who did not respond well to clozapine. Obviously, some clozapine side effects require immediate discontinuation due to medical reasons (e.g., agranulocytosis, cardiorespiratory abnormalities, and severe hypotension), in which case the patient should be closely monitored for the development of rebound psychosis. Occasionally, hospitalization may be considered for safe and rapid withdrawal from clozapine. Rebound psychosis is managed in the same manner as acute psychosis.

A sample schedule for the elective discontinuation of clozapine of a patient maintained on clozapine 400 mg daily is given in Table 11.5. If clozapine is discontinued due to lack of efficacy, the patient may tolerate a more rapid discontinuation rate. The drug manufacturer recommends weekly WBC monitoring for four weeks after clozapine has been stopped.

Techniques to Detect or Minimize Serious Clozapine Side Effects

Agranulocytosis

Since most occurrences of agranulocytosis are reported between two weeks and four months of initiation of clozapine, clinicians or patients

TABLE 11.5. Clozapine: Elective Discontinuation Schedule

Day	Total Dose/Day
0	400 mg (maintenance dose)
1	350 mg
2	300 mg
3	250 mg
4	200 mg
5	175 mg
6	150 mg
7	125 mg
8	100 mg
9	75 mg
10	50 mg
11	25 mg
12	25 mg
13	12.5 mg
14	12.5 mg

who want to be extra cautious may choose to obtain a WBC more frequently than required by the drug manufacturer. For example, the WBC could be obtained every Monday and Friday during the most vulnerable period. After the first four months, the frequency of WBC monitoring may be decreased to the minimum required weekly schedule. A list of major adverse events related to clozapine is given in Table 11.6.

Seizures

Since seizure risk is dose-dependent, it is prudent to consider a prophylactic anticonvulsant for patients who need to be on doses of clozapine greater than 500 mg per day. The seizure risk at this dose or higher is estimated at 5 percent. It is likely that the seizure risk is greater than 5 percent at a dose of 900 mg per day, which is the maximum approved dose of clozapine. Valproate, lamotrigine, amotrigine (Lamictal), or gabapentin (Neurontin) are preferred for seizure prophylasis. An EEG (after the clozapine dosage has been stabilized) can be obtained to rule out the presence of subclinical seizure activity, and may be desirable if clozapine dose exceeds 500 mg per day. Carbamazepine and phenytoin are best avoided due to possible additive effects on bone marrow.

TABLE 11.6. Adverse Effects Related to Clozapine

Serious Events	**Other Events**
Agranulocytosis Hypotension Cardiac Arrest Respiratory Depression	Sedation Dizziness Seizure Salivation Tachycardia Weight Gain Fever Constipation Hypotension Nausea/Vomiting Headache Leukocytosis

Reference: Sandoz Pharmaceuticals: *Clozaril–Management of Adverse Effects*, 1993.

Respiratory Depression and Respiratory Collapse

Avoid benzodiazepines early in treatment, especially when clozapine is first administered. Give a low dose of clozapine (12.5 mg) on the first day, particularly in the elderly. Institute slow dosage escalation if sedation is a problem. A benzodiazepine may be safely introduced after the first several days of clozapine initiation.

Management of various side effects such as hypersalivation, excessive sedation, dizziness, fever, and leukocytosis, are described in a booklet published by Sandoz, *Clozaril–Management of Adverse Events* and is presented in summarized and modified form in Table 11.7.

Starting Clozapine–To Hospitalize or Not

In principle, clozapine can be started on an outpatient basis. Patients who are in control, reliable, and not acutely symptomatic are particularly good candidates for consideration for initiation of clozapine in an outpatient setting. However, the practical reality is that in most cases those patients who are selected for clozapine therapy are acutely symptomatic with symptoms that are poorly controlled on traditional antipsychotic medications. These patients typically need inpatient treatment regardless of clozapine initiation. Patients whose symptoms are stabilized on a traditional antipsychotic and who have intolerable side effects attributed to traditional antipsychotics are another group of patients who could benefit from clozapine treatment. The process of tapering off the traditional antipsychotic and initiating clozapine involves many complex patient-management, procedural, and medical aspects, some of which are listed below:

- The likelihood of relapse increases if the existing antipsychotic is abruptly stopped or rapidly tapered off.
- A relapse might make the patient immediately noncompliant, resulting in further deterioration.
- A careful titration of clozapine dose, with frequent monitoring of vital signs, is essential during the first three to six days to enhance the chances of successful outcome.
- The clozapine dose cannot be rapidly increased should the patient become acutely psychotic, necessitating immediate intervention, that is difficult for the outpatient.
- Though ideally clozapine is to be used as a single medication, in actual clinical practice, most patients need adjunctive medications (including adjunctive low-dose, high-potency traditional antipsy-

chotics or a low dose of risperidone) for optimal outcome. This is crucial during the first several days of clozapine initiation.

- The most common side effects of clozapine, such as dizziness, tachycardia, nausea, hypersalivation, sedation, constipation, and orthostatic changes need medical supervision, management, and frequent reassurance to overcome or to be tolerated by the patient.
- The clozapine titration schedule during the first three to six days is fairly complex. An example of a fairly rapid initiation schedule is given below (standard initiation schedule is given in Table 11.2):

	AM	Noon	PM	HS
Day 1	---	12.5 mg	12.5 mg	12.5 mg
Day 2	12.5 mg	12.5	25	25
Day 3	25	25	25	50
Day 4	25	25	50	75
Day 5	25	25	50	100

Obviously, any major side effects or complications necessitate a slower schedule. A slower schedule still is fairly complex with an increased risk of relapse. As is evident, a seriously ill psychiatric patient would have difficulty complying with such a schedule on his or her own.

- The dose of the existing traditional antipsychotic preferably should not be abruptly discontinued, but must be gradually tapered off. An example follows:

	Haloperidol Dose
Day 1	10 mg HS
Day 2	8 mg HS
Day 3	6 mg HS
Day 4	4 mg HS
Day 5	2 mg HS, then discontinue

Again, severely and chronically mentally ill patients who are fairly dysfunctional (patients who comprise the clozapine target group) will have great difficulty in adhering to these complex schedules during the clozapine initiation phase.

- If the existing antipsychotic is of low potency (such as chlorpromazine or thioridazine), it should preferably be discontinued before clozapine is introduced because medical reasons, such as risk of hypotension, excessive sedation, and cardiorespiratory problems increase the chances of the patient becoming symptomatic during the first three to six days (which are necessary to bring the clozapine dose to a low therapeutic range of 100-200 mg).

- Highly skilled clinical measures such as reassurance, support, persuasion, insistence, perseverance, and close attention to detail are typically needed during the first three to six days to get many patients to complete the clozapine titration process. Some patients may even require emergency intervention to control agitation, including seclusion and restraints during clozapine initiation phase.
- The complex clozapine titration schedule and the gradual tapering-off schedule of the existing antipsychotic are difficult for most severely mentally ill patients to implement as outpatients, unless supportive, responsible, and capable family members or clinical staff are available to closely supervise the treatment in an outpatient setting.
- Many complications and problems, some of which are listed, can threaten the chance of a successful outpatient clozapine-initiation process. This leads to the erroneous conclusion that clozapine was either ineffective or intolerable, when proper clozapine treatment as an inpatient could overcome most of the initial complications, thereby enhancing the chance of a successful outcome.
- Poor initiation could lead to improper abandonment of clozapine, which could be a potentially life-saving therapeutic intervention.
- Clozapine initiation as an outpatient would have to be fairly slow to avoid medical risks as listed earlier. However, slow initiation places the patient at high risk for a relapse that will require control of the acute relapse and all of the complications associated with a relapse, such as refusal to accept treatment, need for involuntary proceedings, refusal of clozapine, and a greater risk of suicide. Obviously, a longer period of hospitalization would generally be required should the patient experience a relapse.

Initiating clozapine can be compared to initiating insulin therapy for a newly diagnosed Type I diabetic. Diabetes will have varying degrees of "brittleness," and this creates different levels of difficulty in controlling each patient's basic disease process. Diabetic patients have varying insulin requirements; therefore, adjusting their dosage based on frequent blood sugar monitoring becomes a quite active and critical clinical process. If done poorly, dosage adjustment can result in harmful extremes of hypoglycemia and/or ketoacidosis. Prescription of a compatible diet is also important. Proper management of complications and absence of negative experiences during the introduction of insulin therapy enhance com-

TABLE 11.7. Clozapine Side-Effect Management Chart

Side Effects	Management Suggestions
Seizures: Grand mal, myoclonic jerks, and cataleptic-like events. Preexisting seizure disorder is not a contraindication to clozapine. Can occur at any time. Dose dependent. 5 percent risk for doses >500 mg/day. Increased risk in patients with history of closed head injury.	Avoid rapid dosage escalation. Use divided doses (TID). Avoid combining with other drugs that lower seizure threshold. Do EEG, neurological consultation. Decrease dose. Start anticonvulsant for treatment of seizures. Avoid carbamazepine/phenytoin. Consider prophylactic anticonvulsant if dosage exceeds 500 mg per day.
Hypotension: Systolic blood pressure <90 mm Hg. Occurs in 9 percent; more common in elderly. Collapse occurs in 1/3,000. Can occur in the first four weeks. May subside over time.	Avoid rapid dosage escalation. Monitor blood pressure and pulse QID supine and standing. Instruct patient to stand slowly. Start first dose at 12.5 mg. Give major dose at bedtime; wear support stockings. Avoid concurrent benzodiazepines. If persistent and severe, consider fludrocortisone acetate 0.1 mg BID-TID with medical clearance and monitoring. Avoid epinephrine because of possible reverse epinephrine effects.
Sedation/Drowsiness: Presents with weakness, fatigue, lethargy, and hypersomnia. Occurs in 30 to 35 percent in the first four weeks. May improve over time.	Give major portion at bedtime. Increase dose slowly. Avoid activities requiring alertness. Add caffeine. Avoid other sedating drugs. For severe sedation, may try dextroamphetamine 5 to 10 mg or methylphenidate 5 to 10 mg AM and noon.
Dizziness/Vertigo: A sensation of unsteadiness with a feeling of movement within the head or external world. Occurs in 19 percent. Can occur at any time during treatment, usually as a result of orthostatic hypotension. Elderly patients are at particular risk while therapy is being initiated.	Slow dosage titration. Monitor blood pressure supine and standing. Advise patient to stand up slowly from sitting or lying positions. Use caution while engaging in activities requiring balance and coordination.
Hypersalivation: Can be profuse during sleep. Occurs in 40 percent. Appears within four weeks and may subside over time.	Prop up pillow. Encourage patients to sleep on their side, use a towel to cover pillow. If severe, consider an anticholinergic or clonidine transdermal patch 0.1 to 0.2 mg per week temporarily.

Side Effects	Management Suggestions
Tachycardia: Heart rate >120 per minute, or heart rate >100 per minute, and patient is symptomatic (sweating, dizziness, chest pain) or coronary risk factors present. Early in treatment, can persist. Tolerance can develop.	Avoid rapid dosage escalation. Reduce caffeine intake and cigarette smoking. If asymptomatic, with no coronary risk factors (obesity, hypertension, smoking, diabetes, family history of CAD, or previous history of CAD) observe two weeks. If patient is younger than 30 years old, is healthy, with no medical problems or CAD risk factors, and no contraindications to beta-blockers (asthma, bronchospastic disease, diabetes, hypoglycemia), can begin atenolol (Tenormin) 25 to 50 mg per day. If tachycardia persists, switch to pindolol (Visken) 5 mg po daily. May increase to 5 mg BID, then 10 mg BID if necessary. Cardiac evaluation to rule out heart disease. Reduce clozapine dose if other interventions not effective.
Constipation: Occurs in 15 percent. Dose-dependent. May improve over time. Rarely, can progress to obstipation or ileus.	High fiber diet. Eliminate other anticholinergic drugs. Increase fluid intake, encourage physical activity. Docusate sodium (Colase) 200 to 300 mg per day. Psyllium hydrophilic mucilloid (Metamucil) one dose/day. Vigorous early treatment can prevent complications.
Weight Gain: Can be from 2 to 25 pounds and persistent. Occurs in about 15 percent. More common in younger patients.	Exercise, watch diet, dietary counseling. If severe and persistent, consider cautious trial on low doses of fenfluramine at 10 to 20 mg two hours before supper.
Leukocytosis: Low incidence. Appears within first four to eight weeks and gradually subsides. Can be dose dependent.	Rule out infection, medical illnesses, eosinophilia, NMS, and other etiologies of leukocytosis. Usually benign. Dosage decrease may improve leukocytosis. Continue to monitor for infection.
Headache: Occurs in 7 percent. Transient, subsides over time.	Analgesic treatment. If persistent, rule out other causes.
Hypertension: Frequency 4 percent. Blood pressure >150/90 mm Hg. Usually dose-dependent.	Avoid rapid dosage escalation. Monitor blood pressure four times a day for two weeks. If significant, initiate antihypertensive therapy (atenolol 50 to 100 mg/day, or pindolol 5 to 10 mg BID). Avoid ACE inhibitors which have been associated with agranulocytosis.

TABLE 11.7 (continued)

Side Effects	Management Suggestions
Nausea/Vomiting: Occurs after four to six weeks.	Reduce the dose and titrate more slowly. If severe, give trimethobenzamide (Tigan), metoclopramide (Reglan), or prochlorperazine (Compazine). Supplement fluids via IV route if unable to take fluids orally. Check BUN, creatinine and electrolytes if vomiting is severe and persists over 48 hours.
Urinary Problems: Frequency 6 percent. Incontinence, enuresis, increased frequency and urgency, hesitancy, and urinary retention. Usually improves over time. Can be dose dependent.	For incontinence, consider anticholinergic drugs for urologic applications; for urinary hesitancy and retention, consider bethanechol. Consider desmopressin nasal spray for enuresis.
Delirium/Confusion: Disorientation, confusion, worse at night. Can be dose-dependent.	Rule out medical etiology and polypharmacy. Consider EEG. Rule out anticholinergic toxicity. Decrease clozapine dose.

Source: Adapted with modifications from Sandoz Corporation, "Clozaril Side Effect Management Chart," *Clozaril Treatment Trends*, 4(1), 1995. Used with permission. Also includes data and recommendations derived from the author's clinical experience.

pliance. A successful initiation of insulin greatly improves the chances of avoiding future complications and hospitalizations. For these clinical reasons, insulin therapy is typically initiated in an inpatient setting. Once insulin is properly initiated, subsequent management can be safely carried out as an outpatient. As a final comparison, a poor initiation of insulin therapy does not result in abandonment of that therapy, whereas regarding clozapine, a poor initiation is likely to result in a false conclusion that clozapine was not effective. Therefore, patients may forever abandon a therapy that may truly have been a life saver.

In the author's experience, clozapine is a superior medication for the treatment of selected severely mentally ill psychiatric patients. To take advantage of its unique benefits without letting the many side effects defeat the treatment, it has to be introduced to the patient appropriately. When clozapine is initiated in an inpatient setting, in the author's estimate, the chance of a successful outcome is in the 70 to 80 percent range, whereas if it is started in an outpatient setting, the chance of successful outcome is lower. In most cases three to six days of inpatient stay is sufficient to get the patient to a dose of 100 to 200 mg, with further dosage titration safely and easily conducted on an outpatient basis. The author has virtually stopped the practice of starting clozapine in an outpatient setting due to the unsatisfactory results.

To begin a patient on clozapine as an outpatient in the interest of economy would be penny-wise and pound-foolish, in most cases. In strict financial terms, clozapine treatment is expensive in the short term, but cost effective in the long term. When there is such a flux in the health insurance industry as is evident currently with frequent changes of insurance carriers, utilization review incentives for maximum cost savings, and competitive bidding for utilization review contracts in which the focus is on immediate profit, it would make no business sense for profit-oriented third-party payers to enthusiastically endorse clozapine therapy. In this regard, the treating clinician has become the only professional to advocate for the patients' best interests, both short- and long-term.

In summary, for assuring the best outcome it is recommended that for the majority of patients, clozapine be initiated in an inpatient setting as a general medical practice, regardless of whether or not patients are willing to start clozapine on an outpatient basis.

Summary of Advantages and Disadvantages of Clozapine

Advantages

- Superior effectiveness for positive symptoms of psychoses
- The most effective among currently available antipsychotics for negative symptoms
- Virtual absence of tardive dyskinesia
- May cause regression of tardive dyskinesia and tardive dystonia induced by traditional antipsychotics
- Extremely low incidence of extrapyramidal symptoms and neuroleptic malignant syndrome
- Has antianxiety, antidepressant, and mood-stabilizing properties
- Effective for controlling psychotic symptoms regardless of diagnosis; may be used in schizophrenia, schizoaffective disorder, severe bipolar disorder, delusional disorder, major depression with psychotic features, or any disorder with chronic psychotic symptoms as listed in the text

– Potential enhancement of insight, compliance, and improvement of overall patient functioning and quality of life
– Continued improvement for up to six months, or longer, prior to reaching a plateau
– No elevation of prolactin level and low incidence of galactorrhea, gynecomastia, and amenorrhea (Since it is estimated that about one-third of human breast cancer is prolactin sensitive, there may be at least a theoretical advantage in using clozapine in patients with a history of breast cancer or in those who are predisposed to it.)
– Potential for sedating properties to help insomnia, a common problem in psychotic patients
– Can supersede the need for a variety of adjunctive medications such as mood stabilizers, anticholinergics, antidepressants, and benzodiazepines, suggesting that clozapine has a broad spectrum of therapeutic effects
– The substantial reduction of risk of suicide attempts with satisfactory response to clozapine
– Possible reduction of craving for and abuse of drugs, alcohol, and nicotine, frequently found among psychotic patients
– Striking decrease in relapse and rehospitalization rate
– Potential significant long term cost savings by reducing direct (e.g., reduced rehospitalization rate) and indirect costs (e.g., reduced number of hospital beds and hospital services, and increased productivity)
– FDA pregnancy category B

Disadvantages

– 1 percent incidence of agranulocytosis and consequent need for weekly CBC monitoring for detection of neutropenia–slightly greater risk in females and in geriatric patients–with greatest risk in the first four months of initiating clozapine treatment
– 4 to 5 percent risk of seizures at higher doses, compared to 1 percent risk of seizures with other antipsychotics
– High cost of treatment (average of $5,500 per year on a dose of 350 mg per day and for weekly CBCs)
– May require inpatient stay (in most cases) of three to six days for initiation of treatment, for optimal outcome
– Parenteral or liquid form not available in the United States
– Potential excessive sedation and orthostatic hypotension in some patients, preventing increase to therapeutic range
– Relatively greater incidence of tachycardia, hypotension, and hypersalivation

– One death (due to agranulocytosis) per 8,426 patients treated with clozapine
– Side effects such as somnolence, weight gain, anergia, and a "drugged" feeling can persist in some patients

Administrative Disadvantages

High initial and maintenance cost can be a disincentive to a community mental health center (CMHC), that has a limited budget but cares for a high percentage of patients with chronic mental illness. Such chronic mentally ill patients can significantly benefit from clozapine. Administrators realize that funding decisions are made and their own accomplishments judged based on short-term and immediate budgetary performance, as is true with regard to most business practices. Any cost savings due to a decreased number of readmissions expected from clozapine treatment is likely to be realized only years later. Improvement in a patient's quality of life is difficult to quantify. Often unrecognized, quality of life is likely to occur gradually and slowly after initiation of clozapine treatment. Since there is a considerable turnover CMHC administrators, the person who makes the decision today to allocate funding for clozapine treatment is not likely to receive any recognition for long-term cost savings. In fact, if clozapine treatment causes short-term budgetary constraints, which is quite possible during the first several years, it may adversely reflect on the administrator. Moreover, in most cases any cost savings in the long run will not be realized by the CMHC, but will benefit the state and federal agencies that administer inpatient health insurance for the indigent. To use an analogy, clozapine is like a long-term investment, and hence is unlikely to appeal to short-term investors who are looking for quick returns. All of these factors make it difficult for administrators of CMHCs to become enthusiastic about clozapine unless policymakers have the foresight and wisdom to allocate to CMHCs at least a portion of the cost savings expected to result from reduced hospitalization rate for funding the higher initiation, maintenance, and patient-monitoring costs associated with clozapine therapy.

Another factor is that some inpatient units that are dependent on readmissions of chronic patients are likely to suffer in the long term with clozapine treatment, due to decreased patient census resulting from clozapine's established efficacy in reducing rehospitalization rate. Therefore, strictly from an administrator's standpoint, those inpatient units that primarily rely on treating chronic patients could have potential long-term losses due to encouraging clozapine use. Those who need a reason to discourage clozapine use have agranulocytosis risk to cite as an apparently rational argument against clozapine.

In summary, clozapine is a superior medication for the treatment of a variety of chronic psychotic conditions and selected chronic, severe mental disorders. It is a complicated medication that requires skillful initiation and careful clinical management. Weekly WBC monitoring enables early detection and treatment of agranulocytosis, preventing a fatal outcome in the great majority of patients. Seizure prophylaxis significantly decreases the seizure risk associated with clozapine dose in the higher dosage range. Clozapine treatment significantly decreases suicide risk. The benefits of clozapine therapy far outweigh the risks associated with it.

OLANZAPINE (ZYPREXA)

Olanzapine, an atypical antipsychotic with sertonin-dopamine antagonist (SDA) effects, was introduced in the United States in October 1996. It is available as unscored 5 mg, 7.5 mg, and 10 mg tablets. The elimination half-life is 30 hours. Plasma-protein binding is 95 percent. The major metabolic route is hepatic, necessitating dosage adjustment in the hepatically impaired and in the elderly. The starting dose as well as the optimal dose recommended by the drug manufacturer for treatment of schizophrenia is 10 mg daily. The dosage range is from 5 to 20 mg daily. All or a major portion of the dose may be given at bedtime to enhance sleep and to minimize daytime drowsiness.

Olanzapine is well tolerated by most patients. Many patients reported significant anxiolytic and calming effect. Its low risk of EPS, effectiveness for both positive and negative symptoms, and absence of major side effects should make it a superior antipsychotic compared to traditional antipsychotics. Furthermore, it does not elevate serum prolactin level significantly, an advantage also shared by clozapine and sertindole, but not by risperidone, among the atypical antipsychotics. Since clinical experience so far has substantiated the expectation particularly of fair effectiveness in treating negative symptoms, low EPS, a benign side effect profile, minimal effects on prolactin level, and superior tolerability, olanzapine has the potential to be the frontline general purpose antipsychotic of choice for treatment of schizophrenia and psychotic symptoms.

The common side effects reported for olanzapine are drowsiness, lightheadedness, dry mouth, weight gain, anxiety, and orthostatic hypotension. Occasionally, it can cause agitation or precipitate mania. Most of these side effects typically subside within one to two weeks of starting the medication. However, some weight gain is likely to persist for the duration of olanzapine therapy. A manic reaction usually requires the discontinuation of olanzapine. Rare incidence of hepatotoxicity has also been reported. Therefore, monitoring of liver function after two weeks and a repeat test after two months of starting olanzapine may be performed in patients susceptible to liver enzyme elevation such as patients with hepatic disease or patients who are being treated with potentially hepatotoxic drugs. Most cases of liver enzyme elevations are transient and tend to subside without the need for dosage adjustment. Liver function studies or laboratory tests are neither necessary nor recommended on a routine basis. Generalized edema can also be a side effect occasionally requiring concomitant diuretic therapy.

Since orthostatic hypotension associated with dizziness and syncope can occur in rare patients, the author's practice is to start patients on olanzapine 5 mg and increase to 10 mg after two to three days, particularly for outpatients. A lower starting dose of 2.5 mg or 3.75 mg may be considered for patients with cardiovascular disease and cerebrovascular disease, and for patients taking antihypertensive medications.

Since clinical experience suggests possible effectiveness for treatment of some treatment-resistant schizophrenias, olanzapine could be a treatment option prior to a trial of clozapine which, for general purpose use, is fettered by a 1 to 2 percent risk of argranulocytosis.

As is generally the case with most psychiatric conditions, mild symptoms might respond to low doses and severe and chronic symptoms might need doses at the higher end of the therapeutic range. Olanzapine dosage guidelines based on the author's clinical experience are given below.

Olanzapine Dosage Guidelines

- Conditions with mild psychotic symptoms such as paranoid personality features, schizotypal features, schizoid features, and dementia might respond to doses in the range of 1.25 to 5 mg daily.
- Conditions with moderate psychotic symptoms such as delusional disorders, psychotic symptoms associated with affective disorders, schizoaffective disorders, and bipolar disorder might respond to a dosage range of 5 to 10 mg daily.
- Conditions characterized by severe psychotic symptoms such as the schizophrenias and severe schizoaffective disorder might need a dosage range of 10 to 20 mg daily for adequate response.

Adjunctive Medications

SSRIs, MAOIs, TCAs, bupropion, mirtazapine, trazodone, nefazodone, lithium, valproate, carbamazepine, gabapentin, lamotrigine, and the benzodiazepines may be used if necessary in a combination treatment regimen involving olanzapine.

Antipsychotic Combinations Involving Olanzapine

Some patients may require the adjunctive use of other antipsychotics for optimal symptom control if olanzapine alone is not sufficient to provide satisfactory control of symptoms. It should be emphasized that as a general rule, polypharmacy should be avoided unless necessary and beneficial to the patient. Antipsychotic combinations involving clozapine and risperidone are not uncommon. Low doses of risperidone or traditional antipsychotics can be combined with a therapeutic dose of olanzapine to control breakthrough psychotic symptoms if olanzapine is otherwise well tolerated or provides other unique and significant benefits to the patient. When multiple medications are employed, the patient is at risk for developing side effects from each of the medications independently and additively. The author has no experience in combining olanzapine and clozapine, but it is conceivable that a rare patient may benefit from such a combination.

Whether or Not to Switch to Olanzapine

The general clinical strategy is not to switch if the patient is doing well on clozapine or risperidone, both of which have low risk of causing tardive dyskinesia (TD), although in the case of risperidone the TD risk is considered greater than that of clozapine, but less than that of traditional antipsychotics. Patients who have responded particularly well to clozapine tend to do poorly when switched to other antipsychotics. Therefore, patients functioning well on clozapine should be switched only if necessary and not simply to try a new antipsychotic. The author's practice is to attempt to switch patients taking traditional antipsychotics to atypical antipsychotics even if they are currently doing well because of the inherent potential of traditional antipsychotics to cause TD in a significant proportion of patients after chronic use. Why wait for TD to emerge when it could be irreversible? Atypical antipsychotics, including olanzapine, offer the theoretical probability of low risk of TD. Since olanzapine tends to cause less acute EPS compared to traditional antipsychotics and since olanzapine does not have the leukopenic and epileptogenic potential of clozapine, olanzapine should be a strong candidate for choice as an agent to switch patients to, among the currently available atypical antipsychotics, all of which have various advantages over the traditional antipsychotics as discussed in the sections describing each of the antipsychotics individually. Clozapine is expected to retain its position as the drug of choice for truly treatment-resistant schizophrenia.

Switching from Other Antipsychotics to Olanzapine

In general, gradual taper of the existing antipsychotic with concurrent gradual initiation of olanzapine is the preferred method. If the antipsychotic being discontinued has anticholinergic effects, as for example, chlorpromazine, thioridazine, or clozapine, a slow taper over 7 to 14 days is recommended on an outpatient basis. Adjunctive anticholinergic medication is preferably discontinued over a four to six day period after starting olanzapine. If the patient has been taking a low dose of an antipsychotic in the high-potency category (for example, haloperidol 0.5 to 2 mg, thiothixene 1 to 4 mg, or equivalent) the patient may be safely switched to olanzapine without the need for gradual taper. However, low-potency antipsychotics such as chlorpromazine, thioridazine, and clozapine are preferably tapered off even if the patient has been taking a low dose (for example, chlorpromazine 25 to 75 mg or equivalent). Several switching schedules involving a few of the common antipsychotics are given below:

Haloperidol 10 mg daily to Olanzapine

	Haloperidol	Olanzapine
Day 1	5 mg	5 mg
Day 2	2.5 mg	5 mg
Day 3	2.5 mg	10 mg
Day 4	1 mg	10 mg
Day 5	---	10 mg

Chlorpromazine 300 mg daily to Olanzapine

	Chlorpromazine	Olanzapine
Day 1	200 mg	5 mg
Day 2	150 mg	5 mg
Day 3	100 mg	5 mg
Day 4	75 mg	10 mg
Day 5	50 mg	10 mg
Day 6	25 mg	10 mg
Day 7	---	10 mg

Clozapine 300 mg daily to Olanzapine

	Clozapine	Olanzapine
Day 1	200 mg	5 mg
Day 2	150 mg	5 mg
Day 3	100 mg	5 mg
Day 4	100 mg	10 mg
Day 5	75 mg	10 mg
Day 6	75 mg	10 mg
Day 7	50 mg	10 mg
Day 8	50 mg	10 mg
Day 9	25 mg	10 mg
Day 10	25 mg	10 mg
Day 11	12.5 mg	10 mg
Day 12	12.5 mg	10 mg
Day 13	12.5 mg	10 mg
Day 14	---	10 mg

These switching schedules may be used as flexible guidelines primarily for outpatient applications. The switch may be completed more rapidly in an inpatient setting. For instance, for an inpatient, the switch form haloperidol can be made by stopping haloperidol and starting olanzapine 10 mg from Day 1. Low-potency antipsychotics such as chlorpromazine and clozapine may be tapered off in four and six days, respectively, as an inpatient while olanzapine is increased to the therapeutic dose of 10 mg daily starting on Day 3. The obvious advantage for an inpatient is that if rebound psychosis, cholinergic rebound, or agitation emerge, immediate intervention can be initiated without risking noncompliance, deterioration, or other complications. In the case of an outpatient, slow tapering of the existing antipsychotic and rapid titration of olanzapine to the therapeutic dose minimizes complications from drug withdrawal. Since clozapine tends to cause moderate to severe withdrawal symptoms if abruptly or rapidly discontinued, clozapine should ideally be tapered off slowly and gradually over a 10- to 20-day period depending on the total daily clozapine dose to avoid withdrawal complications. If the patient, a supportive family member, or a day program staff member is not able to supervise the slow clozapine taper and olanzapine titration as an outpatient, inpatient hospitalization should be considered, particularly if the existing clozapine dose is greater than 200 mg daily. It has to be emphasized, however, that olanzapine is not a substitute for clozapine, and that patients who have shown good response to clozapine and are tolerating clozapine well, may do poorly when switched to currently available antipsychotics including olanzapine.

Cost Comparison

Olanzapine 10 mg daily, which is probably the most common starting dosage for treating schizophrenia, costs approximately $220 per month and $2,640 per year, compared to risperidone 2 mg BID costing approximately $180 per month and $2,160 per year, and clozapine 300 mg daily costing approximately $4,500 per year including the cost of weekly CBC. If a patient needs olanzapine 15 mg daily, which may not be uncommon, the cost would rise to approximately $325 per month and $3,900 per year. Olanzapine 10 mg daily, risperidone 2 mg BID, and clozapine 300 mg daily are fairly equivalent, and therefore comparable doses based on the author's clinical experience.

In summary, review of the literature and clinical experience suggest that olanzapine is an atypical antipsychotic with effectiveness for positive and negative symptoms, low risk of EPS, minimal effect on prolactin level at therapeutic doses, and superior tolerability. The insignificant elevation of prolactin level is a distinct advantage over traditional antipsychotics and risperidone. Therefore olanzapine has the potential to become the general purpose frontline antipsychotic of choice among the antipsychotic medications currently available.

Summary of Advantages and Disadvantages of Olanzapine (Zyprexa)

Advantages

- Effective for positive and negative symptoms
- Very low incidence of acute EPS at therapeutic dosage range (dose dependent)
- Probable low risk of tardive dyskinesia (too early to be conclusive)
- Does not elevate prolactin level significantly
- Generally well tolerated
- Once-a-day dosing improves compliance
- Patients can generally be started at an optimal therapeutic dose of 10 mg at bedtime
- Low incidence of sexual dysfunction
- Effective for treatment of first-episode psychosis as well as some treatment-resistant schizophrenias
- Improved efficacy and tolerability decrease relapses and rehospitalizations
- Potential significant long-term cost savings due to decreased illness-related direct and indirect costs

Disadvantages

- Drowsiness, dizziness, dry mouth, and weight gain can be initial side effects
- Mild EPS possible at the higher dosage range
- High cost (substantial for dose above 10 mg daily due to need for multiple pills)
- Tablets are unscored, making it less convenient to divide
- Parenteral and liquid forms not available as of this writing
- Appetite increase and consequent weight gain can be persistant and substantial for some patients
- Can occasionally precipitate mania, requiring discontinuation of olanzapine

SERTINDOLE (SERLECT)

Sertindole is a serotonin-dopamine antagonist (SDA) antipsychotic expected to be introduced in the United States in 1997. It will be available as 4 mg, 8 mg, 20 mg, and 24 mg capsules. Its half-life is three days. Plasma-protein binding is 99.3 percent. Sertindole is effective for both positive and negative symptoms of schizophrenia with virtually no extrapyramidal symptoms in the recommended dosage range. The risk of tardive dyskinesia is therefore expected to be very low, although chronic exposure to sertindole is necessary to confirm this expectation. There are no significant anticholinergic or sedating effects. Like clozapine, it does not elevate prolactin level. It is generally well tolerated by patients.

Its virtual lack of EPS, efficacy for treating both positive and negative symptoms, lack of elevation of prolactin level, and excellent tolerability should make it one of the frontline general purpose antipsychotics of choice, with clear-cut superiority over the traditional antipsychotics. Sertindole is comparable to olanzapine, though olanzapine has an EPS risk that is slightly greater than that of sertindole. Sertindole compares favorably to risperidone, which can cause sustained elevation of prolactin level. Its efficacy in the treatment of treatment-refractory schizophrenia has not been evaluated.

Sertindole can, however, cause mild asymptomatic prolongation of QT interval in approximately 1 percent of patients. There was no episode of torsades de pointes reported among sertindole-treated patients during extensive premarketing clinical trials. It should be mentioned that other antipsychotics, including thioridazine, risperidone, and clozapine, as well as nonpsychiatric drugs such as terfanadine, astemizole, and cisapride, can also cause mild prolongation of QT interval. Patients who may be at risk for prolongation of QT interval are the elderly; patients with bradycardia, preexisting cardiac conduction defects, and congestive heart failure; patients taking TCAs or antiarrhythmic agents; and patients taking medications that inhibit the metabolism of sertindole and thus increase its plasma concentration. Fluoxetine and paroxetine are examples among common psychiatric medications that can interact with sertindole in this manner. A 25 to 50 percent reduction in sertindole dose is recommended for patients taking fluoxetine and paroxetine, whereas a 25 to 50 percent sertindole dose increase may be necessary for patients taking carbamazepine or phenytoin. It is recommended that patients be started on a dose of 4 mg daily with 4 mg increments every two to four days as tolerated up to a maximum dose of 24 mg, a major portion given as a bedtime dose. The effective dosage range in the majority of patients is 12 to 24 mg daily. The gradual titration of dosage to reach the therapeutic dose is to minimize tachycardia and dizziness, which can be initial side effects that typically subside within two to three days of a dosage increase. However, the need for gradual dosage titration makes sertindole unsuitable for controlling acute psychosis unless benzodiazepines and/or other antipsychotics are used adjunctively until sertindole dose can be titrated to a therapeutic range. Lack of sedation and anticholinergic effects are likely to facilitate patient acceptance and tolerability.

Decreased ejaculatory volume can be an initial side effect which tends to improve gradually as the patient continues taking the medication. Decrease in libido, erectile or orgasmic impairment, and retrograde ejaculation have not been reported at an incidence greater than that for placebo. Other side effects include nasal congestion, nausea, rhinitis, postural hypotension, peripheral edema, tachycardia, dizziness, and mild weight gain. Tolerance develops to most of these side effects. Sertindole should be used cautiously with drugs that prolong QT interval (e.g., terfanadine and astemizole), or with drugs that inhibit sertindole metabolism (itraconazole, quinidine, and ketoconazole). Those patients who are at risk for QT prolongation may need EKG monitoring after the dosage titration is completed or after each dosage increment above 12 mg per day, if the physician decides to start sertindole in such a patient. It is also prudent to monitor pulse and blood pressure during the dosage titration period. Routine EKG monitoring is not needed for patients not at risk for QT prolongation. The dosage titration should be slow in the elderly who may be at greater risk for adverse cardiovascular events. If a patient is off of sertindole for more than one week, dose retitration may be necessary to reach a therapeutic dose. Sertindole metabolism may be enhanced in patients taking carbamazepine or phenytoin.

The dosage should be reduced in the elderly and in patients who have hepatic impairment. Renal patients or patients on hemodialysis may not need dosage adjustment. No correlation has been established between sertindole plasma concentration and efficacy.

Sertindole Dosage Guidelines

- Conditions associated with mild psychotic symptoms such as paranoid, schizotypal and schizoid features, and dementia might respond to doses in the range 4 to 8 mg daily.
- Conditions with moderate psychotic symptoms such as delusional disorders, psychotic symptoms associated with affective disorders, schizoaffective disorders, and bipolar disorder might respond to a dosage range of 8 to 16 mg daily.
- Conditions characterized by severe psychotic symptoms such as the schizophrenias and severe schizoaffective disorders might respond to doses in the range of 12 to 24 mg daily.

Adjunctive Medications

Psychotropic medications that inhibit or induce hepatic enzymes CYP2D6 and CYP3A could affect the plasma level of sertindole. Fluoxetine and paroxetine can inhibit sertindole metabolism, necessitating a dose reduction of sertindole. Carbamazepine can induce sertindole metabolism and therefore sertindole dose increase may be necessary. However, most psychotropic medications can be coadministered with sertindole in a combination treatment if necessary, provided dosage adjustment is made to accommodate hepatic enzyme inhibition and induction. In most instances of combination treatment, if fairly low doses of adjunctive medications or low to medium dose range of the primary medications are employed, drug interaction problems due to hepatic enzyme induction and inhibition, or free-plasma drug level variability due to plasma-protein binding effects are usually not of practical clinical concern.

Switching to Sertindole

The general approach is not to switch if the patient is doing well on clozapine, olanzapine, or risperidone. Review the switching guidelines with reference to olanzapine for general clinical principles that should be applicable to sertindole also. However, if the existing antipsychotic has the potential to prolong QT interval, intitiation of sertindole titration may have to wait until the patient stops taking the existing antipsychotic, in order to minimize possible additive effects on QT interval. If agitation emerges during the transition period, benzodiazepines may provide control of symptoms without increased cardiovascular risk. A unique requirement of sertindole initiation is the need for gradual dosage titration to reach a therapeutic dose, similar to clozapine initiation, but different from risperidone initiation, which affords a fairly rapid titration, and olanzapine therapy, which can be initiated at the therapeutic dose. Sertindole requires a starting dose of 4 mg per day with a 4 mg increment every two to four days as tolerated to arrive at the therapeutic dose. For instance, it will take approximately ten days to reach a therapeutic sertindole dose of 16 mg. The existing antipsychotic may be gradually tapered off over a ten-day period concurrent with the sertindole titration period. Clozapine taper, however, should ideally be completed slowly, over a 10- to 20-day period to minimize the chance of emergence of clozapine withdrawal symptoms. Again, refer to the section on olanzapine for clinical guidelines that are also applicable to sertindole.

To summarize, sertindole is an atypical antipsychotic with effectiveness for positive and negative symptoms, virtually no risk of extrapyramidal symptoms at therapeutic doses, and no effect on prolactin level. If clinical experience with large numbers of patients confirms the expectation that the prolongation of QT interval is of no clinical significance in terms of patient morbidity, sertindole would be one of the highly useful antipsychotics due to its many advantages and relatively minor disadvantages. Price information was not available at the time of this writing.

Summary of Advantages and Disadvantages of Sertindole

Advantages

- Effective for positive and negative symptoms
- Virtual absence of EPS at therapeutic dose range (equal to placebo)
- Very low risk of tardive dyskinesia (too early to be conclusive)
- No significant anticholinergic or sedating effects
- Does not elevate prolactin level
- Does not affect libido or sexual performance (reduced ejaculatory volume frequently improves over time)
- Long half-life enables once-a-day dosing, enhancing compliance
- Generally well tolerated
- Improved efficacy and tolerability should decrease relapses and rehospitalizations

- Potential significant long-term cost savings due to decreased illness-related direct and indirect costs
- Possible medication cost savings due to expected availability of convenient 20 and 24 mg capsules

Disadvantages

- Mild prolongation of the QT interval (routine EKG screening/monitoring is not recommended; however, EKG monitoring may be considered in susceptible patients, e.g., the elderly, patient with congestive heart failure, bradycardia, and left ventricular hypertrophy and patients taking TCAs or antiarrhythmia agents); rare incidence of sudden death reported during clinical trials not attributed to arrhythmia induced by sertindole
- Need for gradual upward titration of dose (due to tachycardia and hypotension if started on a higher initial dose, or if dose is rapidly increased)
- Retitration may be needed if patients are off of sertindole for more than one week
- Capsule form makes it inconvenient to divide
- Parenteral and liquid forms not available currently
- Medication cost expected to be high

HALOPERIDOL (HALDOL)

Haloperidol, a high-potency antipsychotic, is available in oral (tablet and concentrate) and parenteral forms. Tablets are available in 0.5, 1, 2, 5, 10, and 20 mg scored forms. Given its long half-life, haloperidol may be given as a one-time dose at bedtime, after the acute phase is controlled. The usual maintenance dose range for a healthy adult is between 5 and 15 mg daily, preferrably given at bedtime. In some patients a maintenance dose as low as 2 mg daily may be sufficient. Typically higher doses such as 10 to 30 mg are necessary during the first several days of treatment of acute agitation related to exacerbation of psychosis. Once the patient's acute symptoms are controlled, the dose of haloperidol should be gradually decreased to a maintenance dose necessary to keep the symptoms under control. The elderly and the debilitated may respond to a dose as low as 0.5 mg daily. Some severely disturbed and treatment-resistant cases may need as much as 100 mg daily during the acute phase of the illness for response. Haloperidol is still the author's antipsychotic of choice for treatment of acute psychotic agitation and acute manic excitement, use as a "chemical restraint" (frequently in combination with lorazepam), and for parenteral use. Its availability in liquid and parenteral forms for IM and IV applications and its excellent safety profile in short-term use are distinct and major advantages. Among traditional antipsychotics, haloperidol is considered the gold standard, much like imipramine among TCAs.

Parenteral preparation intended for IM injection is available as a haloperidol lactate injection, which may be used as an IV push in patients needing rapid control of agitation or delirium, with excellent results and safety. Haloperidol IV is administered one or two times during an episode of agitation, primarily in patients who are hospitalized in medical wards and who are in acute delirium. In the author's experience of administering haloperidol injections at 1 mg to 5 mg IV push in over 300 cases, there have not been any incidences of acute dystonia, neuroleptic malignant syndrome, or cardiac arrythmias.

Haloperidol is also available as a long-acting depot form called haloperidol decanoate, for deep IM injection at three to four week intervals; this must not be used intravenously. Haloperidol has a half-life of 40 hours and is 92 percent plasma protein bound.

Haloperidol in IM form is rapidly effective in controlling acute hostility and combativeness due to psychosis or other reasons. In healthy adults, it is given in 5 mg IM doses every 30 minutes to one hour until severe agitation is controlled. In most cases, 10 to 20 mg will control the agitation. Adjunctive use of a benzodiazepine such as lorazepam 1 mg alternating with haloperidol or concurrently with haloperidol is extremely effective in rapid control of severe agitation, and may decrease the number of haloperidol doses needed for achieving behavior control. The following are effective protocols for an acutely agitated adult patient:

1. Administer haloperidol 5 mg IM immediately and every hour PRN severe agitation.
   Administer lorazepam 1 mg immediately and every hour PRN severe agitation.
   Haloperidol and lorazepam may be administered concurrently.
   The maximum dose of haloperidol is 25 mg per 24 hours.
   The maximum dose of lorazepam is 5 mg per 24 hours.
   Haloperidol/lorazepam doses may be reduced by half for less severe agitation.
2. Administer haloperidol 5 mg IM and every hour PRN severe agitation.
   The maximum dose is 25 mg per 24 hours.
   Administer lorazepam 1 mg IM 30 minutes after haloperidol if patient is still agitated, then every hour PRN severe agitation.

The maximum dose of lorazepam is 5 mg per 24 hours.
Haloperidol and lorazepam may be alternated.
Haloperidol/lorazepam doses may be reduced by half for less severe agitation.

Avoid benzodiazepines in patients at risk for respiratory depression, in patients who ingested sedatives, or in patients with a compromised respiratory status.

The concurrent administration of an antipsychotic and a benzodiazepine is extremely effective for controlling highly excited and agitated patients. Behavioral control is obtained by the second, or at the most the third dose, after which the patient can be switched to oral dose.

Haloperidol IM is useful for rapid response as well as for medicating patients who are either severely agitated or who need medication involuntarily. If patients are cooperative, haloperidol concentrate is available for oral administration. The advantages of concentrate form are (1) faster absorption compared to tablet form, (2) assurance that patients who are superficially cooperative are unable to "cheek" medication when it is in liquid form, and (3) convenient for patients who have difficulty swallowing pill forms.

Haloperidol, being a high-potency antipsychotic, can cause acute extrapyramidal symptoms and dystonic reaction more frequently than low-potency neuroleptics. Common and significant side effects of antipsychotics and their management are discussed in Chapter 12.

Haloperidol is also available in a long-acting depot format as haloperidol decanoate for deep IM administration. Haloperidol decanoate has a half-life of approximately three weeks, and reaches peak plasma concentration after six days. Patients should first be stabilized on oral haloperidol prior to switching to the depot format to rule out any sensitivity reaction, to affirm that haloperidol is effective for the particular patient, and to ensure that the patient can tolerate the medication. Once administered, haloperidol decanoate stays in the body for up to a month, making a sensitivity reaction difficult to treat should it develop. Haloperidol decanoate is given by IM injection at three- to four-week intervals. The usual formula for converting oral dose to depot dose is 10 to 15 times the oral maintenance dose. For example, a patient maintained on 5 mg daily should do well on haloperidol decanoate 60 mg IM once every four weeks. Since it takes about three to four months for haloperidol decanoate to reach a steady state, supplemental oral doses of haloperidol 1 to 2 mg daily may be given during the first one to two months of initiating depot injection treatment. Another option is to administer a loading dose in the first one or two months. The loading dose should be approximately 130 percent of the total calculated maintenance dose of haloperidol decanoate. In the example given above, 130 percent of haloperidol decanoate 60 mg IM is approximately 80 mg IM in the first one or two months. Subsequent to this, the patient can be maintained on 60 mg IM every four weeks.

A patient on a maintenance dose of haloperidol 10 mg po daily may need 10 to 15 times the oral dose, making the decanoate dose 125 mg IM per month. A loading dose at 130 percent of 125 equals approximately 160 mg, which may be given in the first one or two months, with a subsequent maintenance dose of 125 mg IM monthly. Another option is to keep the dosage the same and to give the medication once every three weeks for the first three doses and then increase the interval to the standard schedule of once every four weeks. The maximum recommended IM decanoate dose is 450 mg. It is available as 50 mg per 1 ml ampules and 100 mg per 1 ml ampules. The maximum dose per injection at one site should not exceed 3 ml. If a higher dose is required, the balance should be administered at another site. In clinical practice, haloperidol decanoate 100 mg IM per month is usually sufficient in most cases. The initial dose should not exceed 100 mg even if the conversion ratio indicates a higher dose to minimize initial adverse effects. The balance of the medication may be administered in three to seven days. For instance, if the initial dose is calculated to be 150 mg per month, the first dose should be 100 mg, and the balance of 50 mg should be given after one week. If the initial month's injection is tolerated well, subsequent doses can be administered in one injection, subject to the maximum dose of 450 mg and maximum volume per injection site of 3 ml. Since the loading dose generally tends to cause a greater incidence of side effects, the author prefers other methods of initiating a patient on long-acting depot preparation, unless a loading dose is desirable in a particular clinical context.

The long-acting depot format is excellent for patients who are noncompliant with daily oral intake of haloperidol and for those who are expected to be maintained on antipsychotic medications chronically. In some patients, even missing several doses due to forgetfulness or due to negligence can lead to impairment of judgment and consequent noncompliance with treatment, resulting in a rapid relapse.

Other uses of haloperidol include treatment of Tourette's syndrome, ballism, intractable hiccups, and the chorea of Huntington's disease.

The author's antipsychotic of choice until the introduction of risperidone had been haloperidol because of its many advantages. It is still the first-line antipsychotic when IM and IV administration are needed, and when rapid control of agitation, excitability, or combativeness is necessary. A list of advantages and disadvantages follows:

Summary of Advantages and Disadvantages of Haloperidol

Advantages

- Potent antipsychotic
- Low sedation
- Low anticholinergic side effects
- PO, IM, long-acting depot, and liquid concentrate formats
- May be safely given IV in 1 to 5 mg doses in emergencies (and in medical wards–though not an FDA-approved use)
- Scored tablet form, enabling flexible dose schedule
- Once-a-day administration possible
- Once-a-month depot format (affords longer interval than fluphenazine decanoate and enanthate); beneficial for noncompliant patients
- Minimal cardiovascular side effects
- Fair safety margin in overdose
- Low cost due to availability of generic form (except depot form)

Disadvantages

- Causes extrapyramidal symptoms more frequently compared to low-potency antipsychotics
- Negative symptoms not significantly improved
- Has all the risks associated with traditional antipsychotics, including tardive dyskinesia
- Decanoate preparation has the disadvantage of prolonged adverse effects, in the event of an adverse reaction

THIOTHIXENE (NAVANE)

Thiothixene is a high-potency antipsychotic that is highly protein bound, with a half-life of approximately 24 hours. It is available in capsules for oral administration at doses of 1, 2, 5, 10, and 20 mg strengths, liquid concentrate form, and in parenteral form for IM use. The uses, side effects, and precautions are similar to that of a high-potency antipsychotic such as haloperidol, except for a few reports of lenticular pigmentation and pigmentary retinopathy related to long-term use at high doses.

Thiothixene is effective for the treatment of psychotic symptoms. As is true of all traditional antipsychotics, it is very effective for positive symptoms, but has limited effectiveness for the treatment of negative symptoms.

Thiothixene offers an acceptable option of a high-potency antipsychotic, and as such, some patients may respond to it better than other high-potency agents. The effective dosage of thiothixene in adults for acute treatment is 20 to 40 mg in divided doses, with an average maintenance dose in the range of 5 to 15 mg daily, usually given as a one-time dose at bedtime. Acutely psychotic, agitated, and uncooperative patients could be treated with IM thiothixene for rapid effect, the dosage being 5 to 10 mg IM every four to six hours, until acute symptoms are controlled to the point that patients can be switched to oral medications. Since it is available in a generic form, thiothixene is inexpensive.

The oral dose can be increased to 60 mg daily, but clinical experience shows that most patients can be maintained on 5 to 15 mg daily. Patients with less acute symptoms can be managed on lower doses, such as 1 to 5 mg daily. Thiothixene is not available in long-acting depot form.

Summary of Advantages and Disadvantages of Thiothixene

Advantages

- High-potency antipsychotic
- Effective for positive symptoms
- Low anticholinergic effects
- Capsule, liquid, and IM forms available
- Once-a-day dosing, preferably at bedtime
- Minimal cardiovascular side effects
- Fair safety margin in overdose
- Low cost due to generic availability

Disadvantages

- Causes extrapyramidal symptoms more frequently compared to low-potency antipsychotics
- Negative symptoms are not significantly improved
- Has all of the risks associated with traditional antipsychotics, including tardive dyskinesia

CHLORPROMAZINE (THORAZINE)

Chlorpromazine is a low-potency phenothiazine antipsychotic that is highly protein bound, with a half-life in excess of 24 hours. It is used in doses of 100 to 300 mg for maintenance and doses of up to 1,000 mg for treatment of acute psychosis. The maximum recommended dose is 2,000 mg. It is available in 10, 25, 50, 100, and 200 mg tablets, liquid form, rectal suppositories, parenteral injection format, and extended release capsules in 30, 75, and 150 mg doses. The highly sedating and anticholinergic properties decrease the risk of acute extrapyramidal symptoms, as well as help control highly agitated and excited patients. In most cases, a dose of 100 mg three times a day or less is sufficient to control symptoms without excessive sedation or hypotension. Some patients respond to very low doses such as 10 to 25 mg two to three times a day. Sedation and hypotension are usually the limiting side effects of chlorpromazine, especially after IM administration. Agranulocytosis is estimated to occur in approximately 1 in 2,000 patients on a low-potency phenothiazine, making it desirable to have periodic CBC monitoring and to instruct patients to report signs of infection immediately, particularly during the first four to eight weeks of treatment when most cases of bone marrow suppression occur. The incidence of cholestatic jaundice is estimated at about 2 percent. Photosensitivity, disruption of hypothalamic thermoregulation, lenticular pigmentation, and pigmentary retinopathy also occur. Chlorpromazine has nonpsychiatric uses, such as in the treatment of nausea and vomiting, intractable hiccups, intermittent porphyria, and tetanus. Because of its numerous side effects and risks, it should not be used for the treatment of anxiety for which much safer medications are currently available. Chlorpromazine 25 to 50 mg can counteract the hypertensive crisis due to an MAOI-tyramine interaction; hence, patients on MAOIs may be encouraged to carry chlorpromazine for emergency use.

Chlorpromazine's anticholinergic effects can cause blurred vision, dry mouth, urinary retention, and constipation. Because of its sedative and anticholinergic side effects, it should be used cautiously in the elderly and in patients with cardiovascular disease. In present-day clinical practice, medications such as risperidone, olanzapine, clozapine, and traditional high-potency and medium-potency antipsychotics are favored over chlorpromazine.

Summary of Advantages and Disadvantages of Chlorpromazine

Advantages

- Effective for positive symptoms
- Sedation desirable in highly agitated patients
- Less risk of acute extrapyramidal symptoms due to anticholinergic properties

- Once-a-day administration at bedtime possible up to 300 mg
- Availability in several formats: tablets, sustained release capsules, liquid, rectal suppositories, and parenteral format
- Low-cost generic available

Disadvantages

- Can cause orthostatic hypotension
- Anticholinergic side effects
- Risk of agranulocytosis and cholestatic jaundice, though rare
- More dangerous in overdose, compared to high-potency agents
- Negative symptoms not significantly improved
- Has all the risks associated with traditional antipsychotics, including neuroleptic malignant syndrome and tardive dyskinesia (NMS risk potentially lower than for high-potency drugs)

THIORIDAZINE (MELLARIL)

Thioridazine is a sedating, low-potency phenothiazine antipsychotic with significant anticholinergic effects. It is highly bound to plasma protein and has a half-life of about 10 hours. It is available as liquid form and as 10, 25, 50, 100, 150, and 200 mg tablets. A parenteral form is not available. Common side effects include sedation, orthostatic hypotension, and anticholinergic effects. Extrapyramidal symptoms are relatively fewer compared to high-potency agents. Because of the above-listed side effects, it should be used with particular caution in the elderly and in patients with cardiovascular disease. It can cause retrograde ejaculation, EKG abnormalities such as flattening or inversion of T-waves, and QT prolongation. Its antiemetic property is less than that of chlorpromazine.

The usual adult dosage range for acute treatment is between 200 and 500 mg daily in divided doses, with a maximum of 800 mg per day, above which there is an increased risk of pigmentary retinopathy.

Most patients can be maintained on thioridazine in the range of 100 to 300 mg per day, given as a one-time dose at bedtime. Because of its anticholinergic, sedative, and hypotensive properties, it is not frequently used today as the primary antipsychotic, especially with the advent of risperidone and olanzapine. However, some patients benefit from very low doses such as 10 to 25 mg, taken several times a day. Given its typical neuroleptic side effects and risks, it should not be used for anxiety or insomnia for which other safer medications are available.

Summary of Advantages and Disadvantages of Thioridazine

Advantages

- Effective for positive symptoms
- Low incidence of acute extrapyramidal symptoms
- Sedation beneficial in agitated and excited patients
- Once-a-day administration possible, up to 300 mg at bedtime
- Low cost generic available
- Tablet and liquid forms

Disadvantages

- Can cause orthostatic hypotension, excessive sedation, and EKG abnormalities
- Pronounced anticholinergic actions
- Retrograde ejaculation
- Maximum dose limit of 800 mg per day
- More dangerous in overdose compared to high-potency agents
- Negative symptoms only mildly improved
- Has all the risks associated with traditional antipsychotics, including neuroleptic malignant syndrome and tardive dyskinesia (NMS risk may be less compared to high-potency drugs)
- No parenteral form available

PERPHENAZINE (TRILAFON)

Perphenazine is a high-potency phenothiazine antipsychotic, highly protein bound, with a half-life in excess of 24 hours, enabling once-daily dosing preferably at bedtime for maintenance purposes. It is available in tablet, liquid concentrate, and parenteral forms. Tablets are in 2, 4, 8, and 16 mg strengths. The dosage range for treatment of acute psychosis is 8 mg po TID-QID, but it can be given up to a maximum dose of 64 mg per day, and 10 mg IM every four to six hours, until acute agitation has subsided, usually within 24 to 48 hours. The typical maintenance dosage range is 4 to 16 mg as a one-time dose at bedtime. Liquid form has the advantage of faster absorption, and of preventing "cheeking" of tablets, primarily in inpatient settings.

In addition to possessing all of the risks and side effects associated with a high-potency antipsychotic, perphenazine (being a phenothiazine compound) has certain unique risks such as a slight risk of cholestatic jaundice, photosensitivity, impairment in hypothalamic thermoregulation, lenticular pigmentation, and lenticular retinopathy. However, these adverse events are probably associated more with low-potency phenothiazines such as chlorpromazine (Thorazine) and thioridazine (Mellaril).

Perphenazine is available in fixed combination with amitriptyline (Elavil) in the following strengths, marketed under two brand names, Triavil and Etrafon, and in generic forms.

Fixed Combinations

2/10:	2 mg of perphenazine	+	10 mg amitriptyline
4/10:	4 mg of perphenazine	+	10 mg amitriptyline
2/25:	2 mg of perphenazine	+	25 mg amitriptyline
4/25:	4 mg of perphenazine	+	25 mg amitriptyline
4/50:	4 mg of perphenazine	+	50 mg amitriptyline

Such a fixed combination is convenient for administration and is probably less expensive if the patient requires doses of both medications in one of the fixed ratios as listed above. Generally, a fixed combination is used for milder psychotic conditions with depressive components. Since amitriptyline is highly anticholinergic, the patient may not need concurrent anticholinergic, antiparkinsonian medications. Amitriptyline also provides sedation, antianxiety effects, hypnotic effects, and an increase in appetite. This combination tends to produce a calming effect. However, antipsychotics should not be used if psychotic symptoms or other indications for use of antipsychotics are not present. There are safer medications to treat anxiety, insomnia, hyperactivity, etc. Obviously, when a fixed combination is used, the side effects, risks, and precautions associated with both medications apply.

Summary of Advantages and Disadvantages of Perphenazine

Advantages

- High-potency antipsychotic
- Effective for positive symptoms
- Fairly low sedation
- Low anticholinergic side effects
- Tablet, liquid concentrate, and parenteral forms
- Once-a-day dosing possible

- Low cost due to generic availability
- Fair safety margin in overdose

Disadvantages

- Causes extrapyramidal symptoms more frequently compared to low-potency antipsychotics
- Negative symptoms are not significantly improved
- Has all the risks associated with antipsychotics, including tardive dyskinesia
- Has the unique risks associated with phenothiazines

Additional Advantages of Fixed Combination (Perphenazine and Amitriptyline)

- Convenient
- Economical
- Anticholinergic prophylaxis built-in, due to highly anticholinergic amitriptyline
- Improves depression and anxiety
- Improves sleep if given at bedtime

Additional Disadvantages of Fixed Combination (Perphenazine and Amitriptyline)

- Inflexible dosing
- Fair safety in overdose is defeated due to the presence of TCA
- Not generally useful in acute and severe psychoses when higher antipsychotic dose is needed
- No IM form

FLUPHENAZINE (PROLIXIN)

Fluphenazine is a high-potency phenothiazine antipsychotic, which is highly protein bound and has a half-life of approximately 24 hours. It is used in doses of 2 to 10 mg per day for maintenance treatment and doses up to 20 mg per day for treatment of acute psychosis. The tablets come in 1, 2.5, 5, and 10 mg doses. Fluphenazine is available in scored tablet, liquid, parenteral, and long-acting depot forms. Its potency is comparable to haloperidol. It shares the risks associated with phenothiazines, including rare cholestatic jaundice, photosensitivity, and thermoregulatory disturbance, but the risk is lower in comparison to low-potency phenothiazines. Fluphenazine causes a higher incidence of acute extrapyramidal symptoms but less sedation or hypotension, as is the case with all traditional high-potency agents.

Highly agitated patients can be effectively treated with an IM dose of 5 mg every four to six hours or more often, up to 30 mg per day, prior to switching to an oral dose. Since fluphenazine can precipitate acute dystonia and other acute extrapyramidal symptoms, coadministration of an anticholinergic medication such as benztropine (Cogentin), trihexiphenidyl (Artane), or diphenhydramine (Benadryl) during the first four to eight weeks should be considered. The adjunctive use of a benzodiazepine is extremely effective for controlling an agitated patient. For example, the adjunctive use of fluphenazine 5 mg IM and lorazepam 0.5 mg or 1 mg IM once or twice is sufficient to control most of the severely agitated patients. Patients with respiratory compromise should be given benzodiazepines at very low doses, especially when given concurrently with other medications that cause synergistic sedation, as is true with all antipsychotics in varying degrees. Geriatric patients may respond well on very low doses such as fluphenazine 0.5 to 1 mg, given as a bedtime dose.

The parenteral long-acting depot form is available in two preparations: (1) fluphenazine decanoate, given IM every three to four weeks; and (2) fluphenazine enanthate, given IM every two weeks. The long-acting depot form should be used only after the patient is stabilized on oral or parenteral fluphenazine to assure tolerability and effectiveness. The conversion ratio is 6.25 mg of the decanoate every three to four weeks for every 5 mg of the regular oral daily dose. For example, since most patients are maintained on 5 mg daily, a starting dose of fluphenazine decanoate 6.25 mg every three to four weeks is usually sufficient. For fluphenazine enanthate, the conversion ratio remains the same, but the dosage interval is shorter. Fluphenazine enanthate is given every two weeks. Because fluphenazine decanoate affords a longer interval of three to four weeks between doses, this is preferred by most clinicians and patients, as is the case with haloperidol decanoate. Since it takes two months for the depot preparation to reach a steady state, an extra dose of 2.5 mg of fluphenazine decanoate or enanthate may be given during the first two or three administrations to guard against clinical deterioration in the initial two months after switching to depot injection. Another option is to keep the dosage the same, but administer the medication one week earlier than the standard interval for the first two or three administrations, and then increase the interval to the standard schedule. Generally, it is advisable not to give a loading dose due to the greater frequency of side effects.

As is the case with haloperidol decanoate, the primary advantage of long-acting preparations is assurance of compliance in poorly compliant patients. Patients who have erratic absorption from the gastrointestinal tract also benefit from long-acting depot IM medication.

Summary of Advantages and Disadvantages of Fluphenazine

Advantages

- Potent antipsychotic
- Low sedation
- Low anticholinergic side effects
- Tablet, IM, liquid, and two types of long-acting depot forms
- Scored tablet form, enabling flexible dosing
- Minimal cardiovascular side effects
- Generic form available at low cost

Disadvantages

- Relatively higher incidence of acute extrapyramidal symptoms
- Negative symptoms not significantly improved
- Has all the risks and side effects associated with phenothiazines, including neuroleptic malignant syndrome, blood dyscrasias, and tardive dyskinesia
- Long-acting medication action cannot be stopped immediately, should an adverse reaction occur

TRIFLUOPERAZINE (STELAZINE)

Trifluoperazine is a high-potency phenothiazine antipsychotic, highly protein bound, with a half-life in excess of 24 hours. It is available in tablet, liquid, and parenteral IM forms. The tablets are in 1, 2, 5, and 10 mg doses. The dosage range for treatment of acute psychosis is between 5 and 20 mg, although some patients may require up to 40 mg per day. A common maintenance dosage range is 2 to 10 mg, administered as a once-a-day dose at bedtime. In adults, an IM dose of 2 to 4 mg every four hours, up to 20 mg per day, can be given for rapid control of a severely agitated psychosis, along with adjunctive use of benzodiazepines. Once the agitation has subsided and the patient is more cooperative, oral medication may be given.

Trifluoperazine shares the risks associated with phenothiazines, such as rare agranulocytosis, cholestatic jaundice, photosensitivity, and impairment of thermoregulatory control. These risks are, however, significantly less compared to the low-potency phenothiazines. Since trifluoperazine can cause acute extrapyramidal symptoms including dystonic reaction, concomitant administration of anticholinergic medication is desirable, especially during the first four to six weeks. It has antiemetic properties like chlorpromazine. It is said to be a mildly stimulating antipsychotic at low doses.

Summary of Advantages and Disadvantages of Trifluoperazine

Advantages

- Potent antipsychotic
- Low sedation
- Low anticholinergic side effects
- Tablet, liquid, and IM forms
- Minimal cardiovascular side effects
- Generic form available at low cost

Disadvantages

- Relatively high incidence of acute extrapyramidal symptoms
- Negative symptoms not significantly improved
- Has unique phenothiazine side effects (but less compared to low-potency phenothiazines)
- Risk of neuroleptic malignant syndrome and tardive dyskinesia similar to all traditional high-potency antipsychotics

MESORIDAZINE (SERENTIL)

Mesoridazine is a low-potency phenothiazine antipsychotic. It is an active metabolite of thioridazine, is twice as potent as thioridazine, and has one-tenth the potency of haloperidol or fluphenazine. It is available in an IM form whereas thioridazine is not. In addition, tablets and liquid forms are available. Tablets are available in 10, 25, 50, and 100 mg strengths. Since IM administration is irritating to tissue, the oral form is preferred. It has hypotensive and cardiovascular side effects when administered intramuscularly. Therefore, the author's preference is to use high-potency antipsychotics when IM administration is necessary, combined with benzodiazepines if additional sedation is desired. When given IM, it can also cause increased risk of hypotension and cardiovascular side effects. Mesoridazine has a moderate risk for causing extrapyramidal symptoms and moderate anticholinergic properties. The dosage range for patients with acute and severe psychotic agitation is between 200 and 500 mg per day in divided doses. The maintenance dose is between 100 and 200 mg, given as a single bedtime dose. It can cause QT prolongation and T-wave flattening or inversion. Pigmentary retinopathy is not a particular concern with mesoridazine.

Summary of Advantages and Disadvantages of Mesoridazine

Advantages

- Effective for positive symptoms
- Fairly low incidence of acute extrapyramidal symptoms
- Once-a-day administration possible, up to 300 mg at bedtime
- Tablet, liquid, and IM forms
- Fewer anticholinergic side effects compared to thioridazine

Disadvantages

- Negative symptoms only mildly improved
- Has all the risks associated with traditional antipsychotics, including neuroleptic malignant syndrome and tardive dyskinesia
- Can cause EKG abnormalities

MOLINDONE (MOBAN)

Molindone is a fairly potent antipsychotic with a half-life of approximately two hours, and a duration of action of about 24 hours, enabling bedtime dosing in maintenance patients. It is highly protein bound, as are all antipsychotics. Molindone is available in 10, 25, 50, and 100 mg tablets and in liquid form. The dosage range for treatment of acute severe psychosis is 100 to 200 mg per day in divided doses, while the dosage range for maintenance treatment is between 25 and 75 mg per day as one bedtime dose. Since a parenteral form is not available, acutely agitated patients who need IM medication will have to be controlled on other antipsychotics. Molindone might not cause significant weight gain.

Summary of Advantages and Disadvantages of Molindone

Advantages

- Fairly potent antipsychotic
- Effective for positive symptoms
- Low anticholinergic side effects
- Tablet and liquid forms
- No significant weight gain in most patients
- Relatively less of a decrease in seizure threshold

Disadvantages

- Negative symptoms not significantly improved
- Has all the risks associated with traditional antipsychotics, including neuroleptic malignant syndrome and tardive dyskinesia
- Generic form not available; fairly expensive
- IM form not available

LOXAPINE (LOXITANE)

Loxapine is a medium-potency antipsychotic available in liquid, parenteral IM, and as 5, 10, 25, and 50 mg capsules. The dosage for the management of acute severe psychosis is between 100 and 200 mg per day in divided doses. The maximum daily dose is 225 mg. For very agitated patients, it may be given 25 to 50 mg IM every four to six hours until the patient is cooperative and calm enough to accept medication orally, usually within 24 to 48 hours. The maintenance dose of loxapine is in the range of 25 to 100 mg, preferably as a bedtime dose. One of the metabolites of loxapine is 8-hydroxyamoxapine, which has clinically insignificant antidepressant activity. Loxapine tends to lower the seizure threshold and hence is relatively contraindicated in patients with a history of seizures, or in those who are predisposed to seizures.

Summary of Advantages and Disadvantages of Loxapine

Advantages

- Medium-potency antipsychotic
- Effective for positive symptoms
- Capsule, liquid, and parenteral IM forms
- Fairly low anticholinergic side effects
- Generic available

Disadvantages

- Negative symptoms not significantly improved
- Has all the risks associated with traditional antipsychotics, including neuroleptic malignant syndrome and tardive dyskinesia
- Tends to lower seizure threshold

CHLORPROTHIXENE (TARACTAN)

Chlorprothixene is a low-potency antipsychotic available in liquid, parenteral IM, and in tablet form in doses of 10, 25, 50, and 100 mg strengths. The dosage range for acutely severe psychosis is between 200 and 500 mg per day in divided doses, with a maximum oral dose of 600 mg per day. For rapid control of severely agitated and uncooperative psychotic patients, it can be administered in doses of 25 to 50 mg IM every four to six hours until acute agitation has subsided and the patient is able to accept oral medications, usually within 24 to 48 hours. Maintenance dosage is in the range of 50 to 200 mg, given at bedtime.

Summary of Advantages and Disadvantages of Chlorprothixene

Advantages

- Effective for positive symptoms
- Sedating property beneficial for agitated patients
- Somewhat low risk of acute extrapyramidal symptoms
- Tablet, liquid, and parenteral IM forms

Disadvantages

- Can cause orthostatic hypotension
- Has anticholinergic side effects
- Has all the risks associated with traditional and phenothiazine antipsychotics, including neuroleptic malignant syndrome, tardive dyskinesia, and blood dyscrasias
- Minimal effect on negative symptoms
- Generic not available; fairly expensive

Chapter 12

Antipsychotic Side Effects and Their Management

ACUTE DYSTONIA

Acute dystonic reaction occurs in about 30 to 40 percent of patients treated on fairly high doses of high-potency antipsychotic medication, usually within three to four days of initiating treatment. The incidence of this side effect is less frequent with low-potency antipsychotics such as chlorpromazine, thioridazine, mesoridazine, chlorprothixene, clozapine, and the newly introduced atypical antipsychotics risperidone and olanzapine. As the dose is increased, the risk of acute dystonia increases proportionately for risperidone. The antipsychotics that most frequently cause acute dystonia are fluphenazine, haloperidol, trifluoperazine, thiothixene, perphenazine, molindone, and loxapine. Acute dystonic reaction can take various forms such as oculogyric crisis, stiffness of the tongue and pharynx, rare but serious laryngospasm, torticollis, opisthotonos, and generalized muscular rigidity. It can develop rapidly, and hence can be quite alarming to the patient. Fortunately, effective and immediate treatment is available.

Anticholinergic medications are the treatment of choice. Benztropine (Cogentin) 2 mg or diphenhydramine 25 to 50 mg given IM or IV is effective within five to ten minutes. Patients should be reassured that acute dystonia is a reaction to the medication and that treatment will completely resolve the symptom. Common antinausea medications such as prochlorperazine (Compazine) and metoclopramide (Reglan) also can cause EPS, including acute dystonia.

Since acute dystonic reaction tends to occur more frequently in young males, it is reasonable to routinely give an anticholinergic medication orally along with the antipsychotic during the first several weeks, after which the anticholinergic medication may be tapered off. Although an anticholinergic given orally is effective, acute dystonic reaction should be treated using IM medication because of the 20 to 30 minutes it may take for oral medication to begin to work. The patient who develops acute dystonia should be started on a standing anticholinergic medication and maintained for several weeks.

<u>Common Oral Doses</u>

- benztropine (Cogentin) 1 mg po TID
- diphenhydramine (Benadryl) 25 to 50 mg po TID
- trihexyphenidyl (Artane) 2 mg po TID
- biperiden (Akineton) 2 mg po TID
- procyclidine (Kemadrin) 2.5 mg po TID

<u>Common IM Doses</u>

- benztropine (Cogentin) 2 mg IM
- biperiden (Akineton) 2 mg IM
- diphenhydramine (Benadryl) 25 mg IM

<u>Common IV Doses</u>

- benztropine (Cogentin) 1 to 2 mg IV
- diphenhydramine (Benadryl) 25 mg IV

If a dystonic reaction occurs while a patient is already on an anticholinergic medication, the dose of the anticholinergic should be increased temporarily, or the dose of the antipsychotic decreased. Decreasing the dose is not a practical option in most cases because such an action could interfere with acute symptom control. If the patient cannot tolerate anticholinergic medication, benzodiazepines may be employed for managing acute dystonic reaction and for prophylactic use. The following are some examples:

– lorazepam (Ativan) 1 to 2 mg IM
– oxazepam (Serax) 30 mg po
– diazepam (Valium) 10 mg IM
– clonazepam (Klonopin) 0.5 mg po BID

Although acute dystonic reactions are less frequent with risperidone in low to moderate doses of 1 to 4 mg per day, their frequency approaches that of traditional high-potency antipsychotics when the dose of risperidone exceeds 6 mg per day. In general, at very low doses, the chance of emergence of dystonic reactions is lower compared to high dosage for all antipsychotics. Both the oral and IM routes of high-potency antipsychotics cause the highest incidence of acute dystonia. Haloperidol IV up to 5 mg when administered short-term tends to cause very low incidence of acute dystonia or other extrapyramidal symptoms, for unknown reasons. Acute laryngospasm due to laryngeal dystonia can compromise the airway and is a medical emergency requiring immediate IV or IM administration of one of the anticholinergics, and maintenance of the airway, if necessary.

Other manifestations include protrusion or stiffness of the tongue, pharyngeal dystonia, and trismus. Occasionally, very low doses of high-potency antipsychotics can induce a dystonic reaction; however, the reactions are likely to be mild.

Patients on low doses of antipsychotics, such as haloperidol 0.5 to 2 mg per day or equivalent, may be started as outpatients without concurrent anticholinergic medications. Patients started on haloperidol between 2 and 5 mg as outpatients should be considered for concomitant treatment with anticholinergic medication to prevent acute dystonia. In most cases, if a patient's symptoms require a starting dose of more than haloperidol 5 mg, or and equivalent dose of another antipsychotic, the author prefers to hospitalize the patient briefly and stabilize him or her on medications for safety.

AKATHISIA

Akathisia is a common side effect of all antipsychotic medications, although it is more frequently seen with high-potency antipsychotics, including risperidone. It is rarely seen with clozapine. Akathisia is manifested by symptoms such as muscular restlessness, an urge to keep moving, frequent pacing, and a feeling as though one wants to "jump out of the skin." It should not be confused with psychotic agitation. Akathisia usually develops within one to two weeks after starting an antipsychotic. The higher the dosage, the greater the chance of developing akathisia and the greater the severity. The physician should have a low threshold for detecting akathisia since patients have difficulty verbalizing their discomfort. Akathisia is so common that physicians should actively look for the symptoms and signs in every patient taking antipsychotic medication.

Treatment consists of adding an anticholinergic medication, antihistamine, dopaminergic medication, benzodiazepine, beta-blocker, or clonidine. The following is a list of various medications of potential benefit for treatment of akathisia.

Medications and Doses for Treatment of Akathisia

- benztropine (Cogentin) 1 to 2 mg po TID
- trihexyphenidyl (Artane) 2 to 5 mg po TID
- biperiden (Akineton) 2 mg po BID-TID
- procyclidine (Kemadrin) 2.5 to 5 mg po BID
- diphenhydramine (Benadryl) 25 to 50 mg po TID
- amantadine (Symmetrel) 100 to 200 mg po BID
- lorazepam (Ativan) 0.5 to 1 mg po TID
- clonazepam (Klonopin) 0.5 mg po BID-TID
- alprazolam (Xanax) 0.25 to 0.5 mg po TID
- oxazepam (Serax) 15 mg po TID
- propranolol (Inderal) 10 to 20 mg po TID
- propranolol LA (Inderal LA) 60 to 80 mg po daily
- atenolol (Tenormin) 50 mg po daily
- clonidine (Catapres) 0.1 mg po BID-TID

In most cases, significant improvement of akathisia can be expected with appropriate treatment. Although the ideal approach is to discontinue or decrease the antipsychotic, this is neither practical nor prudent, simply because psychosis will reemerge. Among the medications listed above, an initial trial on an anticholinergic medication is appropriate if parkinsonian symptoms are also present, since this approach may be the most parsimonious. If the patient has only akathisia, the first choice of medication would be a beta-blocker, with anticholinergics as the second choice, and benzodiazepines as the third choice. If any one of the medications for treating akathisia is partially effective, another from a different class can be added to achieve a better effect. Some examples follow:

– Propranolol LA 60 mg daily + lorazepam 0.5 mg po BID
– Benztropine 1 mg po TID + propranolol LA 60 mg po daily
– Benztropine 1 mg po TID + alprazolam 0.25 mg po TID

Switching the patient to a low-potency antipsychotic can sometimes help, if clinically appropriate. Diligent efforts by the physician in prescribing one medication or combinations of two or three adjunctive medications, can improve akathisia significantly to the point that the patient is not in distress. If akathisia is not diagnosed and treated, patients are likely to discontinue the antipsychotic or may even resort to substance abuse (especially alcohol) or increase cigarette smoking (as a means of self-treatment).

PARKINSONISM

Drug-induced parkinsonism or "pseudo-parkinsonism" is a common side effect of antipsychotics. The highest incidence is with traditional high-potency antipsychotics such as fluphenazine (Prolixin), haloperidol (Haldol), and others. It is also seen in association with low-potency antipsychotics. The incidence is low with risperidone (at low doses) and olanzapine, and very low with clozapine. The signs consist of tremor, bradykinesia, mask-like facies, drooling, rigidity, shuffling gait, slow speech, and apathy. As in the case of akathisia, the higher the dosage, the greater the probability of developing parkinsonism and the greater the severity. The symptoms occur usually after the first three to five days of starting treatment. It is more common and more severe in the elderly and in women. Treatment consists of adding an antiparkinsonian drug or amantadine. Some examples are listed here:

– benztropine (Cogentin) 1 mg po TID
– trihexyphenidyl (Artane) 2-5 mg po TID
– biperiden (Akineton) 2 mg po BID-TID
– procyclidine (Kemadrin) 2.5-5 mg po BID-TID
– diphenhydramine (Benadryl) 25-50 mg po TID
– amantadine (Symmetrel) 100-200 mg po BID

Anticholinergic medications tend to cause dry mouth, blurred vision, constipation, urinary hesitation, and tachycardia. Excessive doses can lead to central anticholinergic syndrome consisting of confusion; delirium; dilated pupils; dry mouth; and warm, dry skin. Hence, combining highly anticholinergic low-potency antipsychotics and anticholinergic medications should be attempted cautiously, especially in children and the elderly who are very susceptible to these adverse effects. Amantadine is preferred for the treatment of pseudoparkinsonism if low-potency antipsychotics are used, in order to avoid anticholinergic toxicity, whereas anticholinergic drugs or amantadine may be used with high-potency antipsychotics without such a concern. At lower than 3 mg of risperidone, the incidence of extrapyramidal symptoms is fairly low. Therefore, concurrent medication to treat extrapyramidal symptoms is usually not needed with risperidone.

After several weeks of being on an anticholinergic drug, the dosage should be decreased gradually to see if the patient has become tolerant to the side effects, in which case the anticholinergic drugs can be slowly tapered off. It is also possible in most cases to decrease the antipsychotic dose to a maintenance dose after three to four weeks of being on the higher acute dose, thereby decreasing the severity of the side effects, including extrapyramidal symptoms. Some patients require anticholinergic medications for the duration of the antipsychotic treatment. Elderly individuals who have idiopathic parkinsonism may be very sensitive to high-potency antipsychotics. These patients would be appropriate candidates for risperidone, olanzapine, clozapine, or low-potency antipsychotics. Although low potency antipsychotics, such as thioridazine (Mellaril) or chlorpromazine (Thorazine) at low doses may help parkinsonism, an antipsychotic dose increase is frequently necessary to relieve psychosis, increasing the risk of anticholinergic side effects. Hence, risperidone and olanzapine are good choices as antipsychotic in the elderly, along with amantadine if extrapyramidal symptoms develop.

NEUROLEPTIC MALIGNANT SYNDROME

Neuroleptic malignant syndrome (NMS) is one of the rarely occurring extrapyramidal symptoms due to antipsychotic treatment. If it is not promptly diagnosed and managed, the mortality rate is high; therefore, it is important to be aware of the nature of its presentation and management.

NMS is characterized by fever, rigidity, autonomic instability (tachycardia and hypertension), delirium, drooling, sweating, agitation, leukocytosis, increased liver enzymes, increased CPK (creatine phosphokinase), and myoglobulinuria. All of these symptoms and signs may not be present in all patients with NMS. It tends to occur more in young males with central nervous system (CNS) lesions and in patients on concomitant CNS-acting medications. High-potency antipsychotics, including risperidone, seem to be associated with a higher risk of NMS, compared to low-potency antipsychotics, including clozapine. If recognized and managed promptly, treatment is very effective. It is estimated to occur in about 1 percent of patients treated with antipsychotics, with a higher incidence in susceptible individuals on high-potency antipsychotics. NMS can occur within several days to one month after starting antipsychotic medication or after a major dosage increase.

The mainstays of treatment are stopping the antipsychotic immediately, IV hydration, and supportive measures. The patient is usually admitted to an intensive care unit or general medical unit. Dantrolene (Dantrium) may be given in doses of 50 mg po TID, or 2 to 4 mg/kg per day IM or IV, divided into a TID or QID schedule, until symptoms are resolved. Dantrolene controls muscle rigidity and prevents muscle breakdown. Bromocriptine (Parlodel) is added to this regimen at a dose of 5 mg po every six hours until symptoms have subsided. Another option, if bromocriptine is not tolerated, is amantadine (Symmetrel) in a dose of 100 mg po three times a day.

Fever should be managed with antipyretics and cooling blankets. Other supportive measures including IV hydration and respiratory support, if required, should be available and provided. During the acute phase of NMS, the patient is usually in an intensive care unit or in a medical unit where management is primarily provided by a critical care specialist, internist, or neurologist, with the psychiatrist in a consulting role. However, the psychiatrist should be familiar with the basic diagnostic, acute management, and post-recovery management information to assist other specialists who may not be as familiar with the presentation and management of this syndrome.

The syndrome usually lasts five to ten days. It is prolonged with long-acting depot antipsychotics such as fluphenazine decanoate, fluphenazine enanthate, and haloperidol decanoate. If patients become psychotic, treatment options include temporary use of benzodiazepines, clonidine (Catapres), and ECT. Depot antipsychotics should be avoided in patients who have had one episode of NMS. When an antipsychotic is restarted, a low-potency antipsychotic or an antipsychotic from another class at low doses should be considered, with close supervision by the physician. Thioridazine, risperidone, olanzapine, and clozapine may be associated with a decreased risk of NMS.

TARDIVE DYSKINESIA

Tardive dyskinesia is a side effect of all antipsychotic medications, with the possible exception of clozapine (Clozaril). It usually appears after chronic intake of antipsychotic medication, and may be resistant to remission even if the antipsychotic is withdrawn. It consists of abnormal movements such as oral and lingual dyskinesias, and choreiform movements of the extremities and trunk. Common forms include vermiform movements, twisting, darting and protrusion of tongue, puckering, chewing movements, puffing of cheeks, sucking movements, facial grimaces, and various abnormal choreiform movements of the trunk, hip, ankle, shoulder, and neck. Less commonly, tardive dystonia–consisting of sustained dystonic movements of extremities, trunk, and neck–can coexist. Akathisia and tardive akathisia can also be present, making the clinical presentation more complex. Although any combination of abnormal movements can occur, the most common symptoms are confined to oral-buccal-lingual dyskinesias. Typically, decreasing or discontinuing the antipsychotic can worsen tardive dyskinesia at least temporarily, and increasing the dose can suppress or mask tardive dyskinesia, although eventually the dyskinesia will break through this masking. Total duration of treatment and, to some extent, cumulative dose tend to correlate with the development of tardive dyskinesia. Mild presentations do not interfere with function but may be cosmetically undesirable. Severe forms can be incapacitating.

Anticholinergic medications and anxiety can worsen dyskinetic movements, which disappear while sleeping. Tardive dyskinesia develops usually after one to two years of antipsychotic treatment, though occasionally it can occur after three to four months of antipsychotic treatment. The elderly are more prone to developing tardive dyskinesia early in the course of antipsychotic treatment.

There is some expectation that risperidone (Risperdal), olanzapine (Zyprexa), and sertindole (Serlect) have a lower risk of causing tardive dyskinesia. Because they are relatively new, time will bear out whether or not this is the case. However, because of the permanent nature of tardive dyskinesia, even the probability of decreased risk should generate interest in risperidone, olanzapine, and sertindole as a first-line antipsychotic.

Clearly superior results have been obtained with clozapine, which has caused tardive dyskinesia to regress in some patients. The author has had several patients for whom typical oral-buccal-lingual movements consistent with tardive dyskinesia have retrogressed after clozapine dosage reached the 300 to 400 mg range. It is also believed that clozapine has very little, if any, risk of causing tardive dyskinesia or associated akathisia. Strictly from a tardive dyskinesia risk standpoint, clozapine is superior to all currently available antipsychotic medications. It should be considered in anyone who is expected to need long-term antipsychotic medication. Risks and problems associated with clozapine are discussed in Chapter 11.

There is no uniformly effective treatment for tardive dyskinesia, other than not using antipsychotic medication. However, this is not a practical option if a patient has chronic psychosis; hence, after the patient's acute psychosis is controlled, the physician must discuss with the patient–and if possible with the family–the advantages and disadvantages of being on an antipsychotic medication, with specific reference to tardive dyskinesia. An entry should be made in the patient's chart indicating that these issues were discussed. Obviously, as in any other medical treatment in which there are risks, a balanced presentation along with the physician's recommendations should be given. Patients and family should be told that, given the chronic and debilitating nature of the patient's condition and given the expected deterioration if medication is not taken, the benefits of taking the medication outweigh the risks.

Only patients with chronic psychosis or other severe mental disorders should be prescribed antipsychotics long-term. It is clinically impractical and risky to stop antipsychotic medication to prevent tardive dyskinesia in patients with chronic psychosis. Antipsychotics are also used to treat conditions that are less chronic, such as mania, psychotic depression, severe agitation, etc. For these indications, antipsychotic drugs should be gradually withdrawn as soon as the patient is maintained on a primary medication such as an antidepressant, mood stabilizer, or antianxiety medication, depending on the condition. The risk of tardive dyskinesia usually is not a practical clinical concern with the use of antipsychotic medications for the short term; that is, less than two to three months except in the elderly. If an antipsychotic is expected to be used for more than two to three months, especially at high doses, tardive dyskinesia risk should be discussed with the patient and this should be documented on the patient's chart.

PERIORAL TREMOR OR "RABBIT SYNDROME"

Perioral tremor or "rabbit syndrome" is one of the extrapyramidal symptoms, consisting of rapid rhythmic movement of the lips, usually occurring in patients on high-potency antipsychotic medications. There is usually no involvement of the tongue. Addition of an anticholinergic medication should improve this condition.

CONSTIPATION AND URINARY RETENTION

Constipation can be managed by bethanechol 10 to 25 mg po TID or stool softener and/or laxative. Bethanechol 10 to 25 mg po TID may be used to treat anticholinergic-induced urinary retention. Bethanechol may also improve blurry vision, which typically affects near vision. Refer to Chapter 5 for details.

AUTONOMIC EFFECTS

Hypotension and orthostatic hypotension are common side effects of low-potency antipsychotics such as chlorpromazine (Thorazine), thioridazine (Mellaril), mesoridazine (Serentil), chlorprothixene (Taractan), and clozapine (Clozaril). Patients with cardiovascular disorders and diabetes, as well as the elderly are more prone to this side effect. High-potency antipsychotics do not cause this side effect as often. If hypotension is significant and the patient is doing extremely well on a particular medication for which there is no substitute, sodium chloride supplementation by increasing salt intake may be beneficial. If this is not effective, administration of fludrocortisone (Florinef) at doses 0.1 to 0.3 mg po daily may be considered if there is no heart failure or other disorders that might cause significant fluid retention (e.g., cirrhosis, nephrotic syndrome).

Anticholinergic side effects such as dry mouth, constipation, urinary hesitation, blurred vision, and tachycardia are pronounced with low-potency antipsychotics, especially at high doses. Dry mouth may improve with the use of bethanechol 10 to 25 mg po TID, frequent mouthwash using pilocarpine 1 percent solution, or chewing sugar-free gum. Dry mucus membranes can worsen breathing in people with respiratory problems. Rarely, paralytic ileus has resulted. Additive anticholinergic effects leading to anticholinergic toxicity and consequent delirium can occur if several medications with anticholinergic effects are given concurrently. An example is coadministration of amitriptyline, thioridazine, and benztropine. Drugs with anticholinergic properties can precipitate narrow-angle glaucoma in susceptible individuals.

Antipsychotics, especially low-potency drugs, can cause ejaculatory inhibition and decreased libido. Thioridazine (Mellaril) in particular is known to cause retrograde ejaculation. Medications such as bethanechol (Urecholine) in doses 10 to 25 mg po TID, amantadine (Symmetrel) 100 mg po BID, yohimbine (Yocon) 5.4 mg po BID, cyproheptadine (Periactin) 4 to 8 mg po several hours prior to coitus, bupropion (Wellbutrin) 75 to 100 mg po BID, and methylphenidate (Ritalin) 5 to 10 mg one hour prior to coitus, have occasionally been found beneficial for treatment of sexual dysfunction. However, all of these have a low success rate.

Sedation

Sedation is particularly common and marked with low-potency antipsychotics, but may be desirable in treating highly agitated patients. All antipsychotics, including high-potency drugs, have sedative effects in sufficient doses. After the acute symptoms are controlled, sedative properties can be exploited by giving most or all of the medication at bedtime, thereby enhancing sleep and minimizing daytime sedation. However, with high doses of low-potency antipsychotics, persistent daytime sedation can be a problem in the majority of cases. The author's preference is to use high- or medium-potency antipsychotics in conjunction with benzodiazepines on an as needed basis if sedation is desired.

With the atypical antipsychotic risperidone, about one-third of patients experience moderate sedation, whereas one-third of patients may experience increased activation or alertness, requiring a benzodiazepine at bedtime or switching risperidone to a morning schedule.

Hematological Side Effects

Benign mild leukopenia is occasionally seen with low-potency antipsychotics such as chlorpromazine and thioridazine. Agranulocytosis is extremely rare and believed to occur in approximately 1 in 10,000 patients treated on antipsychotics, with higher incidence in patients taking low-potency phenothiazines; therefore, routine blood test monitoring of WBC is not usually done, except with clozapine for which the incidence is estimated at 1 percent. Patients taking phenothiazines should be advised to report any signs of infection such as fever, sore throat, mouth sores, or weakness, especially in the first four to eight weeks of treatment. For patients on low-potency phenothiazines, occasional CBC monitoring during the first four months should be considered for detection of blood dyscrasias.

Endocrinologic Effects

All antipsychotics, including risperidone, can increase prolactin levels, causing galactorrhea, gynecomastia, breast tenderness, amenorrhea, weight gain, edema, delayed menstruation, and delayed ovulation. Clozapine, olanzapine, and sertindole have very little effect on the prolactin level, and hence may be the only exceptions, among currently available antipsychotics. Decreased libido and inhibition of orgasm are also seen.

Antipsychotic-induced increase in prolactin level rarely exceeds 100 ng/ml. A prolactin level higher than 300 ng/ml strongly suggests other causes such as prolactinomas or a lesion of the hypothalamus or pituitary stalk. For drug-induced hyperprolactinemia presenting with symptoms or signs as listed, treatment considerations include dosage decrease or discontinuation of the offending drug if clinically appropriate, treatment using bromocriptine (Parlodel) 2.5 to 5 mg once or twice daily, amantadine 100 mg BID-TID, or switching to olanzapine or clozapine. A pituitary adenoma should be ruled out if there is clinical suspicion of an etiology other than drug-induced. The most common side effects of bromocriptine are nausea, headache, dizziness, and fatigue; these are most common at the higher dose range.

Risperidone and molindone are not frequently associated with significant weight gain. Other uncommon endocrinologic effects include changes in metabolism resulting in hypoglycemia or hyperglycemia.

Allergic and Skin Effects

Phenothiazines, particularly chlorpromazine (Thorazine), can cause cholestatic jaundice, photosensitivity, and skin rashes. The medication should be discontinued if a rash or jaundice (hyperbilirubinemia) develops. Patients should be warned of increased sensitivity to sunlight and of the need for reducing sun exposure. Patients should be encouraged to use sunscreen if sun exposure is anticipated. Decreased sweating leading to hyperthermia can also result. Patients should be advised to avoid strenuous activity in hot conditions, especially while on low-potency antipsychotics including clozapine. Patients taking highly anticholinergic psychotropic medications, adjunctive anticholinergics, or antipsychotics may be at increased risk for thermoplegia due to anticholinergic-induced hypohidrosis, or neuroleptic-induced impairment in thermoregulation, particularly during prolonged exposure to hot conditions.

Cardiac Effects

Low-potency antipsychotics and clozapine are likely to cause hypotension, especially in high doses. Phenothiazines, especially thioridazine can cause prolongation of QT interval and flattening or inversion of T-waves. Patients already on cardiac medications and on TCAs may be at increased risk. Clozapine can cause sinus tachycardia, which can be managed using beta-blockers with attention paid to hypotension and orthostatic hypotension. Sertindole can cause mild prolongation of QT interval.

Chapter 13

Miscellaneous Clinical Topics

INSOMNIA

Insomnia is a common symptom encountered in primary care and in psychiatric practice. Various psychiatric problems, including anxiety disorders, mood disorders, psychotic disorders, or situational stress can cause insomnia. Many physical disorders such as nocturia, obstructive sleep apnea, and pain can also cause insomnia. In most of these cases, satisfactory treatment of the primary psychiatric condition or the primary medical problem will eventually improve insomnia. However, during the first several weeks after initiating treatment for the primary condition, adjunctive sleep medications may be necessary. In some patients, insomnia is chronic, requiring treatment for more than several weeks. Situational stresses typically cause insomnia, which remits when the stress is addressed in real life or when stress-induced psychological conflicts are resolved in therapy. Insomnia can be classified into three types: (1) initial insomnia, (2) middle insomnia or restless sleep, and (3) terminal insomnia or early-morning awakening. It is important for the clinician to know the exact nature of insomnia in order to recommend an appropriate choice of medication. The ideal hypnotic will have the following characteristics:

- Optimization of sleep without altering normal sleep architecture
- No daytime sedation
- No dependence potential
- No rebound insomnia upon discontinuation
- No tolerance, making it effective for chronic use if needed
- No significant side effects or interactions with other medications

Obviously, there are no hypnotics currently available that meet the above qualifications. However, there are several hypnotics that are effective and safe for short-term use.

An effective medication that is a good overall first choice for treatment of insomnia is the antidepressant trazodone (Desyrel). At doses of 50 to 150 mg at bedtime, it works well as a hypnotic with no risk of addiction, and has hardly any tolerance. It is effective for initial, middle, and terminal insomnia, and at the low dosage employed for treating insomnia it can be used with SSRIs as well as with MAOIs and bupropion. It does not significantly alter the sleep architecture apart from slightly increasing REM latency and decreasing REM intensity and stage 4 intensity—effects produced by most antidepressants to varying degrees. Some patients need only 25 mg of trazodone at bedtime. There are several patients in my practice who sleep well on doses as low as 12.5 mg (one quarter of a 50 mg tablet) at bedtime. At the low dosages typically employed for treatment of insomnia, the effects on sleep architecture are expected to be minimal. Doses greater than 200 mg should be used cautiously if given to a patient on another antidepressant because of increased risk of interaction. Trazodone can be used with bupropion (Wellbutrin), which tends to cause insomnia. Most patients respond to a 50 to 100 mg dose. See Chapter 4 for more details on trazodone. Depending on the exact nature of the insomnia, different medications are more or less effective than others.

Initial Insomnia

In patients who have no difficulty maintaining sleep, but have difficulty falling asleep, a medication with rapid onset of action and fairly short duration of action should be sufficient. The options are the following:

- trazodone (Desyrel) 50-150 mg
- zolpidem (Ambien) 5-10 mg
- triazolam (Halcion) 0.125-0.25 mg
- lorazepam (Ativan) 0.5-1 mg
- chloral hydrate (Noctec) 500-1000 mg
- temazepam (Restoril) 7.5-30 mg
- estazolam (Prosom) 1-2 mg
- alprazolam (Xanax) 0.25-0.5 mg
- oxazepam (Serax) 15-30 mg
- diphenhydramine (Benadryl) 25-50 mg
- hydroxyzine (Vistaril) 25-50 mg

Any of the medications listed above may be effective for initial insomnia. Patients who are at risk for substance abuse may be given medications such as trazodone, diphenhydramine, or hydroxyzine, which have very little abuse or addiction potential. Trazodone is particularly preferable if insomnia is expected to be chronic.

Middle Insomnia

Medication options for patients who have restless sleep are the following:

- trazodone (Desyrel) 50-150 mg
- estazolam (Prosom) 1-2 mg
- temazepam (Restoril) 7.5-30 mg
- lorazepam (Ativan) 0.5-1 mg
- oxazepam (Serax) 15-30 mg
- clonazepam (Klonopin) 0.25-1 mg
- quazepam (Doral) 7.5-15 mg
- hydroxyzine (Vistaril) 25-50 mg
- chloral hydrate (Noctec) 500-1000 mg

Terminal Insomnia

Patients who have early morning awakening may be treated using the following medications:

- trazodone (Desyrel) 50-150 mg
- lorazepam (Ativan) 0.5-1 mg
- temazepam (Restoril) 7.5-30 mg
- clonazepam (Klonopin) 0.25-1 mg
- estazolam (Prosom) 1-2 mg
- flurazepam (Dalmane) 15-30 mg
- quazepam (Doral) 7.5-15 mg
- clorazepate (Tranxene) 3.75-15 mg
- prazepam (Centrax) 5-10 mg

Since flurazepam, quazepam, clorazepate, and prazepam have a long duration of action, they can cause daytime drowsiness, especially with repeated dosing. For this reason, medications with an intermediate duration of action such as lorazepam, temazepam, clonazepam, and estazolam are preferable for the treatment of early-morning awakening. Although trazodone has a fairly short duration of action, it has been found to be effective for the treatment of terminal insomnia. Its many advantages should make it an attractive option, especially if it is needed for chronic use and the patient is at risk for addiction.

Severe Insomnia

Combinations of various hypnotics have complimentary and synergistic effects and hence may be used together for treating severe insomnia. Examples of safe and effective combinations are given below:

– Trazodone 50 mg – Diphenhydramine 50 mg – Hydroxyzine 50 mg	+	Temazepam 15 mg (or any of the short- and intermediate-acting benzodiazepines)

The addition of trazodone, diphenhydramine, or hydroxyzine to a benzodiazepine will help keep the benzodiazepine dose low. Once the underlying cause of insomnia (such as depression, anxiety, or psychosis) is controlled, the benzodiazepine hypnotic may be withdrawn or the dosage further reduced. Table 13.1 lists various medication combinations for the treatment of severe insomnia.

Other Medications for Insomnia

The sedating effects of TCAs (at low doses) may be exploited for the treatment of insomnia, especially if loss of appetite and weight loss are of concern. The latter symptoms are usually not improved on SSRIs or bupropion, which are frequently used as first-line antidepressants in current clinical practice. Examples of TCAs:

- amitriptyline (Elavil) 10-25 mg
- doxepin (Sinequan) 10-25 mg
- trimipramine (Surmontil) 25 mg
- imipramine (Tofranil) 10-50 mg
- nortriptyline (Pamelor) 10-25 mg

Any of the benzodiazepines can be used along with TCAs for a synergistic sedating effect. The low doses of TCAs employed for treatment of insomnia limit anticholinergic and cardiovascular side effects typically associated with TCAs. Low doses of sedating TCAs are excellent for patients at risk for substance abuse. If a benzodiazepine has to be added, the TCA will help to keep the benzodiazepine dose low and yet provide good hypnotic effects with minimal tolerance, even in fairly long-term use.

TABLE 13.1. Medication Combinations for Treatment of Severe Insomnia

Severe Insomnia: Option I

Trazodone	50 to 150 mg HS				
Amitriptyline	10 to 50 mg HS				
Doxepin	10 to 50 mg HS			+	Any benzodiazepine or zolpidem at dosage listed for insomnia
Hydroxyzine	25 to 50 mg HS				
Diphenhydramine	25 to 50 mg HS				

Severe Insomnia: Option II

Trazodone	50 to 150 mg	+	*One of the following:* Low dose of sedating TCA Hydroxyzine Diphenhydramin	+	Any benzodiazepine or zolpidem at dosage listed for insomnia

Note: Option II is necessary only when less complicated interventions fail.

Other Considerations

Risperidone can occasionally cause insomnia, requiring additional medications. Trazodone, TCAs, and benzodiazepines are options in patients on a high-potency antipsychotic, such as risperidone, and SSRIs, which do not have significant sedating effects and thus may not induce sleep. Generally, therapeutic doses of sedating TCAs, low-potency antipsychotics, and clozapine given at bedtime should be sufficient to promote sleep.

Since lorazepam, temazepam, oxazepam, triazolam, and zolpidem have no active metabolites, they are preferable in patients with liver disease or renal failure. Lorazepam, diazepam, and chlordiazepoxide have the advantage that, in a hospital setting, they can be given IM if necessary although IM absorption of diazepam and chlordiazepoxide is somewhat erratic. In rare clinical situations in hospitalized patients these medications may be given intravenously if patients cannot take oral medications and cannot receive IM medications (patients with bleeding disorders or thrombocytopenia, for example). Dosage examples follow:

- Lorazepam 0.5-1 mg in 50 cc of normal saline IV over 30 minutes
- Lorazepam 0.5 mg IV over one to two minutes
- Diazepam 5-10 mg slow IV push over two minutes
- Chlordiazepoxide 10-25 mg slow IV push over two minutes

Respiration should be monitored during and several minutes after IV administration because of increased risk of respiratory depression with IV use.

Insomnia in Substance Abusers

Medications with a low risk of abuse and addiction are preferred for treating insomnia in patients at risk for substance abuse. The following are some examples:

- Trazodone
- Sedating TCAs
- Diphenhydramine
- Hydroxyzine
- Nefazodone

Patients who abuse narcotics and sedatives, including alcohol, frequently have insomnia either as one of the precipitants or as a result of the abuse. In the former case, if their insomnia is not aggressively addressed, they may be tempted to return to abuse of drugs or alcohol to relieve their insomnia. Substance abusers are not only *not* immune to having sleep disorders, they may even be more prone to having sleep problems, compared to other patient groups. Hence, safely getting them off of the drugs of abuse is important and necessary, but not sufficient. Addiction is a complex disease and it is critical to address as many treatable symptoms as possible.

DISSOCIATIVE DISORDERS: ARE THEY FORMS OF ATYPICAL PSYCHOSIS?

Dissociative disorders are characterized by regressive phenomena resulting in fragmentation of integrative processes such as perception, rational thinking, identity, reasoning, judgment, and consciousness, leading to possible bizarre or irrational behavior. These are some of the mental functions that are also impaired in psychosis. Clearly, there are some similarities between psychotic symptoms and dissociative symptoms. The author believes that purely from a psychopharmacological point of view there are practical advantages in approaching dissociative disorders as a form of atypical psychosis with features of anxiety and hysteria. According to the *DSM-IV*, there are five disorders that have dissociative symptoms:

- Dissociative amnesia
- Dissociative fugue
- Dissociative identity disorder
- Depersonalization disorder
- Dissociative disorder, not otherwise specified

The most well-known among the dissociative disorders is multiple personality disorder, named dissociative identity disorder in the *DSM-IV*.

Pharmacological Treatment

Dissociative mental processes may be compared to psychosis in terms of regressive psychological functions. Dissociative symptoms approach the psychotic spectrum if one or more of the following characteristics are present in a patient diagnosed as suffering from dissociative disorders:

- Frequent dissociative episodes
- Great number of identities

- Bizarre behavior or thinking attributed to dissociative episodes
- Significant functional deterioration
- Psychotic symptoms during dissociative episodes

It follows that such patients should benefit from treatment using antipsychotic medications.

Affective or anxiety symptoms should be concurrently treated with appropriate medications. The author's view is that, having successfully treated a number of patients suffering from severe dissociative disorders through the use of medication combinations involving antipsychotic medications, psychotherapy (with the goal of reintegration of personality functions) proceeds much more effectively when the patient is on an antipsychotic medication. Fortunately, with the availability of risperidone and olanzapine, patients should be able to tolerate low doses without typical antipsychotic side effects. For severe cases, one should consider clozapine.

From a biological and neurochemical perspective, dissociative disorders should be seen as an atypical form of psychosis and treatment should be designed accordingly. The body and the brain are the same, regardless of the number of discrete identities one has. A psychodynamically oriented clinician may be able to work with two or more separate identities. However, antipsychotics affect the same brain and help integrate fragmented (dissociated) functions just as they do in psychotic individuals. Normalcy and psychotic thinking are extremes on a continuum, and so are normalcy and dissociation. It is, therefore, conceivable that mild dissociative phenomena are common, go unnoticed, and may not need treatment. Psychotherapy may be sufficient as a treatment approach for mild forms of dissociation, although it is the author's opinion that antipsychotic medication along with psychotherapy is the treatment of choice for dissociative disorder. Mild forms require only very low doses as well as short-term psychotherapy, and severe forms need higher doses along with long-term psychotherapy.

Symptoms of depression, anxiety, obsessive-compulsiveness, and post-traumatic stress disorder can coexist with dissociative disorders, in which case these symptoms will need specific treatments as outlined in other sections of this text.

SOMATOFORM DISORDERS

Somatoform disorders are characterized by the presence of physical complaints, symptoms, or preoccupation with the fear of having a physical illness in the absence of a medical basis. Various types of somatoform disorders are given in the *DSM-IV*, as follows:

– Somatization disorder
– Undifferentiated somatoform disorder
– Conversion disorder
– Pain disorder
– Hypochondriasis
– Body dysmorphic disorder
– Somatoform disorder, not otherwise specified

Most patients who have somatoform disorders are antagonistic to the idea that their condition has a psychiatric basis. Therefore, they neither seek psychiatric treatment nor are eager to be compliant should they begin psychiatric treatment under pressure from a family physician or a family member.

Psychopharmacological treatment of somatoform disorders is effective for a compliant patient. As in all other psychiatric conditions, the choice of medications depends on the specific symptoms of a particular patient. The most important first step is to make reasonably sure that the patient's symptoms have no physical basis. This can be accomplished by referring the patient for appropriate medical consultations if a medical work-up has not already been completed. Previous history of psychiatric disorders, coexisting anxiety, bizarre behavior, or depression should not be a reason to conclude that a patient's physical complaint is psychogenic. The diagnosis of somatoform disorders, for the most part, should be a diagnosis of exclusion for practical purposes, especially in a legally developed society.

Somatoform disorders commonly share obsessive-compulsive features. The treatment implication of such an observation is that antiobsessional medications such as clomipramine (Anafranil) and SSRIs are likely to be primary medications in the pharmacological treatment of somatoform disorders. If any of the somatic complaints or fears reach irrational, delusional, or bizarre proportions, the probability of the existence of psychotic components is high, requiring the addition of low doses of antipsychotics. The choice antipsychotic in such a context is risperidone (Risperdal) at a dose of 0.5 to 2 mg or olanzapine 2.5 to 5 mg daily. Frequently, anxiety and depressive symptoms are present. Fortunately, clomipramine and SSRIs improve not only obsessive-compulsive symptoms but also depression and anxiety symptoms, making these medications the first choice for treatment of somatoform disorders. Since patients with somatoform disorders are very sensitive to side effects, starting doses should be very low, with smaller dosage increments to minimize side effects and to improve compliance. SSRIs should be the first choice due to their favorable side effect profile, followed by clomipramine. Adjunctive use of benzodiazepines on a PRN schedule is employed if clinical anxiety is present, especially during the first several weeks because of the antidepressant latency period.

Since factitious disorders characterized by intentional production of symptoms probably have a treatable compulsive etiology, as do somatoform disorders, clomipramine and SSRIs are the medications most likely to benefit patients with such disorders. Severe somatic preoccupation can reach delusional proportions leading to chronic and severe dysfunction, in which case clozapine might be considered if treatment using other antipsychotics is ineffective.

PARAPHILIAS

Sexual paraphilias may be considered to have a component of obsessive-compulsive characteristics for psychopharmacological treatment purposes. The paraphilias may take numerous forms, but the physician has to conceptualize the symptoms in a psychopharmacological framework so that the most effective medication can be recommended. The following paraphilias are described in *DSM-IV:*

- Exhibitionism
- Fetishism
- Frotteurism
- Pedophilia
- Sexual masochism
- Sexual sadism
- Transvestite fetishism
- Voyeurism
- Paraphilia, not otherwise specified

In addition to possibly having an obsessive-compulsive quality, many of the above behaviors are illegal. They constitute antisocial behaviors for which stigmatism, punishment, or the threat of punishment have beneficial effects in terms of providing necessary external control. However, clinicians have no authority to prescribe or to implement punishment. This is the responsibility of society: parents, teachers, and the judicial system (although the disciplinary authority of parents and teachers seems to be eroding). The clinician's task is to identify possible treatable components and to attempt treatment, with no guarantee of success.

As with any other psychiatric disorder, there can be coexisting symptoms that may need treatment using different classes of medications. Obsessive-compulsive features are commonly seen in paraphilias. If the paraphilias are bizarre in nature, suggest extreme hostility, or have a delusional/psychotic basis, antipsychotic medications are indicated, either as a stand-alone medication or in addition to an antiobsessional medication. Severe paraphilias frequently have a psychotic basis in addition to obsessive-compulsive features. Since these patients are extremely guarded, manipulative, and sneaky, it behooves the clinician to be extremely alert for signs of psychotic thinking, possibly of a schizotypal level of severity, in addition to obvious sociopathic traits. The presence of guardedness and evasiveness should be sufficient to strongly consider adjunctive antipsychotic treatment. The antipsychotic of choice is risperidone or olanzapine, with clozapine reserved for severe and chronic cases that do not respond to risperidone, olanzapine, or other antipsychotics. The use of antiobsessional medication and antipsychotics is described in other chapters of this text in detail.

The physician should guard against letting the patient exploit the pursuit of psychiatric services simply to avoid or minimize legal responsibility and consequences, although people may have a basic legal right to try to evade or minimize legal responsibility and legal consequences.

EATING DISORDERS

Eating disorders may also be viewed as having obsessive-compulsive features for purposes of psychopharmacological intervention. The eating disorders described in the *DSM-IV* are the following:

- Anorexia nervosa
- Bulimia nervosa
- Eating disorder, not otherwise specified

Antiobsessional medications, especially SSRIs, should be the mainstay of pharmacological treatment of eating disorders, including binge-eating behaviors. Since depression, anxiety, mood irritability, and mild psychotic symptoms coexist, it is important to search for these symptoms and to treat them using adjunctive medications if necessary. Pharmacological, behavioral, or medical attempts to force a patient to gain weight should not be made until antiobsessional medication begins to take effect, unless there is a medical emergency in which case tube feeding or parenteral nutrition must be immediately considered. If body image disturbance has a delusional or strange quality, which is often the case, low doses of antipsychotic medication is indicated. Once the obsessive-compulsive components and the psychotic symptoms, if present, are reasonably controlled, direct intervention to increase weight is more likely to be successful. Sedating TCAs at low doses are excellent for this purpose. Some examples follow:

- Doxepin 10 mg po HS
- Amitriptyline 10 mg HS
- Nortriptyline 10 mg HS
- Imipramine 10 mg HS
- Trimipramine 25 mg HS

The presence of perceptual abnormalities resulting in distortions of body image reaching psychotic proportions could be considered a psychotic symptom requiring antipsychotic treatment. This subtle clinical characteristic is often missed by physicians, leading to unsatisfactory outcomes. Another common clinical error made by psychiatrists and other physicians is starting an anorexic patient on a sedating TCA with the apparently sound logic that TCA treatment will increase appetite and subsequently cause weight gain in addition to providing the obvious antidepressant effects. This strategy backfires in most cases. The patient either purges or becomes noncompliant with taking the TCA. This is why unless the distortion in body image, the irrational fear of normal weight, and obsession with thinness are not controlled first, direct efforts to increase weight are likely to be a failure.

The intense and irrational fear of gaining weight even in the context of being underweight is strongly suggestive of mild psychotic thinking, the optimal treatment of which requires the temporary use of very low doses of antipsychotic medication for a successful outcome. In most cases, the antipsychotic can be withdrawn after the symptoms are controlled, and the patient can be maintained on an SSRI. Thus, the initial treatment of severe eating disorders, particularly anorexia nervosa, could benefit from the following medications:

- Antipsychotic (e.g., low dose of risperidone or olanzapine)
- Antidepressant (any of the SSRIs or clomipramine)
- Other medications, as needed, to address specific discrete symptoms

IMPULSE CONTROL DISORDERS

DSM-IV subtypes of impulse control disorders are as follows:

– Intermittent explosive disorder
– Kleptomania
– Pyromania
– Pathological gambling
– Trichotillomania
– Impulse control disorder, not otherwise specified

Impulse control disorders are characterized by an inability to resist an impulse, urge, or behavior that subsequently results in harm to the self or others. Strictly from a psychopharmacological treatment standpoint, there are advantages to viewing them as manifestations of obsessive-compulsive behaviors. Severe forms of impulse control disorders that have serious consequences may suggest a psychotic basis. For example, intermittent explosive disorder and pyromania can progress to the extent that the behaviors could be considered extremely irrational. In these contexts, addition of an antipsychotic must be considered to contain the out-of-control behavior. SSRIs are excellent for control of anger and obsessive-compulsive symptoms. They are the primary medications, along with clomipramine, for treatment of impulse control disorders. Other medications such as lithium, carbamazepine, valproic acid, clonidine, buspirone, propranolol, verapamil, naltrexone, trazodone, and clonazepam may be effective in some cases, especially in intermittent explosive disorder. There are also antisocial components in some disorders such as kleptomania, pyromania, and intermittent explosive disorder, for which patients will benefit from legal sanctions. It is important for clinicians to take care not to allow people to exploit psychiatric diagnoses for avoiding responsibility for illegal behaviors, even if part of the behavior has a psychiatric etiology or consequence. Severe impulse control disorders, which can be chronic and have serious consequences for the patient or others, deserve consideration of a trial on clozapine if other medications fail.

MISCELLANEOUS MEDICATIONS

Disulfiram (Antabuse)

Disulfiram is employed as a deterrent to alcohol use. Disulfiram causes acetaldehyde to accumulate, causing extremely uncomfortable and even serious toxic effects such as nausea, vomiting, flushing, abdominal cramping, sweating, tachycardia, hypotension, and, in rare cases, death secondary to circulatory shock, seizures, and myocardial infarction.

Given the serious toxic effects of an alcohol-disulfiram reaction, disulfiram is prescribed only for reliable, motivated, compliant, and determined alcoholics as part of a treatment program consisting of psychosocial, rehabilitative, and group interventions. It prevents impulsive drinking; it does not prevent planned drinking, since the toxic interaction effects can be avoided simply by stopping disulfiram and waiting one to two weeks prior to drinking alcohol. Disulfiram is very effective for motivated patients who need a "chemical" restraint as an adjunct to their determination not to resume drinking. Without motivation and compliance, disulfiram is not only ineffective, but may also be dangerous.

The usual starting dose of disulfiram is 250 to 500 mg daily for two weeks. Liver function tests should be obtained periodically. A maintenance dose of 125 mg may be sufficient in most patients. Refer to the *PDR* for further details.

Naltrexone (Revia, Trexan)

Naltrexone is an opioid antagonist approved for use in the treatment of alcoholism. Naltrexone at 50 mg daily tends to decrease the relapse rates in alcoholics when used in conjunction with psychosocial and group therapy approaches (such as Alcoholics Anonymous). It controls relapse by decreasing cravings for alcohol and, to some extent, by inhibiting the hedonistic effects of alcohol. The author's experience in treating a number of patients on naltrexone supports the expectations described here. Naltrexone may also be effective as an adjunctive medication in controlling the compulsive self-mutilation behavior frequently associated with borderline personality disorder. It is available as a 50 mg tablet. Although its half-life is only about four hours, its antialcohol effects last longer, enabling once-a-day administration.

Side effects include anxiety, depression, nausea, and anergia during the first several months of treatment. It can cause an elevation of liver enzymes requiring periodic tests to monitor liver function. Administration of naltrexone to patients on opioids can precipitate sudden opioid withdrawal. Naltrexone should not be administered until the patient has abstained from opioids for about seven days.

Since many alcoholics have hepatic dysfunction, baseline liver function tests and biweekly monitoring of liver enzymes are prudent during the first two months of treatment, with a decreased frequency of laboratory monitoring thereafter. Naltrexone costs approximately $150 for 30 pills. If price is not a deterrent, its use should be encouraged in patients with alcohol dependence because of its beneficial effects.

BLOOD LEVELS OF MEDICATIONS

Blood level monitoring of medications is necessary in some instances. Periodic levels of lithium, carbamazepine, and valproate are obtained as standard practice as is appropriate monitoring of CBC, liver functioning, renal functioning, and thyroid profile at varying intervals. For instance, weekly WBC monitoring is mandatory during clozapine treatment while much less frequent monitoring of the WBC is sufficient for a patient on carbamazepine or on a phenothiazine. Recommendations for medically necessary blood tests are discussed in the chapter dealing with specific medications.

Most patients do not require plasma levels. Antidepressant blood levels are available, but are seldom necessary. Fairly meaningful plasma levels are available for desipramine, nortriptyline, and imipramine. These blood levels are frequently overused, which drives up the cost of medical care. The author has occasionally encounterd patients for whom physicians, and in a few cases, even psychiatrists, have been obtaining antidepressant plasma levels routinely every two to three months, which is an unnecessary utilization of tests. Refer to Table 13.2 for a list of costs of various lab tests.

Plasma level monitoring of antidepressants, antipsychotics, and antianxiety medications may be necessary in one of the following infrequent clinical scenarios:

- To confirm suspicion of noncompliance
- To rule out or to assess toxicity
- To assess lack of response, despite taking high doses

It is not necessary to order plasma levels routinely or periodically for antidepressants, antipsychotics, or for antianxiety medications. The dosage of these medications is adjusted primarily based on clinical response, side effects, and general dosing guidelines. Even for nortriptyline, for which there is thought to be a therapeutic window below or above which clinical response declines, clinical monitoring of response is preferable to blood-test monitoring, except in the rare clinical contexts listed.

TABLE 13.2. Prices of Various Blood Levels and Laboratory Tests (as of July 1995)

Test	Price
Lithium level	$36
Carbamazepine level	$64
Valproic Acid level	$62
Clonazepam level	$87
Desipramine level	$90
Nortriptyline level	$92
Imipramine level	$85
Fluoxetine level	$75
Risperidone level	$89
Clozapine level	$92
Thyroid stimulating hormone (TSH)	$72
CBC with differential	$28
CBC without differential	$21
Chemistry panel - 21 (SMAC-21)	$55

Note: Prices are approximate and may vary with different laboratories.

COMMON PATIENT QUESTIONS, ISSUES, AND ANSWERS

The section on patient questions and answers was included for the benefit of primary care physicians and psychotherapists. Patients with emotional difficulties who take antidepressants or other psychotropic medications are likely to pose one or more of these questions. Therefore, the clinician must be prepared to answer them in an informative and constructive manner without becoming defensive or irritated. Some overlap of portions of the answers is unavoidable. Most of the questions are of a factual nature; therefore, the answers are straightforward and written in a style that is addressed to the reader. A few of the questions require tactful and personalized answers; these are presented as though the author is directly addressing the patient.

Do I Have a Chemical Imbalance?

Patients should be told that "chemical imbalance" is a simplified term to describe a complex process that takes place in the brain. Our emotions, moods, and behavior are mediated by the brain, which controls these functions by complex physiological, chemical, and electrical processes. Sadness, anxiety, anger, happiness, etc., are states of mind that the brain can control. In a simplistic manner of speaking, one can tell patients that the presence of clinical depression, mood swings, anxiety, or any other symptoms suggest a chemical imbalance. Sophisticated patients may also be educated regarding the role of various neurotransmitters, such as norepinephrine, serotonin, dopamine, and others implicated in depression and other disorders. A more technical discussion is not usually necessary with these patients. If the patient suffers from psychosis or mania, any detailed discussion should be postponed until the medication takes effect, after which a more meaningful and educational discussion can take place.

Can I Be Tested for a Chemical Imbalance?

Presently available tests are neither valid nor reliable enough for clinical use. The diagnosis of depression or anxiety is made primarily by an evaluation of symptoms. Patients may be told that there are a few blood tests, such as the dexamethasone suppression test and thyrotropin releasing hormone stimulation test, which can be used for diagnosing depression but not for measuring the various "chemicals" involved. The tests are unnecessary except in rare situations. These tests are neither sensitive nor specific for depression or for any other emotional disorders, and their validity and reliability are low. Occasionally patients see TV programs, read science sections in the newspaper, or read a popular book on depression, and are led to believe that these chemicals can be measured and a specific antidepressant that works on the deficient neurotransmitter system can be chosen based on test results. This may be possible in the future, just like choosing a specific antibiotic based on culture and sensitivity studies, but it is not available in the clinical arena presently, nor is it expected to be available in the near future. Other tests such as evoked potentials (EP), regional cerebral blood flow (rCBF), positron emission tomography (PET), single photon emission computed tomography (SPECT), and brain electrical activity mapping (BEAM) are still research tools and have no place in practical clinical psychiatry at present.

Will Depression Return After the Medication Is Stopped?

Patients should be reassured that if they stay on the medication long enough, and if the medication is gradually tapered off, the majority of patients continue to function satisfactorily without relapse. There is a minority who experience eventual relapse, requiring resumption of medication and a subsequent longer maintenance period. The author tells patients that in his experience, about 75 percent are able to function well for long periods of time after stopping medication, and about 25 percent have a relapse. It should be pointed out that there is no method of reliably predicting who can stop the medication without problems and who will relapse. Patients are reassured by highlighting the promising success rate of 75 percent. They are told that they should expect to do well, and that, in the unlikely event that they have a relapse, they should resume the antidepressant and stay on it longer. Given the lack of known permanent side effects induced by antidepressants, it is better to continue the medication than to endure the depression because depression or other emotional disorders carry the risk of suicide and various psychosocial dysfunctions. Even if these percentages are not accurate, patients are still reassured and provided with hope, and no harm is done. In the event that there is a relapse, they are more likely to contact the physician to resume the medication, without feeling even more hopeless.

The question reveals patients' understandable anxiety about their illness and its prognosis. Physicians have a responsibility to allay patients' anxieties and give them hope, while ensuring that, in the minority of patients who relapse, options that are familiar and successful are available. This gives them confidence in the event of a relapse. The percentages given are to be used for patient reassurance, and are based on clinical estimates rather than a proven statistic supported by research. (Refer to sections on depression, anxiety, psychosis, and bipolar disorders for general guidelines on length of treatment for various disorders.)

What Happens to the "Chemical Imbalance" When the Medication Is Stopped?

Patients may be told that for some yet-unknown reasons, the "chemicals" tend to stabilize if antidepressants are taken for a sufficient length of time, and that some patients need to stay on the antidepressants relatively longer than others. Changes in the neurotransmitter dynamics are complex processes, and a precise answer to this question is not known. Clinical observation indicates that a majority of patients on antidepressants do not need to stay on the medication permanently.

Will the Medication Affect My Driving or My Job?

Patients should be reassured that satisfactory treatment of depression using psychotropic medications is expected to improve functioning in all aspects of life, including personal, social, and job functioning. At therapeutic doses, most medications do not affect the skills necessary for driving. If a medication makes a patient sedated or dizzy, obviously that medication will be discontinued or the dosage adjusted to alleviate those side effects. Usually patients themselves or significant others are the best judge of whether or not the patient's coordination, perception, reaction time, and motor skills necessary for driving are affected. Patients should be warned against mixing medication with over-the-counter cold medications or alcohol.

Successful treatment of the psychiatric condition should improve energy level, motivation, concentration, and emotional control, thereby improving job functioning; whereas, untreated disorders can lead to deterioration in personal, social, and occupational functioning. Patients on medication are probably subject to the same accident risks and job stresses as those who are not on psychiatric medications.

Is the Medication Addictive?

Patients should be assured that antidepressants are not addictive in a physiological sense like alcohol and sedatives. However, medications should not be stopped abruptly unless necessary. Some people experience nausea, headaches, diarrhea, anxiety, and dizziness for several days when an antidepressant medication is stopped abruptly. When it is time to discontinue the antidepressant, it is tapered slowly, both to prevent any mild gastrointestinal discomfort and to minimize the risk of relapse often seen when an antidepressant is discontinued suddenly. These are not indications of true addiction, since there is no craving, drug-seeking behavior, or tolerance to the main effect of the medication. Patients should also be told that if the medication is stopped, there is a chance that, in some patients, the symptoms for which they took the medication initially may reemerge. This does not suggest dependence, but rather that they may need to stay on the medication longer. If patients are still not convinced, I liken their situation to that of a person who has high blood pressure. The condition is controlled on antihypertensive medication but the person may have a relapse of the hypertension when the medication is stopped. This shows that this patient needs the medication for proper control of blood pressure, not because he or she is addicted to it. This example or any such "medically" oriented example will reassure almost all patients. Benzodiazepines are technically "addictive." However, when used at low doses occasionally or for short periods of time, benzodiazepines do not cause patient dependence. Refer to Chapter 2 and Table 2.1 for a detailed discussion on the discontinuation of antidepressants.

For What Length of Time Should Antidepressants Be Prescribed?

The length of treatment depends on various factors, such as chronicity of illness in a particular patient, the severity of depression, presence or absence of psychosocial stressors, or number of previous relapses. However, some general guideline should be followed, based on diagnoses.

Length of Drug Therapy in Patients with Adjustment Disorder with Depressed Mood

This diagnosis, by definition, is related to a stressor that precipitated the symptoms, and hence, in most cases is time limited. In these cases, antidepressants are recommended for six to eight months, after which the medication may be discontinued if the stress that apparently precipitated the symptoms has abated. If the stress is still operating, the author's recommendation is to continue the antidepressant until the stress subsides.

Length of Drug Therapy in Patients with Dysthymia

Dysthymia is a term for low-grade chronic depression. Since the natural course of dysthymia is chronic, the patient should be maintained on an antidepressant for one to two years prior to attempting to discontinue the medication. If a patient's symptoms relapse after the antidepressant is discontinued, the patient should be restarted on the same medication and should be maintained for two to three years prior to another attempt at discontinuation. In general, the antidepressant dosage needed for treatment of acute stages of depression and for maintenance are the same. For example, if a patient did well on fluoxetine 40 mg, the maintenance dose is also 40 mg. In some cases, it is possible to decrease the dose of the medication slightly during the maintenance period. It is possible and even desirable to decrease the dose of most psychotropic medications during the maintenance period. Such medications include antipsychotics, mood stabilizers, and, to some extent, antianxiety medications.

Length of Drug Therapy for Patients with Major Depression

If a patient had a severe episode of depression, one should be more cautious when discontinuing the antidepressant. The more severe the episode, the longer the maintenance treatment period. For example, a patient who had to be hospitalized with a suicide attempt and other serious symptoms should be maintained on the antidepressant for at least one year.

Patients with recurrent depression should be maintained on antidepressants indefinitely, as should be patients whose depressions required full trials on more than three or four antidepressants or ECT for resolution of symptoms, even if the patient had only one episode of depression.

Length of Drug Therapy for Patients with Depression as a Component of Bipolar Disorder

One of the few cases in which the dose of antidepressants should be reduced during the maintenance period is in documented cases of manic depression (bipolar disorder, depressed) where the risk of the patient cycling to mania is a particular concern. In most cases of documented bipolar disorder, the patient will be on prophylactic or adjunctive mood stabilizers such as lithium, carbamazepine (Tegretol), or divalproex sodium (Depakote), which protect the patient from a manic episode. In the occasional instance when a patient cycles into a manic phase, the antidepressant should be stopped, and aggressive control of mania should be attempted.

Patients should be advised that discontinuation of the medication too soon increases the chances of rapid relapse, whereas the chances of a recurrence of symptoms are decreased if patients stay on the medication for four to six months or longer, depending on individual factors.

How Should Antidepressants Be Discontinued?

As a general rule, antidepressants should be discontinued gradually to minimize the risk of relapse. A tapering period of approximately one month for every six months the patient had been on the antidepressant is suggested as a general guideline. For example, if a patient was on an antidepressant for 18 months, a period of 3 months of gradual taper of the dose is recommended prior to discontinuation. Three to four weeks of taper is recommended for a patient who has taken an antidepressant for four to six months. If the medication must be stopped for late onset of adverse effects or for lack of efficacy, the medication may be discontinued rapidly. Some patients who are on MAOIs develop nightmares, severe anxiety, and agitation upon abrupt discontinuation. Therefore, gradual taper over one to two weeks is recommended for MAOIs. Mild withdrawal symptoms consisting of nausea, diarrhea, dizziness, lightheadedness, and anxiety are observed when trazodone, nefazodone, TCAs, and serotonergic medications are discontinued. No significant withdrawal symptoms have been found after stopping bupropion (Wellbutrin). Antidepressant withdrawal symptoms are uncomfortable and of concern to patients, but are not serious, except for MAOI withdrawal, as described. Refer to Chapter 2 and Table 2.1 for further details regarding discontinuing antidepressants and for information on the latency period for emergence of antidepressant discontinuation syndrome.

Can I Take the Medication As Needed?

Patients should be told that antidepressants are not effective when taken as needed. They cannot be compared to acetaminophen (Tylenol), aspirin (Anacin), or cold medications. It usually takes 7 to 21 days for the antidepressant medication to become effective. The patient should be helped to understand that the medication should ideally be taken for several months to get the optimal benefit and that several dosage adjustments or even changes of medication may be necessary before satisfactory symptom control is achieved. Even the relatively faster-acting antidepressants such as bupropion (Wellbutrin) and venlafaxine (Effexor) are not effective if taken on a PRN basis.

Can I Get Pregnant While Taking the Medication?

The standard advice should be to try to discontinue all psychiatric medications prior to pregnancy, if possible. If a patient becomes pregnant while on psychiatric medication, safe and rapid taper of the medication is advised. Patients should be informed that the first three months of pregnancy are the most critical in terms of risk of teratogenicity is concerned, and that if their symptoms relapse anytime during pregnancy, medication will be considered after carefully weighing the risks and benefits at the particular time the relapse occurs. Patients should be reassured that most psychiatric medications have low teratogenic potential, but no guarantees as to the safety of the fetus can be given. The issue is complicated by a certain incidence of fetal abnormalities occurring in nature without the mother or fetus being exposed to any known exogenous substances. If a fetus were to have a birth defect, and if the mother happened to be on an antidepressant medication, how can one say whether or not the defect is due to nature or due to the medication? A more important concern is exposing the fetus to unnecessary drugs. Informed consent stating that the risks, benefits, and alternatives have been discussed and were understood by the mother should be obtained prior to beginning medication treatment while the patient is pregnant. However, if there is an emergency or if the patient is incompetent due to acute psychosis or mental retardation, such discussion of risks and benefits should be directed to a responsible family member or guardian.

In nonemergency situations, a second opinion from another physician, stating that the benefits outweigh the risks and that there is a need for treatment based on an analysis of risk to benefit ratio, should be obtained for medical/legal reasons. The physicians, whose job it is to deal with people's problems, are at high risk when some people seek to blame someone for a misfortune. Unfortunately and paradoxically, physicians must protect themselves from the very patients whom they are trying to help. Fortunately, the author has had the opportunity to treat a number of patients with various diagnoses on medication during pregnancy without any teratogenic events to date. Lithium, carbamazepine (Tegretol), and divalproex sodium (Depakote) are best avoided in the first trimester. Patients with manic symptoms who need to be on a mood stabilizer are probably safer on verapamil or high-potency antipsychotics. Extensive use of benzodiazepines or other sedatives should be avoided. TCAs have a fair safety record in pregnancy. Serotonergic antidepressants are new, but probably share risks similar to TCAs in pregnancy. Antipsychotics are not known to pose particular risks to fetal development.

Patients who have had several severe episodes of depression, mania, or psychosis and are maintained on medications will be taking a substantial risk if they stop the medications. There is an especially high risk for those who have one of the psychoses, such as schizophrenia, paranoid disorder, or schizoaffective disorder, in whom discontinuation of antipsychotics could promptly lead to a relapse. Thus, risks of discontinuing medication should be discussed with the patient and concerned family members.

In the author's opinion, if a patient has a severe emotional disorder that is barely controlled on medication, the patient should not stop the medication at any time, regardless of pregnancy status. Even more prudent should be the decision on the part of the patients who have uncontrolled chronic severe mental illness to neither have children nor adopt children. The stresses and responsibilities involved in rearing children can precipitate a worsening of their condition, resulting in an increased potential for hospitalizations and a higher probability of a very insecure rather than a nurturant family atmosphere both for the patient and the children. Physicians should not refrain from giving advice based on clinical knowledge in the best interest of the patient.

Can I Take This Job?

Occasionally, patients ask the physician's opinion, based on clinical knowledge of their condition, whether or not they should accept a particular job. There are certain general guidelines that are important.

Patients who have Bipolar Disorder with a propensity for mania should avoid jobs that get them emotionally excited, or jobs in which there is potential for excessive stimulation, frustration, or changes, such as commission sales jobs, public speaking, or jobs requiring extensive travel. These patients require stability in their lives. Similarly, patients who have psychosis or bipolar disorder should avoid working variable shifts, which can disrupt the sleep cycle and can precipitate exacerbations. Patients recovering from alcohol dependence obviously are better off not working in a bar or nightclub.

Can I Drink While Taking the Medication?

In general, it is best to completely abstain from drinking. Alcohol can contribute to depression, in addition to impairing sleep and causing a potentially serious interaction with medications resulting in possible enhanced effects of alcohol, and antagonism toward the beneficial effects of the medication. Patients who have depression, mania, or psychosis can worsen their condition by drinking. Many suicides in susceptible individuals occur while under the influence of alcohol. (Similarly, it is common knowledge that many homicides and accidents occur while people are intoxicated.)

Alcohol improves social anxiety and decreases inhibition, which is one of the reasons people drink. However, the risks and problems associated with it are not worth the limited benefit. My practice is to routinely instruct patients not to consume any alcoholic beverages and make it a point to mention that wine, beer, and champagne are included in the prohibition.

Can I Drink Coffee?

Patients should be questioned about the extent of their consumption of coffee, one cup of which contains approximately 60 to 80 mg of caffeine. Coffee tends to suppress sleep stages 3 and 4, thereby affecting the most restful sleep period. A patient who has been drinking four or more cups of brewed coffee daily is likely to have increased anxiety, restlessness, and altered sleep architecture. Patients may not only fail to recognize the harmful effects of coffee on sleep, but may even believe that coffee is helping them sleep. This is probably reinforced by the fact that mild sleep disruption occurs temporarily after coffee intake is discontinued. In fact, what is taking place is caffeine withdrawal with symptoms such as mild irritability, anergia, dysphoria, and headaches. Patients should be reassured not only that these symptoms will subside but also that the sleep quality will improve in four to six days if they avoid coffee. The amount of caffeine intake should be part of an initial intake evaluation. Patients will not volunteer this information unless specifically asked.

Can I Take Over-the-Counter Medication for Cold and Allergies?

There is a standard warning on cold and allergy preparations to not mix with antidepressants. I suspect that this warning is primarily intended for MAOIs and to some extent for TCAs and SSRIs. Mixing cold and allergy medications (with some exceptions, such as diphenhydramine, guaifenesin, loratadine, terfanadine, and astemizole) with MAOIs can be dangerous due to serotonergic crisis or delirium, and mixing these with TCAs and trazodone synergistically increases sedation. However, with serotonergic medications and bupropion, increased sedation due to synergistic action should not be a major concern, except that terfanadine and astemizole are contraindicated with fluvoxamine and nefazodone because of concern regarding emergence of cardiac arrhythmias. Still, it is prudent to advise patients to watch for excessive sedation. Adverse effects consisting of serotonin syndrome due to interaction between decongestants and SSRIs are possible but rare, and patients should be cautioned regarding this potential.

I Don't Have Depression; I Have Anxiety. Why Are You Giving Me an Antidepressant?

It is important to educate patients about the relative advantages and disadvantages of antidepressants and antianxiety medications. The following points regarding antidepressant use for treating anxiety may serve as a guide.

Advantages of Antidepressants for Treatment of Anxiety

Mild depressive symptoms often coexist with anxiety. Among the advantages of using antidepressants for the treatment of anxiety are the following:

- Antidepressants have antidepressant and antianxiety effects.
- They prevent anxiety from manifesting, if taken regularly.
- The newer antidepressants, primarily SSRIs, have fewer side effects compared to the older TCAs and MAOIs and are more amenable for use in the treatment of anxiety disorders.
- They have no significant addictive or tolerance potential.
- They can be used for longer periods compared to antianxiety medications.

Disadvantages of Antidepressants for Treatment of Anxiety

- They take one or two weeks to become effective.

Advantages of Antianxiety Medications for Treatment of Anxiety

- They are effective immediately for the reduction of anxiety.
- They are excellent for occasional use.

Disadvantages of Antianxiety Medications for Treatment of Anxiety

- Addiction and tolerance potential is high.
- They can cause depression and cognitive impairment.
- They are not indicated for prolonged use.
- They do not prevent anxiety, unless taken regularly at fairly high doses.
- Dosage escalation can be a problem with prolonged use.

When properly educated and reassured, most patients will accept an antidepressant as the primary medication for the treatment of anxiety. If patients are still not convinced, the following example may be given. Just as acetaminophen (Tylenol) and aspirin, which can be used for two indications (i.e., for pain and for fever) so, too, can antidepressants be used for different purposes. They can treat both depression and anxiety. In virtually all cases, patients accept the choice of medication when they are educated using facts and simple examples.

I Am Afraid To Take Prozac.

Some patients are highly influenced by newspapers, TV, radio, tabloids, and magazines. The media may sensationalize psychiatric medications because of newsworthiness. At times, unbalanced and unscientific information is highlighted in these sources. Soon after fluoxetine became available, it was linked to several homicide defenses, in which it was blamed for precipitating homicide. Scientific studies have shown no correlation between antidepressants and homicide. Clinical experience has demonstrated that antidepressants, including fluoxetine, decrease depression, anger, and hostility, and consequently decrease suicidal and homicidal ideation. Interestingly, it was reported several years ago that fluoxetine was used in defending a charge of prostitution. The argument was that fluoxetine caused nymphomania by increasing libido, which drove the defendant to satisfy her increased sexual appetite by engaging in prostitution. In clinical experience, having treated over several thousand patients on fluoxetine, I have come across only a single case of slightly improved sexual functioning while taking fluoxetine. On the contrary, fluoxetine and most other antidepressants cause decrease in libido and inhibition of climax in the majority of patients. The point is, a defense claim in a legal case is hardly a source of accurate clinical information for patients. Unfortunately, these interesting defenses make good headlines for the news media.

Patients need reassurance regarding the safety of medications, including fluoxetine, when used as prescribed under the supervision of a physician. Clinicians can reassure patients by informing them that fluoxetine is as safe as any other SSRI and that there is no scientifically or clinically validated association between fluoxetine and increased homicidal risk. Given fluoxetine's well-known effects of decreasing anger and hostility, it is more likely that the individual who was taking fluoxetine when the murder was committed could have been more vicious, or could have had even more victims had he or she not been on fluoxetine.

Again, a medical example might easily provide clarification and reassurance to the patient. Death is an inherent risk associated with heart disease. Patients could still die while taking medications to treat heart disease. It would be ridiculous to suggest that the patient died *because of* the heart medication. Similarly, most severe psychiatric disorders carry a certain inherent risk of suicide and, in some cases, a risk of homicide. The psychiatric medication may not always be effective in successfully treating the psychiatric disorder. Just as in the medical example referring to heart medications, it is unfair to blame the psychiatric medication for failing to be effective against potential inherent complications associated with a disorder. The difference is that, since psychiatric disorders do not have well-defined anatomic correlates (as does heart disease) and therefore rely on clinical, functional, and psychosocial conceptualizations that make them less "concrete" compared to heart disease, psychiatric disorders, psychiatric medications, and even the field of psychiatry remain vulnerable areas for opportunistic individuals or groups to exploit and attack with impunity. This could change when biochemical, physiological, and anatomic correlates for psychiatric disorders are identified in the future. There is no rational, scientific, or medical basis for blaming a medication for self-destructive or criminal behavior committed by people except in the extremely rare case in which a severe delirium was induced by the improper use of drugs.

Most people probably had something to eat before committing suicide or homicide. Could a defendant claim that food was responsible for the commission of a homicide? Yes. It is the right of any defendant to present a defense and it is the ethical responsibility of any good defense lawyer to present whatever defense might result in the best outcome for the defendant. However, physicians must rely on scientific facts, as well as their own clinical experience and judgment. They have a further obligation to educate and reassure patients based on scientific findings and observations. Moreover, when disturbing side effects result from any medication, the responsible course of action is to notify the prescribing physician and/or to immediately stop the medication. With some reassurance from the physician, most patients accept fluoxetine without further concerns. They should be reassured that if a medication causes side effects, it can be stopped at any time and the side effects will resolve rapidly.

Don't You Think Anyone Who Has Gone Through What I Have Gone Through Would Be Depressed? Why Do I Need to Take Medication?

My response when patients pose this question is as follows:

"Your depression is quite understandable. However, the symptoms that we enumerated are interfering with your life. Let me give you an example. Pneumonia can be caused by bacteria for various known reasons. Does that mean that because the causes of pneumonia are understandable, you don't have to treat it? You still need treatment. If symptoms are not treated, they can worsen and cause further complications."

Nearly all patients will accept assurance of the need for treatment when a simple "medical" example is used. They can relate to this much more easily than a discussion of neurotransmitters and mind-body interaction.

How Does the Antidepressant Work?

One sample answer is the following:

"Our emotions and feelings are affected by various chemicals in the brain called neurotransmitters. In a highly simplified manner of speaking, the antidepressant balances the chemicals in the brain, thereby controlling excessive emotions. Antidepressants work with the chemicals that are already in the brain. In order to make it more understandable to you, I have simplified what is a very complex process in the brain."

Most patients will be satisfied with this answer. For curious patients, a more detailed explanation of the mechanism of antidepressant action with the names of specific neurotransmitters may be educational and reassuring.

I Don't Want to Give Control to a Drug; I Want to Deal with the Problems on My Own.

There are several variations of this. Some patients say they do not want to depend on a drug to solve their problems. Others feel that medications will only mask their problems and will prevent them from finding solutions to tackle their problems. The following explanation may be offered:

"Your symptoms (such as insomnia, lack of energy, and hopelessness) are presently interfering with your optimal functioning. You cannot let these symptoms continue to disrupt your life. They are easily treated with the use of medications. There are psychological issues, conflicts, and stresses that may have brought on the symptoms. Once your symptoms are under control, these psychological issues need to be analyzed, understood, and resolved. Along with medications that I will prescribe for you, I will refer you for psychotherapy which is equally important, for full recovery. The medications will give you better control of your emotions and symptoms, and will help you participate more fully in therapy and to benefit more from it. Medication is expected to help you to function at a higher level more rapidly, which will give you more energy to work on your psychological issues with your therapist. Medication is usually for temporary use, anywhere from four to eight months in most cases, after which it can be gradually tapered off. Let me give you an example. You know that untreated fever and infection can cause serious medical complications. Therefore, aspirin and an antibiotic are immediately started to treat fever and infection. However, balanced nutrition, exercise, a healthy lifestyle, and proper hygiene are essential for facilitating full recovery, preventing future infections, and promoting health. In addition, vaccination can prevent certain infections. However, these interventions would not rapidly control an active infection; hence, you need medication to quickly control infection and accompanying fever. Psychiatric medication can be compared to the use of antibiotics and aspirin for controlling fever and infection, whereas psychotherapy is analogous to the more fundamental long-term and preventive interventions listed here. As you can see from this example, both medication and psychotherapy are essential to ensure a satisfactory outcome and optimal long-term functioning. Let me refer you to a therapist, but start the medication so you will begin to feel better soon."

Most patients are satisfied and encouraged by this kind of explanation, which takes only a minute. If a patient is still not convinced, additional explanation is necessary. If the patient is still ambivalent, referral to a therapist is made, with instruction to return if and when the patient agrees to a trial of medication.

Does Depression Run in the Family? Will My Children Get It?

"Your genes come from your parents. You share your genes with your children. Hence, there are genetic similarities among blood relatives. Just as physical characteristics are genetically transmitted, psychological attributes also run in the family. A person's environment also has a considerable impact on depression. There is some genetic vulnerability to emotional disorders, but psychosocial stressors usually bring the depression to the surface. So, if psychosocial stressors can be avoided, depression may not manifest, even if there is a family history. However, in a present day society, it may be impossible to avoid psychosocial stressors. The genetic vulnerability to depression is transmitted in varying degrees in different relatives; hence, your children may or may not be vulnerable. Even if one of your relatives becomes depressed, there is effective and simple treatment available. So the concern regarding passing the depression or anxiety on to your children should not be a major worry."

By posing this question, patients are asking for some facts and some reassurance, both of which are provided in simple language in this response.

How Can You Diagnose Depression After Talking to Me for Just a Few Minutes? You Don't Even Know Me.

This statement or variations of this statement may represent a lack of rapport, distrust, devaluation of the clinician, and hostility in varying degrees. Such patients need considerable explanation, reassurance, and psychological support. It might also suggest underlying paranoia and perhaps a narcissistic or hypomanic grandiosity related to the belief that their problems are so special that it takes a brilliant clinician and considerable time to evaluate them and to suggest treatment.

The approach to deal with concerns raised by this question is not to give a direct answer to the question. For example, you would not tell the patient that you are well trained at prestigious institutions, are highly experienced, and that you can diagnose depression in a few minutes, even if these assertions are true. The approach I use is to present a summary of the symptoms leading to the diagnostic impression and then explain why the patient needs the treatment and how treatment will be of benefit. This approach is nonconfrontational, goal-directed, and conveys a professional but supportive and empathic stance. If such an approach does not work, further explanation and reassurance may be given. As a last resort, I give this example:

"When you take your car to the garage for repair, the mechanic asks a few questions regarding the problem, and starts fixing your car. The mechanic typically does not need to know which roads the car traveled, who drove the car, or where the car was bought. Obviously, people are more complicated than cars, and hence there is a lot of significant information about an individual. However, you have given me the essential information to get the treatment started. As we go along, I will ask for additional information when needed. Please do not hesitate to bring up information that you think is important and please ask questions as they arise. So let us start the treatment."

It is the rare patient who does not respond favorably to these explanations. Using the example of car repair brings the patients to a practical and down-to-earth perspective with which they can easily identify. Stating that people are more complex than cars neutralizes any feelings that comparison to an automobile is devaluing to them. If the patient still refuses treatment or is argumentative, the clinician may not, in fact, be able to get the patient to accept treatment during that visit. A resistant patient may need several sessions to establish sufficient rapport as well as a psychotherapy referral before being willing to accept medication treatment. In a patient with excessive guardedness, hostility, and mistrust, using a short-term, low-dose antipsychotic, such as risperidone 0.5 mg po daily for two to three weeks might be beneficial if and when the patient accepts treatment.

How Long Does It Take for the Medication to Start Working?

Antidepressants typically take one to three weeks to show response. Most patients on SSRIs should show some response by the end of the second week. Some antidepressants such as bupropion and venlafaxine tend to show response more rapidly. Since TCAs and MAOIs have to be gradually titrated up over a period of seven to ten days to reach a low therapeutic dosage range, a total of two to four weeks is generally needed for TCAs and MAOIs. Since SSRIs are frequently started at a low but effective therapeutic dosage range, their response time is comparatively less.

Antianxiety medications work almost immediately; hence, they are often used for quick response, on an as needed basis. Buspirone, an antianxiety medication, takes 10 to 14 days to begin to work when taken regularly.

Antipsychotics work fairly rapidly. Some of the psychotic symptoms such as agitation and confusion improve within 24 to 48 hours, whereas symptoms such as delusions, hallucinations, disorganized thought, and negative symptoms take longer to respond. Mood stabilizers such as lithium, carbamazepine, and valproate take one to two weeks to be effective. For chronic conditions such as cyclothymia or severe bipolar disorder, the latency period may be longer.

Medication Is Like a Band-Aid; I Don't Need a Band-Aid.

Psychiatric conditions, if not treated effectively and in a timely manner, can continue to affect one's life and get worse to the point of needing hospitalizations. Although the symptoms may not be considered serious now, the symptoms are beginning to have a major impact on almost every aspect of your life. The psychiatric evaluation has determined that your current difficulties deserve treatment that includes medication and therapy. The medication is expected to help you conquer your symptoms and enable you to be fully functional rapidly, as well as prepare you to benefit more from therapy. These are very important benefits that you can expect from the medication treatment. Therefore, you should start the recommended treatment without delay.

What Is the Best Medication for Depression? I Want the Best Medicine There Is.

There is no one medication that will work for everyone. A medication that worked extremely well for one individual could cause intolerable side effects or may not be effective for someone else. Similarly, a medication that was not effective for a particular patient might work very well for another patient. Yet medication choice is not a random or trial-and-error process. The choice of a medication for a particular patient is based on many important factors including the specific symptom profile, medication features, past history of response to medications, medical history, etc. One of the primary purposes of the psychiatric evaluation is to gather clinical information that is necessary for the process of choosing a medication that will most likely help you at the first attempt. If the first medication does not work for you or causes side effects that do not subside, another medication will be recommended, again based on clinical guidelines and the features of various medications. Essentially the medication that works for an individual is the best medication for that particular individual.

The Pharmacist Told Me This Medicine Is for Schizophrenia (or, The Pharmacy Gave Me a Medication Profile Sheet Which Indicated That This Medicine Is for Seizures), So I Didn't Take the Medication.

Patients frequently obtain additional information about their diagnosis and medications from other sources. Pharmacies provide standard information on medications for patient education purposes. Typically a medication profile sheet provided by the pharmacy includes a summary of FDA-approved indications, and major side effects. As previously mentioned, most psychiatric patients have a certain degree of ambivalence toward psychiatric medications. This is heightened when a medication is prescribed for a non-FDA approved indication, which is fairly common in medical practice. For instance, carbamazepine (Tegretol, Epitol) is frequently prescribed for a patient with bipolar disorder. A pharmacy sheet will list the FDA-approved indications of epilepsy and trigeminal neuralgia. If the patient is not informed about the off-label uses of carbamazepine, some patients might be reluctant to take the medication. Another example is when a very low dose of an antipsychotic (such as risperidone 0.5 mg or olanzapine 2.5 mg) is prescribed for mild suspiciousness, hostility, agitation, or irrational guilt, which could accompany severe depression. Short term use of low-dose antipsychotics is extremely beneficial for such patient problems. In this context, the formal diagnosis could be major depression, but the patient information sheet provided by the pharmacy may state that the medication is indicated for psychotic disorders or schizophrenia. Patients will understandably be perplexed and might even refuse to take the medication. The best approach to deal with this problem is to routinely anticipate this and to educate the patient at the time the medication is first prescribed. A sample instruction could be as follows:

"Let me mention that risperidone is prescribed for you at a low dose to control your irrational fears, anger, guilt and difficulty in thinking. At much higher doses this medication can be given for other conditions such as schizophrenia, mania, and Tourette's disorder. You don't have any of these conditions. The pharmacy might give you a patient information sheet which could list these or other indications for this medication. Please don't become nervous or fail to take the medication after reading the information sheet. Doctors sometimes use the same drug for treating a variety of conditions. The patient information sheet contains standard information, and does not specifically address your particular problem or treatment, and therefore may not be entirely relevant to you."

Patient compliance problems and many evening phone calls can be avoided with a simple preventive instructional presentation of the general nature as given here.

My Therapist Told Me I Should Work Through My Emotions and That Medications Will Blunt My Feelings.

It is true that one of the expected and desired goals of treatment using medications is to rapidly and efficiently control excessive emotions and feelings people have, so that they are able to function optimally within a matter of several weeks. If the medication blunts all emotions and makes people feel like a "zombie," then the medication choice needs to be reevaluated. The medication should help people to experience normal emotions and feelings. Generally speaking, medication treatment works rapidly. Psychotherapy is extremely beneficial in tackling and resolving various psychosocial, interpersonal, family, and occupational conflicts that might have precipitated the symptoms in the first place or were brought on by the symptoms. In fact, the ideal treatment for virtually all psychiatric conditions is a combination of psychotherapy and medication. It is also important to note that appropriate control of symptoms significantly facilitates the therapeutic process because patients are then able to discuss, analyze, understand, and resolve their conflicts and issues without becoming overwhelmed and choked by symptoms such as crying, anger, and anxiety. Patients should not be tempted to forego psychotherapy simply because their symptoms are controlled on a medication. A medication cannot resolve the various psychosocial conflicts that might persist or emerge in a person's life. In order to improve the chances of eventually discontinuing the medication and to learn more effective coping skills, psychotherapy is essential. In brief, medication helps people to become functional and regain control rapidly, and benefit more from psychotherapy. A mistake some patients make is that when they obtain fairly rapid relief of symptoms from medications, they discontinue their psychotherapy. The effort and time it takes to persist with psychotherapy are well worth it because of its potential to enrich one's life in the long term and to prevent future psychiatric problems.

The Package Insert That Came with the Medication Sample Has Two Pages of Side Effects (or, I Read the PDR in the Library–This Medicine Has Two Pages of Side Effects). I Am Scared To Take This Medication, So I Didn't Take the Medication.

The PDR lists all side effects including common, rare, minor, and serious. Patients should be routinely informed regarding the most common and significant side effects and of the fact that most patients do not experience any of the major side effects. Even if a patient has a side effect, usually the side effect subsides over five to ten days (depending on the specific side effect). If the side effect is pronounced or persistent, the medication can be safely discontinued.

Patients with obsessional, paranoid, and hypochondriacal tendencies particularly are overwhelmed when they see the long list of side effects and cautions. For this reason, the author frequently advises these patients to wait several weeks after starting the medication before they review the

PDR. If the patients are insistent on reading the PDR prior to trying the medication, considerable reassurance is necessary to overcome the fear and resistance these patients could experience. Lowering the starting dose could at times be reassuring. An ambivalent patient should be expressly encouraged to call the physician before the next scheduled appointment if any side effects emerge, so the physician can evaluate the side effect immediately and intervene. Most patients are reassured by this approach.

Is There a Blood Test to Diagnose Manic-Depression?

The diagnosis of manic-depression is based on the pattern, severity, and frequency of mood changes, a description of which is elicited in the psychiatric evaluation. A thyroid hormone level is frequently obtained to detect any thyroid abnormalities which can make the mood swings worse. However, currently there are no blood tests or other laboratory tests that can diagnose bipolar disorder.

All I Had Was Mania. I Was Never Depressed. Why Do You Diagnose Manic Depression?

Patients with typical manic depression (the current *DSM-IV* diagnosis of bipolar disorder) have had episodes of both depression and mania. In the majority of patients, manic depression initially presents with a depressive episode. In the absence of a history of a previous episode of mania the diagnosis of depression is made and treatment of depression is initiated. If that patient subsequently becomes manic, the diagnosis is then changed to manic depression. The treatment is also altered accordingly. However, there are some people whose initial presentation can be with a manic episode. While most of these patients are at high risk for eventually experiencing episodes of depression, there may be a minority of patients who only have manic episodes and no depressive episodes. These patients are also diagnosed with manic depression. I suppose a diagnosis of "unipolar mania" might best describe these patients, but this is not a formal *DSM-IV* diagnosis.

How to Respond to Questions Regarding Patients' Short-Term or Long-Term Disability and Functional Capacity: Questions Raised by Employers

Many patients being treated for emotional disorders are unable to function in their jobs and may need statements from prescribing physicians regarding diagnosis, course, treatment, prognosis, and assessment of functional capacity, regardless of whether the prescribing physician is a psychiatrist or a nonpsychiatrist. Any physician who treats emotional disorders should become familiar with completing these forms in a manner that is objective and factual. If physicians make claims that they are unable to substantiate, patients risk losing benefits and physicians place their credibility in question. The treating physician's primary obligation is to the patient. As a result, the clinician should be as supportive to the patient as possible without giving opinions that are unreasonable.

The following is a discussion of issues commonly raised by employers. Physicians must assess the patient's capacity to perform a particular job or component skills in a job, after studying a detailed job description that is attached to the questionnaire. Some companies ask the physician which jobs the patient can and cannot perform. My way of dealing with these requests is not to directly respond to these questions because physicians are not experts in evaluating the suitability of an individual for any specific job or task. It is much more meaningful and within the physician's competence to list the areas of impairment in a patient and to let the employer or the disability evaluator apply the clinician's findings to the patient and the job. It is wise not to get involved in making recommendations as to which specific tasks the patient can and cannot perform. A useful statement format is given here. Obviously, specifics will vary in individual cases.

> My evaluation reveals that the patient's emotional stability, energy level, motivation, concentration, interests, sleep, and logical thinking capacity are impaired. On this basis, he would be unable to perform any job requiring optimal levels of the above functions. The patient is presently under my treatment. It is expected that if and when treatment is successful, the patient will return to his previous level of functioning. I anticipate that it will take approximately two to three months for treatment to have maximum effect.

Many of the conclusions in psychiatry are based on patients' statements and self-reports. There are no lab tests or X rays to objectively diagnose or quantify depression, anxiety or suicidality, for example. Since the physician is not an investigator, it is necessary to rely on a patient's history. Hence the physician's conclusion and opinion, in many situations, should also be noted to be based on patients' reports. For example, if a patient reports that he or she is suicidal, no mental health professional should refute that. Whereas, this is different in other specialties. For instance, if a patient claims that a particular bone is broken, immediate and accurate affirmation or refutal of that assertion is possible with an X ray. Reliable and valid objective testing of subjective feelings and thoughts is not available in psychiatry. While psychological testing has the aura of objectivity, it is truly subjective. Psychological tests are standardized. Standardization and objectivity are two different concepts that are often confusing to people.

TREATMENT OF SPECIAL PATIENTS

Any patient who is a celebrity, a public figure, or who is newsworthy could be considered a "special" patient. Included in this group are politicians, entertainment professionals, notorious criminals, etc. Physicians and various health professionals are also usually treated with special consideration.

It is sometimes necessary to make special arrangements to provide psychiatric treatment to special patients. Since many of them are recognized by others, arrangements should be made to assure, within reason, that the visit to the psychiatrist will be confidential. In the case of a physician patient who practices in the local community, there is always a chance that a mutual patient could be in the waiting room. To deal with these situations, when necessary, I have offered to see special patients at a neutral location, or in the patient's home or office, depending on individual circumstances. In addition to such arrangements, it is common practice to give a professional courtesy discount of 25 percent to other health professionals, and in some cases, complimentary service to individuals who are direct professional or personal acquaintances. Examples include friends, neighbors, and other health professionals who are personally known through referrals, patient care, consultations, etc.

However, the clinician must be vigilant so that no special arrangements or "discounts" are made in terms of clinical assessment, judgment, and treatment recommendations. Thus, if a special patient needs to be involuntarily committed based on clinical findings, the special status of the patient must not be allowed to interfere with the clinician's decision. If the clinical evaluation shows that the patient is likely to be noncompliant, and for this or other reasons the patient is not likely to benefit from treatment, the clinician should not hesitate to refuse further services. He or she should give the relevant reasons, just as one would deal with any patient who is likely to be noncompliant.

It is important to remember that all patients, including special patients, have similar anatomy, physiology, and neurochemistry. The basic psychological dynamics are also similar. The clinician must be on guard against being influenced by the occasional narcissistic gratification inherent in being the professional providing services to a special patient. Such a temptation if not understood and managed can lead to compromises and poor judgment in clinical evaluation and management decisions. Efforts to do more usually are neither effective nor desirable. Hence, the basic approach when dealing with special patients is to treat them just like any other patient from a clinical standpoint but to give special treatment in nonclinical matters (such as appointments, house calls, etc.) in order to accommodate their unique needs.

Let me illustrate these points by citing an example from another specialty. An appendectomy is done the same way, regardless of whether the patient is special or not, because anatomy and physiology are sufficiently similar in all individuals. If changes are made in the surgical technique, for example, suturing slower than usual, having extra surgeons to assist, giving more fluids or blood than necessary, delaying or hurrying the procedure, etc., complications are more likely to occur. Hence, the surgical team has to forget the special nature of the patient on entering the operating room. Similarly, psychiatric assessment and treatment should be based strictly on clinical material. Refer to Table 13.3 for a list of clinical errors made by mental health professionals when treating special patients.

Any therapy boundary violation is likely to lead to disruption of treatment. If the special patient happens to be socially prominent, the clinician may be tempted, by virtue of human nature, to accept invitations for social or sports events, etc. The secondary prestige the physician experiences in these situations is ephemeral since the disruption of treatment that usually accompanies such overinvolvement is likely to lead to a negative outcome. In the long run, this has the potential to tarnish the reputation of the clinician, especially when it is the negative outcome that gets publicity. Social stigma associated with mental health treatment is still prevalent in varying degrees in different geographical locations. Moreover, one of the fundamental duties of the clinician is to maintain confidentiality of treatment, regardless of the outcome. It is unlikely that patients receiving mental health services will boast of their treatment and openly recommend the clinician, unlike other medical specialties such as surgery, cardiology, or plastic surgery, where social stigma is not a factor. For these reasons, it may even be desirable for a mental health clinician to keep a low profile socially. In other medical specialties, especially plastic surgery, social exposure may even be a marketing necessity, but this is clearly not the case in psychiatry today.

The mental health clinician does not gain much, other than possible professional fees, in treating a special patient. In general, the many diffi-

TABLE 13.3. Clinical Errors Made by Clinicians in Treating Special Patients

- Minimalization or underdiagnosis of the severity of problems
- Failure to properly assess potential for harm to self or others
- Reluctance to administer medication involuntarily when clinically indicated
- Reluctance to diagnose psychosis
- Reluctance to prescribe antipsychotics
- Avoidance of dealing with noncompliance
- Excessive use of sedatives
- Failure to strictly monitor sedative use
- Change of diagnosis for nonclinical reasons
- Excessive social involvement, acceptance of gifts, etc.
- Overenthusiasm and overinvolvement
- Reluctance to recommend hospitalization and to insist on hospitalization when clinically indicated
- Failure to discharge from practice when patient is chronically noncompliant or when the patient refuses important treatment recommendations
- Excessive and inappropriate use of telephone consultations instead of the standard face-to-face visit
- Discussion of the case with colleagues socially
- Psychiatric rationalization and treatment provided for essentially criminal conducts

culties inherent in dealing with a noncompliant special patient and extra efforts involved in scheduling and in assuring confidentiality make the task of treating a special patient a challenge that usually has low personal benefit-to-effort ratio when compared to treating an average patient.

However, there is tremendous personal and professional satisfaction associated with treating a compliant special patient, especially if the outcome is successful, despite the greater administrative efforts involved. It is one of the indications of ultimate professional recognition and confidence when another medical professional or a special patient chooses the clinician for provision of treatment.

Chapter 14

Office Management of Severe Disorders: General Clinical Concepts

There are many instances in a busy office practice when patients present with symptoms severe enough to benefit from hospitalization. Third-party payers may refer a severely ill patient directly to the office for emergency psychiatric evaluation and management. The physician is under more pressure in today's managed care environment to treat as outpatients very ill patients who only a few years ago would have been routinely admitted. In the past, when third-party payment for psychiatric hospitalizations was fairly liberal, hospitalizations were often the option for patients who could have been treated satisfactorily as outpatients. Even when hospitalization is possible from a third-party payment or self-pay standpoint, many patients prefer to be treated as outpatients or may refuse hospitalization for other reasons. In some of these instances, a patient's symptoms may not meet the clinical criteria for involuntary commitment, especially if the patient is cooperative in receiving treatment as an outpatient. The physician may have no choice but to begin treatment as an outpatient. The choice of the physician to refuse to treat a patient who is noncompliant with treatment recommendations is an option that may need to be exercised at times. In most situations, however, the physician will initiate treatment in the office. Although hospitalization may be the ideal choice for numerous patients, the present reality is that hospitalization may not be possible.

Third-party payers, especially managed care companies, understandably expect the physician to treat increasingly sick patients effectively in the office. For all of these reasons, the physician should be well-versed in rapid management strategies for treating severely emotionally disordered patients in the office. Specific management strategies of various acute cases presented in the office are discussed in the clinical case section (Part II).

The most important first step in managing severely ill patients is accurate diagnosis, which is obviously important in all conditions regardless of the severity. However, there are certain symptoms that can complicate the clinical picture and put the patient at risk if they are not recognized immediately and managed. Examples of these are suicidality, psychosis, coexisting mania, abuse of alcohol or drugs, and homicidality. These symptoms, when present, require intensive and aggressive management with medications, as well as supervision by caring family members.

Suicidal ideation need not be a sufficient reason to hospitalize a patient. However, if a patient is extremely suicidal with intent or plan and refuses treatment, emergency hospitalization is necessary. If a supportive family member or responsible friend is available to supervise the patient during the first week of treatment, and if the patient is cooperative with outpatient treatment, it is possible to manage the patient in the office. In nearly all of these situations, rational and balanced polypharmacy, as described in this text, is usually necessary. The choice of medications depends on specific symptoms, as outlined in other sections of this text as well as in the clinical case section. Medication should not generally be withheld until the results of laboratory tests are obtained unless toxicity or other medical etiology is suspected. Clinical experience has shown that the yield from most laboratory studies is low in a patient presenting with typical psychiatric symptoms. Hence, it is crucial to start medication immediately in patients who are in severe distress. Concurrent with medications, it is beneficial to begin psychotherapy especially for any severely distressed patient. So that medication adjustments can be made frequently, if needed, the patient should be monitored by the physician every two to three days in the office until distressing symptoms such as psychotic thinking, agitation, homicidality, suicidality, and insomnia are improving or under control. Patients and significant others should be encouraged to call the physician to report any deterioration, or problem with the medication.

Since severely depressed patients commonly have irrational thinking and feelings of guilt, it is prudent to use low doses of antipsychotic medication during the first one to two weeks. The presence of psychotic features does not necessarily require hospitalization. However, it is of utmost importance to have a low threshold in identifying even mild psychotic symptoms, and to start treatment specifically to address the psychosis. In these cases, at the very least, a combination of an antidepressant and an antipsychotic is required. Coexisting mild psychosis is frequently missed by the physician, resulting in clinical deterioration or lack of improvement. If there is even a suspicion of the presence of psychotic symptoms, the cautious approach would be to prescribe a very low dose of an antipsychotic during the first one or two weeks of office treatment for severe depression. Exposing the patient to a low dose of an antipsychotic for one or two weeks should not cause significant long-term neuroleptic side effects, particularly if risperidone or olanzapine, which have relatively few side effects, is used. The dose needed is in the range of risperidone 0.5 mg or olanzapine 2.5 mg per day. The low dose of antipsychotics affords considerable protection to the patient from self-directed or other violent acts seen in some severe depressions during the first two weeks while the antidepressants are taking effect. The antipsychotic may be withdrawn after the antidepressant begins to be effective.

In most cases, the beginning of medication treatment should not be contingent on the availability of results of baseline or screening laboratory studies or psychological testing, which, if necessary, can be obtained later. As discussed earlier, psychiatric diagnosis, for most practical purposes, remains a clinical diagnosis. A clinical practitioner should have sufficient confidence in the diagnosis during the first visit to start treatment. In some cases, the diagnosis may have to be revised as more information becomes available during the course of treatment. For example, bipolar disorder and psychotic disorders frequently present with depressive symptoms. For this reason, the clinician must think like a detective and diligently search for other more malignant processes in patients complaining of the common presenting symptoms of depression and anxiety. There must also be a willingness to alter treatment as needed in response to new information; this makes the treatment course a very dynamic process.

Depression and homicidality are a dangerous mix, requiring immediate treatment using antipsychotics to rapidly control the externally directed hostility, even though homicidal ideation and depression are not associated with typical psychotic thinking. Since antidepressant medication takes one to two weeks to begin to be effective, the patient needs something that will immediately and effectively decrease hostility and agitation. Frequently, a combination of antipsychotics and benzodiazepines is very effective, allowing time for the antidepressant to start working, while protecting the patient and others. Once the antidepressant medication begins to become effective, other medications may be slowly tapered off. SSRIs are particularly effective for control of depression-based anger and hostility. Anger and hostility related to underlying psychosis can be made worse by antidepressants. Violence is always a grave sign, requiring aggressive and intensive management.

There is a fundamental difference in the initial medication intervention in managing severe depression as compared to psychosis. Antidepressant medication is typically started at a low therapeutic dose with a gradual dosage increase for the treatment of severe depression. Associated symptoms are managed by prescribing adjunctive medications for rapid relief. The immediate benefit to the severely depressed patient is not obtained from antidepressants. Adjunctive medications provide rapid relief and are critical in the first several weeks of treating a severely depressed patient. In the case of a severely depressed individual with considerable anxiety, insomnia, and anorexia, treatment with an antidepressant has a latency period of one to three weeks. Adjunctive medications will immediately control the additional symptoms. The antidepressant dosage is gradually increased until a response is seen and the dosage is maintained at the effective level. For example, imipramine is usually started at 50 mg and gradually increased to 300 mg if needed. Similarly, fluoxetine is started at 20 mg and slowly increased up to 80 mg. It is not customary to start a patient on imipramine 300 mg or fluoxetine 80 mg.

The clinical strategy in treating acute psychotic conditions is different. Psychotic patients are usually started on fairly high doses of antipsychotics for rapid control. After the psychosis is controlled, the dose is slowly decreased and the patient is kept on a maintenance dose that is typically less than the effective dose used initially. For instance, it is not unusual to give haloperidol 20 mg or the equivalent daily to a psychotic patient during the first two to four days of treatment, and then to gradually decrease the dose to a maintenance dose of haloperidol 5 to 10 mg or equivalent. The clinical significance of this is that when severely depressed patients are treated in the office, aggressive management using adjunctive medications is necessary so that hospitalization can be prevented. It is the adjunctive medications that "hold" a patient for the first several weeks necessary for the antidepressant response to manifest. In contrast, antipsychotic medication (for an acutely psychotic patient) is started at moderate to high doses for rapid control and becomes effective much faster than an antidepressant.

The traditional approach to treating a severely depressed patient has been to hospitalize the patient, start an antidepressant, and wait for the antidepressant to work. By using a medication combination as discussed in the text and in the case-study section, many severely depressed patients can be safely managed in the office. Mild psychosis requires only low doses of antipsychotic medications and can also be safely managed in the office.

If the patient is in a hospital inpatient unit where protection is afforded, antipsychotic medication during the first several weeks may not be necessary. Paradoxically, outpatient treatment of severe disorders has to be psychopharmacologically more aggressive because the patient is more dependent on the medication for control of internal impulses and behavior.

With prompt and aggressive office management and the use of a combination of medications, many hospitalizations can be prevented. Obviously, patients who are out of control, uncooperative, or intoxicated cannot be managed in the office.

The choice of combinations of medications is based on presenting symptoms, clinical reasoning, and psychopharmacological principles. The medications should be complementary, and together improve all of the symptoms without side effects. When more than one medication is started at the same time, there is a greater risk of emergence of a side effect or an allergic reaction and therefore greater difficulty in identifying the medication responsible for the reaction. In most cases, the nature of side effects can help identify the medication responsible for causing the side effect. However, it is harder to identify the medication if an allergic reaction such as a rash is the problem. For a patient with severe symptoms, this risk is negligible compared to the benefits. However, for a patient with a fairly routine diagnosis and in whom immediate control of symptoms is not necessary, a sequential trial of medication is sufficient and avoids these risks.

PART II: ONE HUNDRED TEACHING CLINICAL CASES

Chapter 15

Simple Cases

INTRODUCTION TO CASES

The 100 clinical cases are classified into three categories as follows: simple cases, moderately complex cases, and complex cases. The first paragraph of each case summarizes the presenting complaints and symptoms derived from the interview of the patient, collateral history, mental status examination and, in some cases, psychological test results. Since the main theme of the text is practical treatment guidelines, detailed historical information and a separate section on mental-status examination are omitted. Patients typically do not volunteer that they have ideas of reference, paranoia, dissociative episodes, obsessive-compulsive tendencies, mania, hypomania, hallucinations, or a thought disorder unless they have had psychiatric training. These are conclusions and formulations arrived at by the clinician after studying information from multiple sources as listed above. In some cases the information presented in the beginning paragraph of each case was obtained after several patient visits. A unique aspect of psychiatric evaluation is that patients do not divulge all of the information during the first visit. They are more forthcoming with information after they feel comfortable with the clinician. This is particularly true for patients with Axis I problems complicated by an Axis II diagnosis and for patients who have "sensitive" symptoms or history including suicidal and homicidal ideation and history of abuse.

The cases emphasize a variety of aspects related to treatment. The specific dose of medications and treatment course are given in some detail. The section titled "Comments" primarily discusses management issues.

CASES 1 TO 32

Case #1

Presenting Symptoms: The patient was a 64-year-old female. Symptoms consisted of extreme fear of storms and rain, wind, tornadoes, and being in an elevator. Whenever exposed to any of these situations or when anticipating them, the patient experienced diarrhea, dry mouth, sweating, palpitations, and fright. Paroxetine 20 mg was tried but stopped due to excessive fatigue. The patient had been seen by a physician who placed her on a trial of sertraline 50 mg and lorazepam 1 mg PRN for three weeks with no effects. She discontinued the medications prior to scheduling an appointment with me. She denied substance abuse, smoking, or caffeine intake. Her current medications were estrogen 1.25 mg for estrogen supplementation and Simvastatin 10 mg for hypercholesterolemia. Her family history was unremarkable for psychiatric disorders except for a daughter who the patient reported to be depressed.

Current Diagnosis: Specific phobia

Current Treatment: 1. clomipramine 75 mg HS
2. alprazolam 0.5 mg BID PRN anxiety
3. psychotherapy

Treatment Course: The patient was started on clomipramine (Anafranil) 25 mg for the first three days, then increased to 50 mg at bedtime, along with alprazolam (Xanax) 0.5 mg TID PRN. When seen for follow-up after two weeks, the patient reported moderate improvement in the phobic symptoms. The dose of clomipramine was increased to 75 mg at bedtime. After two weeks, there was remarkable improvement in all phobic symptoms and in anticipatory anxiety. Once the clomipramine was increased to 75 mg, the patient no longer felt the need to use alprazolam. She has endured several rainstorms without being overwhelmed during the last three months. The patient now sees a counselor once a month and sees me once every three months for medication follow-up.

Comments: Antidepressant medications should be used as a first-line medication for all anxiety disorders, including phobias. Because of their favorable side effect profile, selective SSRIs are the first choice among antidepressants. In this particular case, paroxetine and sertraline were tried, but had to be discontinued. Clomipramine was not only tolerated well by the patient, but she had an excellent response to it. For reasons that I cannot recall, fluoxetine, fluvoxamine, and venlafaxine were not tried, but would have also been excellent choices. All TCAs and MAOIs such as phenelzine and tranylcypromine are very effective for anxiety disorders. However, the latter group of medications are not first-line medications in current clinical practice since the advent of SSRIs.

High-potency benzodiazepines are extremely useful as adjunctive medications when used on a PRN basis. They should not be the primary medications for the treatment of anxiety disorders unless the patient cannot tolerate SSRIs, TCAs, and MAOIs.

Case #2

Presenting Symptoms: The patient was a 23-year-old male with complaints of anxiety, anxiety attacks at a frequency of about one per day, obsessive worrying, increased emotional sensitivity, occasional spontaneous crying, anticipatory anxiety, agoraphobia (avoided eating in public), and occasional depressed mood. These symptoms had been present for about three months. He denied substance abuse, smoking, or caffeine intake. He reported no medical problems other than frequent heartburn. He had no family history of psychiatric disorders.

Current Diagnosis: Panic disorder with agoraphobia
Depressive symptoms

Current Treatment: 1. paroxetine 30 mg AM

Treatment Course: The patient was started on paroxetine 20 mg AM and ranitidine (Zantac) 150 mg at bedtime. When seen after three weeks, anxiety symptoms had improved moderately. Ranitidine was discontinued after the first three weeks. The dosage of paroxetine was increased to 30 mg AM with significant improvement in all anxiety and depressive symptoms. The patient is seen for follow-up once every three to four months.

Comments: Depressive symptoms frequently accompany a primary anxiety disorder such as panic disorder. One could have opted to treat this patient on alprazolam or any of the high-potency benzodiazepines, or imipramine or any of the TCAs. Any of the SSRIs probably would have given equally satisfactory results. Because of the problems associated with benzodiazepines (see section on treatment of anxiety) and TCAs, an SSRI was chosen as the first-line medication.

When patients report dyspepsia or symptoms suggestive of gastric hyperacidity, it is helpful to start them on an H2 blocker for one to two weeks, especially when initiating SSRIs, which can exacerbate gastric irritability. A low dose of high-potency benzodiazepine or beta-blocker for PRN use could have been prescribed for anticipatory anxiety and for use in agoraphobic situations. Since the patient responded well to paroxetine alone, it was fortunate that adjunctive benzodiazepines or beta-blockers were not needed. Although psychotherapy was recommended at the second office visit, the patient felt that he did not need it.

Case #3

Presenting Symptoms: The patient was a 15-year-old female with complaints of irritability, anger attacks, excessive emotional sensitivity, depressed mood, feelings of hopelessness, suicidal ideation without intent or plan, crying episodes, anergia, and anhedonia. These symptoms had been present for several years, but had worsened during the past two to three months with no known precipitants. She denied drug and alcohol abuse, smoking, and caffeine intake. She also denied any previous psychiatric treatment. The patient had no medical problems. She was taking oral contraceptives. Her father suffered from manic-depression and substance abuse.

Current Diagnosis: Major depression, moderate, single episode
Dysthymia

Current Treatment:
1. paroxetine 30 mg AM
2. trazodone 25 mg HS
3. psychotherapy once every one to two weeks by the referring psychologist

Treatment Course: The patient was started on fluoxetine 20 mg AM and felt better for the first five days after which depressive symptoms returned. Dosage was increased to 40 mg AM two weeks after the initial visit. Since she experienced racing thoughts, restlessness, and insomnia on this dose, her mother requested that the dosage be decreased to 20 mg, which was not sufficient to control depressive symptoms. I increased the dose to 30 mg, which again caused racing thoughts, restlessness, anxiety, and insomnia. At this point, I decided to discontinue fluoxetine and try sertraline 50 mg AM, which I discontinued after several weeks because of persistent nausea and heartburn. Next paroxetine 20 mg AM was started, with significant improvement in symptoms and no major side effects, except insomnia, for which trazodone 50 mg was tried. Since trazodone 50 mg produced daytime drowsiness, the dose was decreased to 25 mg. The dose of paroxetine was eventually increased to 30 mg AM for optimal improvement.

Comments: This patient had symptoms suggestive of major depression superimposed on dysthymia. Paroxetine was found to be effective without major side effects following trials on fluoxetine and sertraline that were not successful.

The choice of an antidepressant within a major class of antidepressants is based on guesswork in most cases. Another patient with similar symptoms could respond well to fluoxetine or sertraline. However, there are certain general guidelines based on medication and side-effect characteristics, as outlined in Chapter 2. The use of these guidelines could improve the chances of selecting the most effective antidepressant for a particular symptom pattern. In general, SSRIs or bupropion are chosen as the first-line antidepressants because of their favorable side effect profiles. The goal of the physician is to prescribe the best antidepressant for the particular patient so that symptoms are treated without having to change medications. Since depressed patients are easily frustrated and tend to give up quickly, they should be counseled that it is both likely and understable if they become frustrated. However, they should not allow their frustration to interfere with continued efforts to find the appropriate antidepressant. Patients should also be assured that the antidepressant that is right for them will be found sooner or later. Such supportive instructions enhance compliance, especially when dealing with teenagers, some of whom are not inherently motivated, but are pressured by their parents to seek treatment.

Also of note, depression can be a side effect of oral contraceptives. Although a change of the oral contraceptive is an option, an antidepressant is frequently necessary if depressive symptoms are of a moderate or greater severity.

Case #4

Presenting Symptoms: The patient was a 40-year-old female with complaints of anorexia, irritability, anxiety, panic attacks, occasional crying episodes, excessive emotional sensitivity, obsessive worrying, initial and middle insomnia, feelings of hopelessness, and anhedonia. These symptoms worsened several months ago due to family conflicts and work stress. She tried nortriptyline two years ago, but stopped after three months because of increased agitation and hostility. She denied drug and alcohol abuse and caffeine intake. The patient's mother had a diagnosis of manic-depression and her son had attention deficit hyperactivity disorder.

Current Diagnosis: Adjustment disorder with depressed mood
Dysthymia

Current Treatment:
1. paroxetine 20 mg AM
2. doxepin 25 mg HS
3. bupropion 100 mg AM and noon
4. psychotherapy with a psychologist

Treatment Course: The patient was started on paroxetine 20 mg AM, doxepin 10 mg HS, and lorazepam 1 mg HS. Her depressive symptoms and sleep improved, but there was no improvement in her appetite when seen two weeks later; hence, doxepin was increased to 25 mg HS and lorazepam decreased to 0.5 mg HS. Her appetite improved satisfactorily on this regimen. Lorazepam was discontinued because she was sleeping well on doxepin alone. However, she complained of anergia and impaired sexual functioning for which bupropion 100 mg AM was added with some improvement in these symptoms. The dose of bupropion was further increased to 100 mg AM and at noon which improved her energy level and sexual functioning to a satisfactory level. The patient is functioning well in her job and as a mother without any significant side effects.

Comments: This patient had a height of 5 feet, 7 inches, and a weight of 105 pounds. She had complained of chronic anorexia and wanted to gain weight. One of the side effects of tricyclic antidepressants (TCAs) is weight gain. Since this side effect is evident even at low doses, one of the convenient and effective medication strategies to increase appetite is to place the patient on a low dose of a TCA. If the patient also has insomnia, a sedating TCA such as doxepin or amitriptyline at 10 to 25 mg is useful, whereas if sedation is not desirable, one may choose a less-sedating TCA such as desipramine or nortriptyline at 10 to 25 mg HS. If a patient also has dyspepsia, the H2 blocking properties of doxepin can be exploited. This is an example of taking advantage of the side effects of a medication to treat a specific symptom, thereby enhancing patient comfort.

Sexual dysfunction is a common side effect of all antidepressants, particularly the SSRIs. An exception to this is bupropion. Trazodone, mirtazapine, and nefazodone do not interfere with sexual functioning significantly. A list of various adjunctive medications that can be tried to treat SSRI-induced sexual dysfunction is given in Chapter 3.

This patient complained of persistent anergia. Other depressive symptoms completely resolved. Hence, it was decided to add bupropion initially at 100 mg AM, later increased to 100 mg AM and at noon for optimal effectiveness. Anergia improved significantly. Sexual dysfunction improved only moderately after the addition of bupropion. Most patients accept the sexual dysfunction as a "trade off" if their presenting symptoms are significantly improved. In many patients, sexual functioning improves by itself over several months. However, in some patients sexual functioning is sufficiently impaired such that either change of medication or specific treatment to alleviate the problem is indicated. TCAs, except for clomipramine, impair sexual functioning less in comparison to selective serotonin reuptake inhibitors. The sexual side effects of MAOIs are similar to those of SSRIs. In this patient, given her anergia and absence of a history of substance abuse, the clinician could have chosen a stimulant, such as methylphenidate 5 to 10 mg BID or dextroamphetamine 5 to 10 mg AM.

Fluoxetine, with its mildly stimulating properties, could have improved depressive symptoms and anergia in this patient. Sertraline and venlafaxine could also have been effective. Among TCAs, imipramine would have provided effective antidepressant effects, along with moderate sedation, appetite stimulation, and relatively less impairment of sexual functioning, avoiding the need for adjunctive doxepin and perhaps bupropion. Similarly, mirtazapine would have been a reasonable choice especially regarding its lack of impairment of sexual functioning and its appetite-enhancing effects. These options are presented to emphasize that there is more than one method of treating the patient depending on the physician's orientation, experience, and judgment, and the patient's preferences.

Some of the other medication interventions may be even better tolerated and more parsimonious for the patient. However, in actual practice, it is not possible for the physician to try all options before selecting a medication or combination of medications. Medication choices are made based on patient symptoms, clinical judgment, and medication characteristics.

Once the patient achieves sufficient weight gain, doxepin may gradually be withdrawn. If insomnia recurs, choices are trazodone 25 to 100 mg HS or one of the benzodiazepine hypnotics.

Since bupropion lowers seizure threshold, its dose should be kept low when used adjunctively in combination with other antidepressants. (Refer to details on use of bupropion in the section on antidepressants.)

Case #5

Presenting Symptoms: The patient was a 53-year-old female. She was admitted to an inpatient psychiatric unit with severely depressed mood, frequent crying, suicidal ideation, severe insomnia, anorexia, feelings of hopelessness and worthlessness, and anhedonia. The symptoms emerged several months before the initial evaluation and worsened with no acute precipitants. She denied drug and alcohol abuse and caffeine intake, and smoked one pack of cigarettes per day. She denied previous psychiatric treatment and denied any family history of psychiatric disorders. The patient's medical history was significant for mitral valve replacement due to rheumatic fever as a child, and for a history of peptic ulcer. She was on Warfarin 5 mg daily, and has been taking over-the-counter antacids PRN.

Current Diagnosis: Major depression, severe, single episode

Current Treatment:
1. fluoxetine 20 mg AM
2. doxepin 50 mg HS
3. individual therapy by counselor as needed

Treatment Course: The patient was discharged from the hospital in improved condition after seven days of inpatient treatment on fluoxetine 20 mg AM, doxepin 25 mg HS, and clonazepam 0.5 mg PRN for insomnia. As an outpatient, doxepin was increased to 50 mg HS to improve sleep and appetite. Clonazepam was discontinued. Fluoxetine was stopped by the patient, but after two months the medication was restarted because depressive symptoms began to reemerge. The patient has done well on fluoxetine 20 mg AM and doxepin 50 mg HS for several years now. She has not needed antacids since starting doxepin. She is now seen in the office every six months for medication follow-up.

Comments: The H2-blocking properties of doxepin can be exploited for patients with dyspepsia if other side effects, such as sedation and appetite stimulation, are also beneficial to the patient. There is no definitive answer as to how long a patient should stay on an antidepressant. Maintenance antidepressant treatment should be individualized to the patient's needs, as in all areas of medicine. General guidelines are six to twelve months for the first episode, and more than twelve months for recurrent depression. For dysthymia, which by definition is a chronic condition, several years of antidepressant treatment may be beneficial prior to discontinuation.

The maintenance dose of an antidepressant is generally the same as the effective dose used for the acute treatment of depression. However, many patients do well on lower doses, especially if the dose used for the acute treatment phase was on the high end of the dosage range. For those who are already on a fairly low dose, further dosage decrease during the maintenance phase may not be effective. Ideally, antidepressants should be gradually tapered off over a period of several weeks—especially those that have a short half-life. Refer to Chapter 13 for details regarding the length of treatment on antidepressants.

Since fluoxetine is highly protein bound, it can displace other protein-bound drugs such as anticoagulants. The coagulation status should be monitored more closely during initiation of treatment, although this has not been a practical problem in the author's experience. In general, when the patient is on medications that have a narrow therapeutic index, it is a good practice to monitor the serum level or other indexes more closely until dosages are stabilized.

Case #6

Presenting Symptoms: The patient was a 29-year-old female, with complaints of obsessive preoccupation that her children would soon die from a disease. She also presented with anxiety, irritability, anger outbursts, and periodic depression. The irritability and anxiety symptoms had been present for many years. The obsessional symptoms emerged after a recent interstate move due to a job transfer. She denied drug and alcohol abuse, smoking, and caffeine intake. She had counseling off and on in the past for moodiness, anxiety, and excessive anger. The patient's mother suffered from manic depression, and her maternal grandfather had had a "nervous breakdown." She denied any medical problems.

Current Diagnosis: Obsessive-compulsive disorder (OCD)
Dysthymia

Current Treatment: 1. paroxetine 20 mg AM
2. Counseling with a therapist was recommended; to date the patient has not followed up on this.

Treatment Course: The patient had psychotherapy periodically for years, with short-term improvement, yet she was very reluctant to try medication. She did not feel that further psychotherapy was needed, although a referral had been made. Reluctantly, she agreed to try medication. She was started on fluoxetine 10 mg, which had to be discontinued after two weeks because of increased anxiety and restlessness. On her second visit, paroxetine 20 mg was started. After two weeks, she reported significant improvement in her obsessional, anger, and mood symptoms. The only side effect was significant impairment in libido and sexual functioning. The following medications and dosages were tried serially to treat the sexual dysfunction without success:

- bupropion 75 mg AM and at noon
- trazodone 50 mg HS
- amantadine (Symmetral) 100 mg BID
- bethanechol (Urecholine) 25 mg TID
- methylphenidate 5 mg BID

The patient was offered a change of medication to try to overcome sexual side effects. Her improvement and confidence on paroxetine were now so strong that she decided to bear with the sexual side effects, rather than risk relapse by changing medications. She has now been on paroxetine for six months, and she wants to continue on it indefinitely.

Comments: Nearly all patients who have obsessive-compulsive symptoms also have symptoms of depression, but the clinician must systematically look for them. From a treatment standpoint, the identification of obsessive-compulsive symptoms is important because SSRIs and clomipramine are preferentially effective, whereas for depression without obsessive-compulsive symptoms, all antidepressants are fairly equally effective with equivalent dosages, with the difference being in the side effect profile.

Medication and psychotherapy work together, perhaps synergistically. Although this patient has been somewhat disappointed with psychotherapy in the past, it is the author's view that psychotherapy could help her more when her distressing symptoms are under control on medication. This would enable her to work on more fundamental conflicts, motives, fears, anxieties, coping skills, and relationship issues, without being overwhelmed or distracted by symptoms. In general, medication and psychotherapy work better together than either alone. This is valid even for disorders that are primarily biological because illness has psychosocial consequences.

Antidepressants frequently cause sexual dysfunction, such as decreased libido, decreased pleasurable body sensations, inhibition of orgasm, inhibition of ejaculation, impotence, and, in rare cases, an active dislike of physical intimacy. The medications used to treat SSRI-induced sexual side effects have a low success rate. This issue is discussed in more detail in Chapter 3. Since SSRIs and clomipramine cause sexual dysfunction at varying degrees, a change of antidepressant is a reasonable option. Perhaps fluvoxamine, sertraline, or one of the other SSRIs would have been less offensive in this regard. Bupropion, mirtazapine, trazodone, and nefazodone are relatively free of sexual side effects, with bupropion causing the least sexual dysfunction. However, these four medications are not particularly effective for obsessive-compulsive symptoms in the author's experience. For depression characterized by apathy, anergia, hypersomnia, hyperphagia, or psychomotor retardation, bupropion could be one of the first-line medications because of its stimulating properties.

Clomipramine is probably the most effective medication for obsessive-compulsive symptoms among the medications currently available, but its TCA side effects and epileptogenic potential make it a second-line medication compared to SSRIs. Although all SSRIs are expected to be equally effective for the treatment of obsessive-compulsive symptoms, only fluoxetine, fluvoxamine, paroxetine, and sertaline among SSRIs are currently FDA-approved for the treatment of obsessive-compulsive disorder.

Case #7

Presenting Symptoms: The patient was a 46-year-old female with complaints of anger outbursts, irritability, depressed mood, extreme moodiness, occasional crying episodes, perfectionistic tendencies, initial insomnia, feelings of hopelessness, anorexia, and anhedonia. She has had episodic depression during the last ten years, for which she was treated in

1973 with amitriptyline and in 1993 with nortriptyline. These resolved her depression but caused persistent dry mouth and constipation. The symptoms worsened following her mother's death a year ago. She denied drug and alcohol abuse, smoked one-half of a pack of cigarettes per day and drank two to three cups of regular coffee daily. Her brother had a history of depression. The patient's medical history was remarkable for migraine headaches, for which she was on Atenolol.

Current Diagnosis: Adjustment disorder with depressed mood
Dysthymia

Current Treatment:
1. paroxetine 30 mg AM and 15 mg at noon
2. nortriptyline 25 mg PRN for premenstrual dysphoria
3. zolpidem 5 mg HS PRN for insomnia
4. psychotherapy with the referring therapist

Treatment Course: The patient was started on paroxetine 20 mg AM, amitriptyline 10 mg HS, and lorazepam 0.5 mg HS. Except for insomnia, the patient reported improvement. Amitriptyline was discontinued and replaced with trazodone 50 mg HS, resulting in satisfactory improvement in insomnia. A month later, the patient again complained of insomnia, prompting an increase of trazodone to 100 mg HS, which resulted in improvement in insomnia. One month later, depressive symptoms in a milder form resurfaced. Hence, paroxetine was increased to 30 mg AM. She was able to stop trazodone and lorazepam. About three months later, she complained of breakthrough symptoms of depression, dyspepsia, premenstrual dysphoria, and initial insomnia. The dose of paroxetine was increased to 30 mg AM and 15 mg at noon. Additionally, she was started on nortriptyline 25 mg PRN for premenstrual dysphoria, ranitidine 150 mg HS (for one month), and zolpidem 5 mg PRN insomnia. She has done well on the above medications for the last six months.

Comments: Breakthrough depression in a patient who is on an antidepressant that was effective requires upward adjustment of the dose, if possible. The dosage can be decreased slightly after the acute depression is controlled.

Premenstrual dysphoria responds well to TCAs; SSRIs are also effective. By increasing the dose during four to six days premenstrually, most patients obtain relief. The sedative effects of TCAs, when used on a PRN basis as in this case, are beneficial.

SSRIs commonly cause dyspepsia or worsen it; hence, H2 blockers may be needed for short-term treatment. Among the H2 blockers, cimetidine (Tagamet) tends to inhibit liver enzymes that also metabolize SSRIs, resulting in increases in SSRI plasma levels. This is usually not a problem at standard starting SSRI doses. Because of this interaction, ranitidine or one of the other H2 blockers is preferred when antidepressants and H2 blockers have to be coadministered.

Many patients with depression or anxiety seen by the psychiatrist or family physician respond well to a simple regimen consisting of a single antidepressant medication. The improved safety and the relatively low side effects associated with SSRIs have made the treatment of uncomplicated anxiety and depressive symptoms fairly simple, hence easily manageable for the primary care physician.

Case #8

Presenting Symptoms: The patient was a 65-year-old male with complaints of compulsive picking of the skin of the sole of his right foot for the last 15 years, causing frequent bleeding. He also suffered from perfectionistic tendencies, depressed mood, feelings of hopelessness, and anhedonia. The depressive symptoms were recently precipitated by conflicts with his wife of the last five years and conflicts with his adult children. He denied drug and alcohol abuse and smoking. He drank two cups of regular coffee daily. He denied previous psychiatric treatment and a family history of psychiatric disorders. His medical history was significant for hypertension for which he was on verapamil SR 120 mg daily.

Current Diagnosis: Obsessive-compulsive disorder
Adjustment disorder with depressed mood

Current Treatment: 1. fluoxetine 20 mg HS
2. referral to a psychologist

Treatment Course: The patient was started on fluoxetine 20 mg AM. Significant improvement was reported by the patient when seen after two weeks. Since he complained of yawning and drowsiness during the daytime, fluoxetine was switched to bedtime, resulting in improvement in these side effects. After one month of starting fluoxetine, there was near complete resolution of his compulsive and depressive symptoms. He has now been maintained on the same dose for nine months. He is seen in the office every three to four months for medication follow-up.

Comments: Fluoxetine is typically started in the morning because its stimulating properties can interfere with sleep. In some patients, however, fluoxetine causes drowsiness. The standard approach in these cases is to switch fluoxetine to bedtime. This patient had an excellent response to a low dose of fluoxetine. Usually, higher doses are required for the treatment of obsessive-compulsive disorder. Compulsive self-mutilating behavior could at times respond to naltrexone 50 mg daily, or a combination of an SSRI and naltrexone.

SSRIs can cause dyspepsia, diarrhea, anxiety, restlessness, and headache, which usually subside after four to seven days. If patients are educated regarding these side effects and their self-limiting nature, they are less likely to stop the medication unless the side effects are severe and unremitting. Various medication interventions to treat these side effects, if they persist, are given in Chapter 5.

Case #9

Presenting Symptoms: The patient was a 49-year-old female with complaints of depressed mood, obsessive worrying, perfectionistic tendencies, irritability, excessive emotional sensitivity, anger outbursts, anxiety, anergia, occasional crying episodes, hyperphagia, feelings of hopelessness, and anhedonia. She denied drug and alcohol abuse, had stopped smoking three years ago, and drank one to two cups of coffee daily. These symptoms were precipitated by a divorce five years ago and more recently by financial difficulties. She had been on nortriptyline 75 mg HS for four years prior to the first visit. She denied a family history of psychiatric disorders. She was taking levothyroxine for hypothyroidism and estrogen supplements. Thyroid tests, including TSH, were within the normal range.

Current Diagnosis: Major depression, moderate

Current Treatment:
1. venlafaxine 50 mg BID
2. lorazepam 0.5 mg PRN anxiety or insomnia (taken once or twice a week, on average)
3. continued psychotherapy with referring therapist

Treatment Course: Because of hyperphagia, obesity, and the presence of depressive symptoms while on nortriptyline, the patient was offered a switch to fluoxetine 20 mg AM, which was started the following day. Nortriptyline was tapered off over a period of one week. Lorazepam 0.5 mg HS was started for insomnia, which was anticipated during the initial period of stopping nortriptyline. The dose of fluoxetine was increased to 40 mg after one month since the patient had residual symptoms of depression. She did well for several months; then, some of the depressive symptoms reemerged, necessitating a recommendation to increase the dose to 60 mg daily. Since the patient did not have third-party coverage for medication and had financial difficulties, she requested a trial on a less expensive antidepressant with characteristics similar to fluoxetine. Fluoxetine was discontinued and she was started on venlafaxine 25 mg BID, later increased to 50 mg BID, which satisfactorily eliminated depressive symptoms. She has now been maintained on the above regimen for three months.

Comments: TCAs and MAOIs typically cause an increased appetite and resultant weight gain, whereas SSRIs and bupropion are fairly devoid of weight gain as a side effect. Frequently, there may be a slight decrease in appetite during the first several months of starting on an SSRI or bupropion. For this reason, it is appropriate to switch patients on a TCA or an MAOI to an SSRI or bupropion if weight gain is a major side effect, even if the medication is otherwise satisfactory. The initial appetite suppressant properties of SSRIs usually do not persist beyond the first several months; still, they do not cause a dramatic increase in appetite. TCAs typically aid sleep. Hence, when tricyclic antidepressants are withdrawn, the patient will need a hypnotic medication temporarily.

Cost is a major consideration for some patients due to various practical reasons. Fluoxetine is available in 10 and 20 mg capsules. The usual effective dosage range is between 20 and 60 mg per day, with the most common dosage being 20 mg to 40 mg per day. A patient needing 60 mg daily requires three 20 mg strength capsules, as in this case, costing approximately $155 per month. Some of the other SSRIs are available in comparatively high dosage strengths with a great range of dosages and a more favorable price range. An example is venlafaxine, which is available in 25, 37.5, 50, 75, and 100 mg strength tablets. Another example is nefazodone, available in 100, 150, 200, and 250 mg strength tablets. This patient was eventually maintained on venlafaxine 50 mg twice a day. Since the tablet form is available, a 100 mg tablet was prescribed, which could be divided, thereby further reducing the cost to approximately $40 per month. This resulted in a savings of about $115 per month as compared to the cost of fluoxetine.

There is considerable interindividual variation as to the equivalency in dosage among various SSRIs; hence, it should not be construed that fluoxetine 60 mg is equivalent to venlafaxine 100 mg. For another patient, venlafaxine may not be effective, a different dose of venlafaxine may be needed, or fluoxetine 20 mg may be sufficient to treat the symptoms, changing the cost calculations. The physician should be aware of such cost considerations and cost differences among medications in order to help the patient achieve the most effective symptom control in the most economical manner. (Refer to Table 1 in the Introduction for cost comparisons of various antidepressants.)

Generally, tablets offer greater flexibility because they can be easily divided. Some of the more resourceful patients have been able to open fluoxetine capsules, divide the powder form of the medication, and take smaller doses mixed in fruit juice or honey. This would make sense only when lower than the available fixed-dose capsule strength is needed. It should be noted that fluoxetine is available in a liquid form, enabling precise dose titration. However, the liquid form is generally more expensive than the capsules. For most tablet forms, the cost of a higher strength is only slightly greater than a lower strength. Notable exceptions among psychiatric drugs are risperidone and clozapine, for which the cost of a higher strength tablet is proportionately greater than a lower strength, making less attractive the money-saving strategy of buying a higher strength tablet and dividing it to get the desired dose. Nevertheless, even with these latter medications, some cost savings are still possible when higher strength tablets are divided.

Case #10

Presenting Symptoms: The patient was a 45-year-old female, with complaints of depressed mood, irritability, anxiety, hyperphagia, crying episodes, excessive emotional sensitivity, restless sleep, poor concentration, feelings of hopelessness, and anhedonia. She had had many episodes of depression in the past. Her symptoms worsened a month prior to the first visit, precipitated by work stress, as reported by the patient. She denied drug and alcohol abuse and smoking. She drank five to six cups of regular coffee daily. She had been tried on fluoxetine for six months in 1992 with suboptimal improvement. The patient's mother had had several bouts of depression. The patient denied any medical problems.

Current Diagnosis: Major depression, moderate, recurrent
Dysthymia

Current Treatment:
1. venlafaxine 50 mg BID
2. continued psychotherapy with the referring therapist
3. decrease in daily coffee intake to two cups or less

Treatment Course: The patient was initially started on venlafaxine 37.5 mg BID and temazepam 15 mg HS. After two months, the dose of venlafaxine was increased to 50 mg BID, on which she has been maintained for one year now with excellent results. Temazepam was discontinued three months into the treatment, with no adverse effects. The patient is seen every four months for medication management.

Comments: Venlafaxine has a broad spectrum of activity by virtue of its balanced norepinephrinergic and serotonergic effects, and in this respect, is similar to imipramine. However, it causes gastrointestinal side effects, such as dyspepsia and nausea, slightly more commonly than most other antidepressants. This tends to subside over a period of one week in most patients. Its broad spectrum of activity should make it a good choice of an antidepressant, regardless of whether or not the depression is preferentially responsive to serotonergic or norepinephrinergic effects. (Refer to the section on antidepressants for dosing guidelines and other practical information.)

Case #11

Presenting Symptoms: The patient was a 29-year-old female with a history of anxiety attacks at a frequency of five per day, depressed mood, feelings of hopelessness, and multiple vague somatic complaints. At the time of her first visit to my office, the symptoms had been well controlled on bupropion 100 mg TID since 1991 and clonazepam 1 mg TID since 1990. She had moved from another state and wanted to continue the above medications. History revealed that various medications, including tricyclic antidepressants, fluoxetine, sertraline, trazodone, and lithium had failed to adequately control depression and anxiety until bupropion was tried. The patient's sister had bipolar disorder. Medical problems reported by the patient were "pseudo-obstruction of the gastrointestinal tract," and chronic bladder infections.

Current Diagnosis: Major depression, mild
Panic disorder

Current Treatment:
1. bupropion 100 mg TID
2. clonazepam 1 mg TID
3. referral to a psychotherapist

Treatment Course: The patient has been maintained on these medications since 1993, when she was first seen. She is currently seen once every five to six months for medication follow-up.

Comments: Since the patient had been doing well on both a subjective and objective basis, there was no clinical reason to recommend a change of medications. Clonazepam was not sufficient to control anxiety. Other antidepressants along with clonazepam were unsuccessful, whereas bupropion and clonazepam provided satisfactory improvement. Bupropion is not very effective, in the author's experience, for controlling anxiety symptoms. In general, other antidepressants are preferable as first-line medications for the treatment of anxiety. This case was included to show that there are exceptions to general principles when dealing with individuals and their responses to medications and that in a complex specialty such as psychiatry, the physician must have considerable flexibility with regard to treatment options. Although this case is somewhat complicated by the concurrent use of clonazepam and bupropion, the author is satisfied after a review of the chronology of various medication trials, that this combination was of clear benefit in improving this patient's depression and anxiety.

Case #12

Presenting Symptoms: The patient was a 45-year-old male with complaints of excessive worrying, increased anger, anxiety, moodiness, irritability, feelings of hopelessness, and episodic binge drinking consisting of six to twelve beers every two to three weeks. He denied drug abuse, smoking, and caffeine intake. He also denied any acute precipitants. This patient's past psychiatric history was significant for outpatient counseling and participation in Alcoholics Anonymous. His father had had an anxiety disorder. The patient denied any major medical problems.

Current Diagnosis: Dysthymia
Alcohol abuse

Current Treatment:
1. paroxetine 30 mg AM
2. naltrexone (Revia) 50 mg HS
3. referral for drug and alcohol counseling and Alcoholics Anonymous

Treatment Course: The patient responded well to sertraline 50 mg AM, which he took for two months. It was discontinued because of sexual dysfunction. He was started on bupropion 100 mg BID, which did not result in sexual dysfunction. He reported that his depressive symptoms improved but that his anxiety worsened. He took bupropion for about six months and stopped on his own. He did not return for his three-month follow-up visit and dropped out of treatment. About eight months later, he presented to the office complaining of the same symptoms that initially brought him to me. Since anxiety remained a major complaint, paroxetine 20 mg AM instead of bupropion, was tried. This time, he was also started on naltrexone 50 mg HS for treatment of the alcoholism. Liver function tests obtained after one month of starting naltrexone were normal. The dose of paroxetine was increased to 30 mg after one month, with complete resolution of depressive and anxiety symptoms. Sexual dysfunction returned, but the patient chose to stay on paroxetine. He receives outpatient drug and alcohol counseling and participates in Alcoholics Anonymous.

Comments: All antidepressants are effective for depression and anxiety. Some SSRIs tend to cause anxiety during the first week of treatment, but this anxiety usually subsides completely over seven to ten days. SSRIs cause sexual dysfunction in about 60 percent of patients. Bupropion is devoid of sexual side effects, but does not typically improve anxiety symptoms. It is common for patients to drop out of treatment as this patient did. However, they return when symptoms return and become unmanageable. In most cases, they will stay in treatment longer during the second or third go-around. Naltrexone can be used as an adjunctive medication as part of a comprehensive alcohol rehabilitation program. Patients should not be led to believe that the medication in the absence of counseling and Alcoholics Anonymous is sufficient treatment for alcoholism. The occasional monitoring of liver function tests is recommended while on naltrexone.

All SSRIs, particularly paroxetine, have excellent antianxiety properties when used daily, in addition to their obvious antidepressant effects.

Case #13

Presenting Symptoms: The patient was a 74-year-old male with complaints of anxiety, depressed mood, severe insomnia, anergia, irritability, anorexia, anhedonia, and occasional feelings of hopelessness. These symptoms had been present for many years. He took amitriptyline for several months 20 years ago. He denied drug and alcohol abuse, smoking, and caffeine intake. He described his mother as "moody." This patient's medical history was significant for benign prostatic hypertrophy, back pain, peptic ulcer, emphysema, and mitral valve prolapse. He was being treated with propoxyphene/acetaminophen PRN and sucralfate (Carafate).

Current Diagnosis: Dysthymia

Current Treatment: 1. clonazepam 0.5 mg HS
2. diphenhydramine 50 mg HS

Treatment Course: This patient was placed on sequential trials of low doses of amitriptyline, doxepin, imipramine, nortriptyline, fluoxetine, paroxetine, sertraline, and alprazolam. He was unable to tolerate the above medications for various reasons. His sleep normalized on the combination of clonazepam 0.5 mg HS and diphenhydramine 50 mg HS. He did not wish to try other medications. He refused a referral to see a therapist for counseling. The patient is now seen once every six months for medication follow-up.

Comments: Anticholinergic medications can cause urinary outflow obstruction, especially in patients who have prostatic hypertrophy; hence, they should be used cautiously and at low doses. Rarely, the physician comes across a patient whose symptoms do not respond to antidepressants or who cannot tolerate various medications, despite diligent efforts in trying different medications. Even in these cases, some relief can be given to the patient by improvement of one or more symptoms. In this case, resolution of insomnia on clonazepam and diphenhydramine satisfied the patient sufficiently to continue treatment indefinitely. It seems that he is able to deal with his depressive symptoms much better when he is able to have a good night's sleep.

For a number of reasons, some patients choose not to pursue psychotherapy. This patient would have had a better overall outcome if he had complied with the recommendation for counseling.

Case #14

Presenting Symptoms: The patient was a 44-year-old female with complaints of frequent panic attacks, anxiety, anergia, and occasional depressed mood. These symptoms worsened recently due to marital problems. She denied drug and alcohol abuse, smoking, and caffeine intake. She had tried amitriptyline and desipramine a year ago, with moderate improvement, but these were discontinued due to excessive weight gain. The patient's father had panic disorder and her grandmother had bipolar disorder. The patient took estrogen supplements. Her medical history was significant for mitral valve prolapse, fibromyalgia, and chronic fatigue syndrome.

Current Diagnosis: Panic disorder without agoraphobia
Marital problems

Current Treatment:
1. fluoxetine 60 mg AM
2. alprazolam 0.5 mg TID PRN
3. referral to a psychotherapist

Treatment Course: The patient was initially started on fluoxetine 10 mg AM and alprazolam 0.5 mg TID PRN for severe anxiety. Since there was no improvement and no worsening after two weeks, fluoxetine was increased to 20 mg AM. Mild improvement was reported two weeks later. The dose of fluoxetine was increased to 40 mg AM. When seen a month later, the patient felt moderate improvement in panic attacks, anxiety, and anergia. The dose of fluoxetine was again increased to the current dose of 60 mg AM, which satisfactorily resolved all of the symptoms. The patient has been using alprazolam only occasionally after increasing fluoxetine dose to 60 mg.

Comments: Anxiety disorders, including panic disorder and obsessive-compulsive disorder, respond nicely to antidepressants. However, patients with panic disorder can be sensitive to the stimulating properties of antidepressants; hence, the starting dose is usually lower than the standard starting dose used for the treatment of depression or OCD. SSRIs should be the first-line antidepressants for treatment of anxiety, primarily due to their favorable side effect profile and safety in overdose. Among the SSRIs, fluoxetine and venlafaxine are relatively more energizing compared to others. Since this patient had anergia as a symptom, fluoxetine was chosen as a first try. Although she was started on a low dose of 10 mg to reduce the risk of overstimulation, she eventually needed 60 mg to control panic attacks, anxiety, and anergia, suggesting that there is considerable individual variation in dosing–even for treatment of panic disorder. It is important to prescribe a benzodiazepine for PRN use because antidepressants have a latency period of one to three weeks to be effective. Moreover, some antidepressants can worsen anxiety during the first week of treatment. Patients should be educated regarding this, and instructed to use the benzodiazepine for acute anxiety. Benzodiazepines are a poor choice as the primary medication for anxiety disorders, including panic disorder and generalized anxiety disorder, for reasons discussed in Chapter 7.

Buspirone can improve mild to moderate anxiety in some patients when taken for two to three weeks. It is not effective for PRN use for treatment of acute anxiety. It is primarily used as an adjunctive medication rather than as a primary medication for treatment of anxiety and depressive disorders.

Depression usually coexists with anxiety disorders. It is rare to see, upon careful evaluation, a patient with an anxiety disorder who does not have depressive symptoms.

There seems to be some correlation between panic disorder and mitral valve prolapse. However, the correlation, if any, has no practical bearing on treatment, which consists of antidepressants as primary medication and low doses of benzodiazepines or beta-blocking drugs as secondary medication for PRN use. However, if the patient is at risk for substance abuse, sedatives are best avoided.

Patients with chronic fatigue syndrome and fibromyalgia have anergia as a prominent symptom. Many of them have typical depressive symptoms as well. Stimulating antidepressants such as bupropion, fluoxetine, venlafaxine, desipramine, protriptyline, and tranylcypromine may be beneficial in these patients. Adjunctive use of stimulants is also a fairly effective strategy.

Case #15

Presenting Symptoms: The patient was a 39-year-old female with complaints of depressed mood, excessive worrying, anxiety, irritability, crying episodes, initial insomnia, anergia, feelings of hopelessness, perfectionistic tendencies, and anhedonia. These symptoms had been recently worsened by family conflicts. She denied drug and alcohol abuse. She smoked one pack of cigarettes per day and drank two cups of coffee daily. This patient denied any major medical problems.

Current Diagnosis: Major depression, mild
Dysthymia

Current Treatment:
1. paroxetine 30 mg half tablet AM
2. trazodone 50 mg half tablet HS
3. lorazepam 0.5 mg HS PRN insomnia
4. referral to a psychotherapist

Treatment Course: This patient was started on paroxetine 20 mg AM, lorazepam 0.5 mg po HS, and trazodone 25 mg HS. She reported satisfactory improvement in all symptoms when seen three weeks later. She was advised to take trazodone daily, and to take lorazepam 0.5 mg only if needed for insomnia. The patient requested to be placed on paroxetine 30 mg tablets, which can be cut in half to obtain two doses of 15 mg each, thereby saving some medication costs. Symptoms remained under control on the 15 mg dose.

Comments: About one-half of the patients treated for depression respond to the first antidepressant tried. The effective use of combination of a low dose of trazodone and a low dose of a benzodiazepine is again shown in this case. Lorazepam was eventually used by the patient only occasionally. The combination of medications resulted in rapid relief of the patient's symptoms. Tablet forms have the advantage of being able to be divided, rendering smaller doses. This is more cost-effective than purchasing the smaller dose tablets. One exception is risperidone, for which the greater-strength dose is priced proportionately higher. The greatest savings can be had with venlafaxine, which is available in five different strengths, and with nefazodone and paroxetine, which are available in four different strengths.

Case #16

Presenting Symptoms: The patient was a 58-year-old male with complaints of depressed mood, poor concentration, anergia, poor recent memory, irritability, feelings of hopelessness, excessive emotional sensitivity, early morning awakening, and anhedonia. These symptoms emerged after he suffered a left-hemisphere stroke six months previously. He denied drug and alcohol abuse and smoking. He drank one cup of coffee daily. The patient had a bout of depression eight years ago and was treated using a tricyclic antidepressant. He had been on phenytoin for a seizure disorder secondary to his stroke.

Current Diagnosis: Organic mood disorder, depressed

Current Treatment: 1. sertraline 100 mg half tablet AM daily
2. ergoloid mesylates (Hydergine) 1 mg po TID

Treatment Course: The patient was started on sertraline 25 mg AM and temazepam 7.5 mg HS. He reported mild improvements without any side effects when seen three weeks later. Satisfactory improvement in depressive symptoms occurred on sertraline 50 mg AM. Since insomnia also resolved, temazepam was discontinued. However, the patient continued to complain of poor memory consisting of impaired retention of names, phone numbers, and recent events. Hence he was given ergoloid mesylates (Hydergine) 1 mg TID. The patient reported mild improvement in memory. He is now seen once every four months for medication management.

Comments: Depression characterized by symptoms such as apathy, irritability, and "emotional incontinence" is fairly common after a stroke. These symptoms respond well to antidepressants. Since this patient had a seizure disorder, TCAs and bupropion are relatively contraindicated, whereas SSRIs and MAOIs are less of a problem. Medium or long half-life benzodiazepines are the preferred hypnotics in patients who are at risk for seizures because of their smooth offset of action. Hypnotics with short half-lives, such as zolpidem and triazolam, should be avoided in seizure-prone patients.

Ergoloid mesylates are at times beneficial in improving memory in patients with mild dementia. Recently, tacrine (Cognex) was approved for treatment of cognitive decline seen in dementia associated with aging or in primary degenerative dementia. Donepezil (Aricept) is another drug that was recently approved for slowing the cognitive decline in demented patients. Reportedly, donepezil has less side effects compared to tacrine. Although this patient's impairment in memory was related to his stroke, the ergoloid mesylates proved to be of some help, according to the patient's subjective report. Hydergine is typically given at a dose of 1 mg po TID. It usually takes about two to three weeks to see a response. Its effectiveness has not been universally endorsed. It is devoid of major side effects. A slight decrease in blood pressure and heart rate is occasionally seen.

Benzodiazepines can make the memory problem worse; hence, long-term use should be avoided if possible in patients with cognitive impairment, particularly memory problems.

Case #17

Presenting Symptoms: The patient was a 40-year-old male with complaints of poor attention, poor concentration, moodiness, distractibility, anxiety, circumstantial thinking, and depressed mood. He denied any acute precipitants. He also denied drug and alcohol abuse and smoking. He drank two cups of coffee daily. This patient denied any previous psychiatric treatment. His father had bipolar disorder. The patient denied any major medical problems.

Current Diagnosis: Attention deficit disorder (ADD)
Dysthymia

Current Treatment: 1. methylphenidate 10 mg BID
2. fluoxetine 20 mg AM

Treatment Course: The patient responded well to methylphenidate, which dramatically improved the symptoms of ADD. Since depressive symptoms persisted, fluoxetine was started at 10 mg AM. This was eventually increased to 20 mg AM, which resolved depressive symptoms. He is seen every three months for medication management.

Comments: All stimulants have some antidepressant effects and all antidepressants improve attention deficit symptoms, to some extent; however, stimulants are the most efficacious for treating ADD, and antidepressants are the preferred medications to treat depressive symptoms. When ADD and depression coexist, both a stimulant and an antidepressant may be necessary for the best outcome. Because of overlapping symptoms and medication effects, it is prudent to start the patient on one medication (that is, either a stimulant or an antidepressant) so that the effects of medications on each condition can be assessed, even when it is obvious that both ADD and depression coexist. The effect of stimulants on ADD is rapid and dramatic in most cases, whereas the effect of antidepressants is gradual and more modest. Tolerance to stimulants is usually not a problem in patients with ADD.

Case #18

Presenting Symptoms: The patient was a 33-year-old male with complaints of frequent flashbacks, occasional startle response, excessive sensitivity to noise, irritability, depressed mood, insomnia, anxiety, nightmares, and preoccupation with an explosion accident that the patient was involved in about one year ago, which precipitated the symptoms. He denied drug or alcohol abuse. He smoked one pack of cigarettes per day and drank one to two cups of coffee daily. This patient denied any history of psychiatric treatment. He was taking ibuprofen occasionally for headaches that had become more frequent since the accident.

Current Diagnosis: Post-traumatic stress disorder (PTSD)
Consider adjustment disorder with depressed mood

Current Treatment:
1. paroxetine 30 mg AM and 15 mg at noon
2. buspirone 10 mg TID
3. trazodone 50 mg HS
4. referral to a psychotherapist

Treatment Course: This patient was started on paroxetine 20 mg AM, trazodone 50 mg AM, and buspirone 5 mg TID. Over a period of two months, the dose of paroxetine was increased to 30 mg AM, 15 mg at noon, and buspirone to 10 mg TID with remarkable improvement in anxiety and depressive symptoms. After six months, the patient felt he did not need to continue the medications; thus, they were gradually stopped. About four months after stopping the medications, the symptoms relapsed. When he returned for treatment, he was started back on the same medications with moderate improvement of symptoms.

Comments: PTSD symptoms tend to respond well to antidepressants. Since anxiety is a prominent symptom, buspirone is particularly effective for long-term use. Trazodone is effective for insomnia and nightmares. If other symptoms such as paranoia, ideas of reference, or severe anxiety persist, additional medications such as antipsychotics or benzodiazepines may be necessary at low doses for short-term use. Patients with PTSD frequently have associated depressive symptoms; hence, an antidepressant medication is nearly always needed as one of the medications in the treatment of PTSD.

Buspirone is an excellent adjunctive medication in disorders with prominent anxiety symptoms. Because of the one- to three-week latency period for buspirone's antianxiety effects to become evident, low doses of benzodiazepines may be beneficial initially. Buspirone works well with all antidepressants except MAOIs.

Case #19

Presenting Symptoms: The patient was a 40-year-old female with complaints of depressed mood, frequent crying, feelings of hopelessness, anxiety, anergia, insomnia, irritability, occasional anger outbursts, and anhedonia. These symptoms gradually worsened over the last ten years, but became significantly exacerbated after a recent hysterectomy. She denied drug and alcohol abuse and smoking. She drank one to two cups of coffee daily. The patient's mother had severe depression and paranoia. The patient had been taking estrogen supplements since her hysterectomy six months ago.

Current Diagnosis: Major depression, moderate, single episode
Dysthymia

Current Treatment: 1. venlafaxine 100 mg BID
2. trazodone 100 mg HS

Treatment Course: At the first visit, this patient was started on venlafaxine 37.5 mg BID with meals, and eventually increased to an effective dose of 100 mg BID. Since the patient complained of insomnia, trazodone was added at 50 mg HS and several months later was increased to 100 mg HS. The combination of venlafaxine and trazodone effectively treated the depression and the insomnia. The patient has been on the medications for one year.

Comments: About 50 percent of patients with depression respond well to the first antidepressant tried when the medication choice is based on practical considerations outlined in Chapter 1. Venlafaxine is truly a broad-spectrum antidepressant because of its fairly potent serotonergic and norepinephrinergic properties, much like imipramine, but without tricyclic antidepressant side effects.

Case #20

Presenting Symptoms: The patient was a 30-year-old male with complaints of frequent panic attacks, depressed mood, anergia, social withdrawal, irritability, and excessive worrying. He had been taking clonazepam 1 mg BID for eight months, prescribed by another psychiatrist. He denied drug and alcohol abuse. He smoked one pack of cigarettes daily and drank one cup of coffee per day. The patient's mother had anxiety attacks, and his father suffered from alcoholism. The patient denied any major medical problems.

Current Diagnosis: Panic disorder
Dysthymia

Current Treatment: 1. paroxetine 30 mg AM
2. clonazepam 0.5 mg BID PRN
3. referral for psychotherapy

Treatment Course: The patient was continued on clonazepam 1 mg BID. Paroxetine 20 mg AM was started at the first visit. When seen two weeks later, he reported moderate improvement. He was able to decrease the clonazepam to 0.5 mg BID. The dose of paroxetine was increased to 30 mg AM. A month later, the improvement in symptoms continued. Clonazepam was decreased to 0.5 mg once or twice a day to a PRN schedule.

Comments: All benzodiazepines at appropriate doses are effective for controlling anxiety. They are attractive and tempting to physicians and to patients because they are almost immediately effective and maintain the efficacy for the first three to four weeks at the starting dose. Frequently, the dose has to be increased every two to three months to control breakthrough anxiety, to some extent due to partial tolerance. The author has seen many patients over the years who have been taking up to 2 to 3 mg of clonazepam TID and alprazolam 2 mg TID-QID prescribed by psychiatrists for treatment of panic and other anxiety disorders. However, they were still experiencing breakthrough anxiety symptoms. Higher doses of these medications will probably control the breakthrough symptoms temporarily for several months before yet another dosage escalation becomes necessary. At high dosage, patients are physiologically dependent on the medication. For these reasons, generally, benzodiazepines or other sedatives should not be used as long-term medications even for chronic anxiety disorders. Antidepressants are much superior to benzodiazepines for the long-term treatment of all anxiety disorders because of lack of tolerance, absence of physiological dependence, and more complete and prophylactic control of symptoms.

Clonazepam in particular should be withdrawn very slowly to prevent emergence of withdrawal seizures, although this precaution is applicable to all sedatives.

It is frequently observed that the prescribing of antidepressants decreases or eliminates the need for benzodiazepines in the treatment of anxiety disorders, including panic disorder and post-traumatic stress disorder.

Case #21

Presenting Symptoms: The patient was a 29-year-old female with complaints of depressed mood, anger outbursts, irritability, excessive emotional sensitivity, moodiness, anxiety, severe insomnia, hyperphagia, perfectionistic tendencies, poor concentration, distractibility, difficulty completing tasks, restlessness, anhedonia, and feelings of hopelessness. These symptoms, at a lesser level of severity, had been present since age 18, but they recently worsened without any precipitants. She denied drug and alcohol abuse and smoking. She drank one cup of coffee daily. The patient had been taking bupropion 150 mg TID and trazodone 150 mg HS for one year, at the time she was first seen at my office. Previously she had tried fluoxetine, nortriptyline, and thioridazine from other physicians. Both parents suffered from depression. The patient has been taking levothyroxine 0.05 mg for hypothyroidism. Thyroid profile was within the normal range.

Current Diagnosis: Major depression, moderate
Dysthymia
Consider mild attention deficit disorder

Current Treatment:
1. venlafaxine 75 mg TID
2. temazepam 15 mg HS
3. trazodone 100 mg HS
4. referral to psychotherapy

Treatment Course: Bupropion was discontinued since the patient was symptomatic despite being on the highest dose (450 mg daily). Venlafaxine was started at 25 mg TID at the time of the first visit and was gradually increased to the current dose of 75 mg TID. The addition of temazepam 15 mg HS, along with trazodone 100 mg HS, markedly improved insomnia with no daytime sedation or "drugged" feeling. Depressive symptoms and ADD symptoms improved on this combination.

Comments: ADD is a clinical diagnosis, as are nearly all diagnoses in psychiatry. There is no biochemical or psychological test that is specific for ADD. Evaluation of clinical symptoms, patient report, collateral information, and behavioral observations are the most important sources of data that will help to make a diagnosis. In children and adolescents, reports of parents and teachers provide crucial and reliable information. If there is still uncertainty, a trial on a stimulant will clarify the clinical picture if ADD is suspected. A good medication response usually confirms the diagnosis, whereas lack of response to a medication does not rule out the diagnosis. Norepinephrinergic antidepressants are particularly effective for treatment of ADD and coexisting depression. Examples are bupropion, desipramine, nortriptyline, imipramine, and venlafaxine. Although bupropion is effective for ADD and depression, it was not effective for this particular patient. Generally, if depressive symptoms are present, a trial on an antidepressant is attempted first. If the antidepressant does not improve ADD symptoms or is only partially effective, a stimulant can be added to the regimen.

Case #22

Presenting Symptoms: The patient was a 39-year-old male with complaints of depressed mood, irritability, insomnia, anorexia, mood swings, anger episodes, and anhedonia, which were resolved on sertraline 100 mg AM at the time he presented at my office. Symptoms such as severe insomnia and anorexia were still present. The patient was referred to my office due to insurance changes. He denied drug and alcohol abuse, smoking, and caffeine intake. The patient complained of occasional heartburn for which he took over-the-counter antacids.

Current Diagnosis: Dysthymia

Current Treatment:
1. sertraline 100 mg AM
2. doxepin 25 mg HS
3. clonazepam 0.25 mg (1/2 of a 0.5 mg tablet) HS
4. referral to psychotherapy

Treatment Course: Sertraline 100 mg was continued since depressive symptoms were well controlled. Doxepin 25 mg was started at the first visit, with satisfactory improvement in anorexia and heartburn, and mild improvement in insomnia. At the second visit, clonazepam 0.25 mg was added, resulting in complete resolution of insomnia. The patient has been maintained on this combination for about eight months.

Comments: TCAs are excellent for adjunctively treating loss of appetite. Preferred TCAs for specific symptoms are listed below.

Examples of Adjunctive Medications and Doses

Loss of Appetite (without insomnia)

- desipramine 10 to 25 mg HS
- nortriptyline 10 to 25 mg HS

Loss of Appetite (with insomnia)

- amitriptyline 10 to 25 mg HS
- doxepin 10 to 25 mg HS
- trimipramine 25 mg HS
- imipramine 10 to 25 mg HS
- maprotiline 25 mg HS

Loss of Appetite (with hypersomnia)

- protriptyline 10 mg AM or noon

Loss of Appetite, Insomnia, and Dyspepsia

- doxepin 10 to 50 mg HS
- amitriptyline 10 to 50 mg HS
- any tricyclic antidepressant at low dose and one of the H2 blockers

Although cyproheptadine (Periactin) can be used for increasing appetite, its antagonism of serotonergic effects can precipitate depression; hence, it should be avoided for routine use in patients being treated for depression.

Case #23

Presenting Symptoms: The patient was a 75-year-old female with complaints of anergia, hypersomnia, decreased motivation, and apathy, for which she had been taking nortriptyline 50 mg HS for a month, prescribed by her family physician. She denied symptoms of depression and any acute stressors. She also denied drug and alcohol abuse, smoking, and caffeine intake. The patient had been taking bumetanide and potassium supplements for hypertension and CHF (congestive heart failure).

Current Diagnosis: Mood disorder, possibly due to CHF or medications, depressive type
Current Treatment: bupropion 75 mg AM

Treatment Course: Nortriptyline was discontinued and the patient was switched to bupropion 75 mg po AM. She reported significant improvement in anergia, apathy, and hypersomnia by the end of the first week on bupropion.

Comments: It is likely that the patient's symptoms were primarily due to her medical condition. Nortriptyline is generally an excellent choice in the elderly, because it does not cause excessive sedation or orthostatic hypotension, compared to its parent compound amitriptyline or one of the sedating tricyclic antidepressants (TCAs); hence, nortriptyline is still one of the commonly used antidepressants, along with imipramine and desipramine, among TCAs. However, SSRIs and bupropion are generally safer than any TCA in the elderly who have cardiovascular problems. Bupropion is particularly effective for symptoms such as those of this patient. Usually, a low dose is sufficient, especially in the elderly.

Case #24

Presenting Symptoms: The patient was a 29-year-old female with complaints of depressed mood, anxiety, excessive worrying, occasional crying, irritability, severe insomnia, perfectionistic tendencies, excessive emotional sensitivity, difficulty making decisions, feelings of hopelessness, and anhedonia. The symptoms had been present for two to three years, with no identifiable precipitants. She denied drug and alcohol abuse and caffeine intake. She smoked one-half pack of cigarettes daily. Her uncle had been diagnosed with bipolar disorder, and her mother suffered from depression.

Current Diagnosis: Dysthymia
Current Treatment: continue therapy by psychotherapist

Treatment Course: At the first visit, the patient was started on fluoxetine 20 mg AM, trazodone 50 mg HS, and temazepam 15 mg HS, which remarkably improved all symptoms within two weeks. Therefore, she was maintained on these medications. A month later, she reported that some of the depressive symptoms slowly resurfaced. Fluoxetine was increased to 40 mg AM, effectively controlling all the symptoms again. Temazepam was discontinued. Since the patient complained of mild sedation during the daytime, attributed to fluoxetine, the schedule of fluoxetine was changed from AM to HS and trazodone was discontinued. Daytime sedation subsided. After about six months of being on fluoxetine, it was tapered off gradually with the hope that the patient would continue the improvement without medication. She has not called my office since stopping the medication, about six months ago. I assume that she is still euthymic.

Comments: It is not unusual to observe a good response to an antidepressant medication during the first two to four weeks of treatment, with subsequent breakthrough of symptoms for no apparent reason. In these cases, a dosage increase frequently resolves the problem. In some cases, it is possible to decrease the dosage after being on a dose for a while without losing efficacy. Increasing medication dosage is not necessary when the initial dose has been effective.

SSRIs are usually started in the morning, preferably after breakfast; however, some patients taking SSRIs in the morning report daytime somnolence, yawning, and sedation. These patients should be switched to bedtime dosing, which could improve their sleep and eliminate daytime somnolence. For the majority of patients, though, SSRIs cause insomnia, which is the reason why they are typically started in the morning in new patients.

Case #25

Presenting Symptoms: The patient was a 31-year-old male with complaints of panic attacks at a frequency of three to four per week, anxiety, insomnia, excessive worrying, and irritability. He denied any acute precipitants. He also denied drug and alcohol abuse. He smoked half of a pack of cigarettes per day, and drank four to five cups of coffee daily. This patient denied any major medical problems.

Current Diagnosis: Panic disorder without agoraphobia
Consider caffeine-induced anxiety disorder

Current Treatment: 1. fluoxetine 20 mg AM
2. trazodone 50 mg HS
3. temazepam 15 mg HS
4. limited intake of coffee and other caffeinated beverages to two cups or less daily
5. referral for psychotherapy

Treatment Course: At the first visit, the patient was started on fluoxetine 20 mg AM, trazodone 50 mg HS, and temazepam 15 mg HS, and was advised to decrease daily coffee intake to two cups or less. When seen after two weeks, all the symptoms improved significantly. Fluoxetine and trazodone are now taken daily. Temazepam is now taken only infrequently, "as needed" for insomnia.

Comments: Panic disorder is best treated using antidepressants. In most cases of panic disorder, an antidepressant alone is sufficient to prevent panic attacks.

Patients who have anxiety disorders are sensitive to the stimulant effects of nicotine and caffeine; hence, consumption of both should be eliminated or at least decreased for optimal treatment outcome. It is not excessively difficult to decrease caffeine intake; however, cigarette smoking is highly addictive and is very difficult to stop, unless the patient is extremely motivated and determined.

Case #26

Presenting Symptoms: The patient was a 40-year-old female with complaints of panic attacks and performance anxiety related to making presentations to a group of colleagues. She denied drug and alcohol abuse and smoking. Her aunt had a "nervous breakdown." This patient's medical history is significant for mitral valve prolapse.

Current Diagnosis: Panic disorder without agoraphobia
Social phobia

Current Treatment: 1. paroxetine 10 mg AM
2. propranolol 10 mg one hour before public speaking, PRN
3. alprazolam 0.25 mg one hour before public speaking, PRN
4. Propranolol and alprazolam may be taken concurrently.

Treatment Course: The patient was started on the above combination of medications. Paroxetine treated the panic disorder symptoms. This patient had a good response to propranolol and alprazolam taken concurrently about one hour prior to a public presentation, as needed, at an average frequency of one to two times per week.

Comments: Beta-blockers or benzodiazepines alone or in combination are extremely effective for occasional use in social phobia if the phobic stimulus is predictable and fairly infrequent. If the phobic stimulus is unpredictable and is present frequently, the addition of an antidepressant to the beta-blocker-benzodiazepine combination can help. Beta-blockers suppress the peripheral manifestations of anxiety, and benzodiazepines improve the subjective feelings of anxiety; hence, the combination has a complementary effect.

Case #27

Presenting Symptoms: The patient was a 13-year-old male with complaints of distractibility, impulsivity, conduct problems, irritability, restlessness, poor comprehension, disobedience, and assaultive behavior. He denied drug and alcohol abuse and smoking.

Current Diagnosis: Attention deficit hyperactivity disorder (ADHD)

Current Treatment: 1. methylphenidate 10 mg AM and 10 at 1 PM
2. imipramine 10 mg HS

Treatment Course: Methylphenidate 5 mg BID was started at the first visit. Moderate improvement was noted the first day of starting the medication. Eventually, the dose was increased to 10 mg BID with optimal improvement. However, the patient reported loss of appetite, insomnia, and anxiety. When imipramine 10 mg HS was added, these symptoms resolved. The patient was switched to methylphenidate slow-release form 20 mg daily AM, but the patient's mother reported that the regular preparation at 10 mg BID was more effective. He was switched back to methylphenidate 10 mg BID. He has done well on this regimen since 1993.

Comments: This patient had symptoms of conduct disorder. However, treatment completely controlled all symptoms, perhaps suggesting that conduct disorder symptoms in this patient were a manifestation of ADHD. Children with ADHD do well on low doses of TCAs when combined with full doses of stimulants. TCAs at high doses can cause a relatively greater incidence of cardiac conduction disturbance in children and adolescents and are best given at very low doses as adjunctive medications.

For some patients, the slow-release form of methylphenidate is not as effective as the regular preparation for unknown reasons.

Case #28

Presenting Symptoms: The patient was a 39-year-old female with complaints of depressed mood, crying episodes, insomnia, bad dreams, loss of appetite, anxiety, anergia, irritability, feelings of hopelessness, and anhedonia. These symptoms had been worsening for the last five months, precipitated by major stressors such as a breakup with her boyfriend because of his infidelity, loss of a job, and conflicts with her teenage son who left to live with his father. She denied drug and alcohol abuse and smoking. She drank one to two cups of coffee daily. The patient had been taking alprazolam 0.25 mg TID for one week, prescribed by her family physician. Her mother suffered from depression, and has been doing well on fluoxetine. The patient has neck muscle spasm for which she has been taking diazepam 5 mg BID PRN for years.

Current Diagnosis: Major depression, moderate, single episode

Current Treatment:
1. paroxetine 60 mg HS
2. bupropion 100 mg AM
3. referral for psychotherapy
4. continued use of diazepam 5 mg BID PRN for neck spasm, managed by her family physician

Treatment Course: Fluoxetine was the logical first choice because the patient's mother had done well on it. The patient was started on fluoxetine 20 mg AM and doxepin 10 mg HS. Alprazolam was tapered off. When seen after two weeks, the patient complained of frequent headaches, thought to be due to fluoxetine; hence, fluoxetine was discontinued in favor of paroxetine 20 mg AM. Paroxetine improved most of the depressive symptoms, but caused somnolence; hence, paroxetine was switched to bedtime and doxepin was discontinued. Eventually, paroxetine was gradually increased to 60 mg HS. Since the patient's initial complaint of anergia persisted, bupropion 100 mg AM was added, with satisfactory response.

Comments: Family history of medication response is not a guarantee that another family member will do well on the same medication for similar indications, although the odds that a family member will respond to the same medication are greater. With the introduction of so many new classes of antidepressants and antipsychotics, there is now less reliance on family history of medication response in medication selection. Rather, more emphasis is placed on symptom characteristics and medication features.

Bupropion at low dose (for example, 100 mg AM) is excellent as an adjunctive medication for improving anergia or apathy in a patient on an SSRI.

Case #29

Presenting Symptoms: The patient was a 65-year-old male with complaints of anxiety, depressed mood, chronic insomnia, a tingling and burning sensation in his extremities, palpitations, vague fears, excessive worrying, and anhedonia. He denied drug and alcohol abuse, smoking, and caffeine intake. The patient had been on chlordiazepoxide 10 mg HS for ten years. His mother had bipolar disorder. This patient had a prostatectomy approximately ten years ago.

Current Diagnosis: Generalized anxiety disorder

Current Treatment: 1. doxepin 25 mg HS
2. chlordiazepoxide 5 mg HS

Treatment Course: The patient was sequentially tried on fluoxetine 10 mg AM, trazodone 50 mg HS, and nortriptyline 20 mg HS at various times. Improvement in sleep and anxiety was noted with doxepin 25 mg HS. After starting doxepin, the patient was able to decrease chlordiazepoxide to 5 mg HS. Further decrease resulted in increased anxiety. He has now been maintained on doxepin 25 mg HS and chlordiazepoxide 5 mg HS for two years.

Comments: For long-term antianxiety effects, low doses of antidepressants are excellent. This patient was on chlordiazepoxide 10 mg HS for ten years when he came to the office with the complaints outlined here. Eventual addition of doxepin not only enabled him to decrease chlordiazepoxide to 5 mg HS, but also resolved the main presenting symptoms. Low doses of antidepressants are usually sufficient if given enough time for the medication to become effective, especially when used to treat anxiety.

Generally, long half-life benzodiazepines such as chlordiazepoxide and diazepam are best avoided in the elderly because of potential for drug accumulation. However, at extremely low doses, such as chlordiazepoxide 5 mg, this is not a major concern.

Case #30

Presenting Symptoms: The patient was an 83-year-old female with complaints of paranoid ideation, ideas of reference, and auditory hallucinations. The patient reported that she had been depressed due to stress secondary to the belief that people had been harassing her. Cognitive functioning was remarkably intact. She denied drug and alcohol abuse and caffeine intake. She had quit smoking 15 years ago. She was taking atenolol for hypertension.

Current Diagnosis: Delusional disorder, persecutory type
Current Treatment: risperidone 0.25 mg (one-quarter of a 1 mg pill) HS

Treatment Course: From early 1992 to 1994, the patient was treated using haloperidol 0.5 mg HS. When risperidone became available in 1994, she was switched to risperidone, initially at 0.5 mg HS and eventually at 0.25 mg HS. The patient's complaint of jaw tightness while on haloperidol completely resolved after switching to risperidone with no decrease in effectiveness.

Comments: The elderly are sensitive to antipsychotic medications; hence, extremely low doses are often effective and sufficient.

Case #31

Presenting Symptoms: The patient was a 13-year-old male with complaints of distractibility, disobedience, frequent lying, fighting, poor grades, anergia, poor concentration, truancy, irritability, impulsivity, restlessness, anger outbursts, and moodiness. The patient smoked marijuana at the rate of one cigarette per week. He denied alcohol abuse. He smoked a half of a pack of cigarettes per day. He denied any acute precipitants. The patient's uncle has bipolar disorder and alcoholism, and his aunt has been diagnosed with depression.

Current Diagnosis: Attention deficit hyperactivity disorder
Marijuana abuse
Consider dysthymia
Conduct disorder
Current Treatment: fluoxetine 20 mg AM

Treatment Course: The patient was first tried on methylphenidate 5 mg AM and at noon, which had to be discontinued due to increased irritability, hyperactivity, and anxiety. Fluoxetine was started at the second visit, resulting in dramatic improvement of all presenting symptoms within ten days. The patient has been doing well for many months.

Comments: Antidepressants are at times more effective than stimulants for treatment of ADHD. This patient had typical ADHD symptoms with overlapping symptoms of conduct disorder, dysthymia, and anxiety.

Among antidepressants, bupropion and venlafaxine are particularly effective for ADHD symptoms, especially if there are overlapping emotional symptoms. One disadvantage of bupropion and venlafaxine is that a multiple dosing schedule is required, making compliance a problem. A stimulating antidepressant such as fluoxetine can also be effective and has the advantage of once-a-day dosing.

The brain-behavior relationships of children and adolescents are governed by similar neurochemical and neurophysiological principles as those of adults. Therefore, medications that are effective for adults should also be effective for children and adolescents for similar indications, subject to variations in dosing. At appropriate doses, all psychiatric medications have the potential to be safely and effectively used in children and adolescents. When children present with treatable symptoms, they should be treated, just as is the case with adults. The earlier effective treatment begins, the better the outcome, as is true with most disorders.

Case #32

Presenting Symptoms: The patient was a 39-year-old female with complaints of panic attacks at a frequency of two to three per week for about three months, obsessive worrying, severe insomnia, and increased generalized anxiety. These symptoms were precipitated by her mother's serious illness about three months previous. She denied drug and alcohol abuse, smoking, and caffeine intake. The patient had been taking alprazolam 0.5 mg TID and buspirone 10 mg TID, prescribed by her primary care physician. The patient's mother suffered from depression. This patient's medical history was significant for radio-iodide treatment for Grave's disease and subsequent thyroid replacement, as well as a peptic ulcer. She was taking levothyroxine and famotidine.

Current Diagnosis: Panic disorder

Current Treatment:
1. paroxetine 20 mg AM
2. alprazolam 0.5 mg one to two per day PRN anxiety
3. referral to psychotherapy

Treatment Course: The patient was started on paroxetine 10 mg AM, in addition to continuing alprazolam and buspirone. She was advised to decrease the dose of alprazolam and to use alprazolam on a PRN basis after paroxetine began to work. Buspirone was discontinued at the second visit because the patient did not feel it was helping. The dose of paroxetine was increased to 20 mg at the third visit. Paroxetine has effectively prevented panic attacks. Alprazolam is now taken very infrequently.

Comments: Antidepressants are excellent for panic prophylaxis. They do not treat panic attacks in progress; hence, antidepressants must be taken regularly for true panic prophylaxis. Benzodiazepines are effective in treating a panic attack in progress, and hence can be taken PRN. However, taking benzodiazepines regularly at fairly high doses can have prophylactic effects on panic attacks. For various reasons described in the text, benzodiazepines are best used infrequently on an as-needed basis for treating breakthrough anxiety, and antidepressants best used regularly for panic prophylaxis.

Chapter 16

Moderately Complex Cases

CASES 33 TO 66

Case #33

Presenting Symptoms: The patient was a 35-year-old male with complaints of depressed mood, anxiety, irritability, outbursts of anger, anergia, restless sleep, feelings of hopelessness, and anhedonia. He also presented with an obsessive preoccupation with and an irresistible impulse to have extramarital affairs, and had a history of numerous extramarital affairs. He saw a psychiatrist approximately a year ago, with similar complaints, but was told that he was a "codependent," and that he had a "sex addiction." He was started on nortriptyline and referred to group therapy for sex addicts, which the patient did not pursue. Mild improvement was obtained from nortriptyline, which he took for one year. He had stopped nortriptyline by the time he was seen in my office. The patient denied drug and alcohol abuse.

Current Diagnosis: Dysthymia
Obsessive-compulsive features

Current Treatment:
1. fluoxetine 20 mg III AM
2. temazepam 15 mg HS
3. trazodone 50 mg HS
4. referral for psychotherapy

Treatment Course: The patient was started on fluoxetine 20 mg AM and temazepam 15 mg HS. When seen three weeks later, he felt slightly better, but still complained of insomnia. The dose of fluoxetine was increased to 40 mg AM, and trazodone 50 mg was added to temazepam 15 mg at bedtime. There was significant improvement in depressive symptoms and moderate improvement in obsessive-compulsive symptoms on this regimen when seen three weeks later. The patient was maintained on this combination for another six weeks. Since the patient still complained of continuing obsessive preoccupation with having extramarital affairs, and since no side effects were reported, the dose of fluoxetine was increased to 60 mg AM. This increase markedly decreased the obsessive preoccupation. The patient has now been maintained on this combination of medications for six months. He is successful in his business and is now a more happily married man. I presently see him in my office once every three months for medication maintenance.

Comments: It is rare to find a patient with distressing obsessions or compulsions who is not depressed or anxious. Addictions, regardless of the focus, tend to have varying degrees of obsessive-compulsive characteristics associated with them. SSRIs and clomipramine are the medications of choice for obsessive-compulsive symptoms. The insomnia, not completely treated with temazepam 15 mg, responded well when trazodone 50 mg was added. Both are low doses and have been very effective, with no daytime sedation or evidence of interaction with fluoxetine. Attempts to skip either trazodone or temazepam resulted in some sleep impairment; hence, it was decided to continue both trazodone and temazepam at night. The patient was encouraged to continue in therapy.

Case #34

Presenting Symptoms: The patient was a 51-year-old woman with complaints of compulsive organizing, checking, cleaning, depressed mood, crying episodes, anergia, hypersomnia, hyperphagia, feelings of hopelessness, anhedonia, and suicidal ideation without intent or plan. The above symptoms had been present for many years, and had worsened after the death of her father five months prior to her first visit to my office. She denied drug and alcohol abuse, smoking, and caffeine intake. She denied previous psychiatric treatment. Her father suffered from alcoholism. Her medical history was insignificant except for estrogen supplements, which she had been taking since a hysterectomy several years ago.

Current Diagnosis: Major depression, moderate, single episode
Obsessive-compulsive disorder

Current Treatment:
1. sertraline 100 mg AM
2. buspirone 5 mg TID
3. continued counseling with the referring therapist

Treatment Course: The patient was started on fluoxetine 20 mg AM, which after two weeks did not improve any of the symptoms. Fluoxetine was discontinued and paroxetine 20 mg was started, which improved anxiety and depression. Paroxetine was increased to 30 mg a month later, after the patient had reported recurrence of anxiety and depressive symptoms. Since no improvement was noted on the increased dose of paroxetine, this was discontinued and sertraline 50 mg AM was started. She was also given alprazolam 0.25 mg TID PRN for anxiety. Trazodone 50 mg was added at bedtime to treat insomnia. Since there was some improvement on sertraline, the dose was increased to 100 mg AM. Although anxiety and depression had improved on sertraline 100 mg, the patient still had compulsive behavior. The dose was again increased to 100 mg AM and at noon. She continued to have some compulsive tendencies. At this time, fluvoxamine became available. The patient expressed an interest in a trial of fluvoxamine, which was started at 50 mg BID and slowly increased to 100 mg BID, but failed to treat the symptoms. Sexual dysfunction had become a concern, which was a side effect of all of the SSRIs tried up to this point. When nefazodone was introduced with the expectation of lack of sexual side effects, the patient wanted to try it. Following the unsuccessful trial of fluvoxamine, nefazodone was started at 100 mg BID. The patient had severe lightheadedness and a "foggy" feeling after several doses, prompting the patient to discontinue nefazodone after two days. She felt that of all the medications tried so far, sertraline had the best effect; thus, she requested to be started back on it. She was started at sertraline 50 mg and increased to 100 mg, resulting in modest improvements in depression and compulsive symptoms. The patient herself discontinued trazodone and alprazolam because her anxiety and insomnia had improved. Further improvement in compulsive symptoms were seen after buspirone (Buspar) 5 mg TID was added as an adjunctive medication.

Comments: The usual approach when a starting dose given for two to three weeks is not effective is to increase the dose unless side effects are present. Typically, most antidepressants have a latency period of about one to three weeks for manifesting clinical response. However, in clinical practice, if there is not even slight improvement in any of the symptoms after being on the usual starting dose of SSRI, the chances of it producing a response at a higher dose is low in the author's view. But if there is mild improvement in some of the symptoms, the clinician may find it worthwhile to gradually increase the dose to the maximum approved dose unless side effects interfere. In this case, further increases in the dose of fluoxetine were not attempted because of lack of improvement in any of the symptoms. Another clinician would be well justified in deciding to continue fluoxetine and give it more time at higher doses. For TCAs and MAOIs, the starting dose is not near the effective therapeutic dose range; hence, a gradual increase in dosage is the rule. Increases in TCA or MAOI dose are made every two to three days until the low range of therapeutic dose is achieved, and then the patient is maintained on this dose for several weeks to assess the effectiveness. With SSRIs, the starting dose is usually at the low end of the therapeutic range; therefore, the common approach is to start the patient on a fixed dose and just wait for several weeks.

Failure to maintain a response to an antidepressant that was initially effective is a frequently encountered phenomenon. The standard approach then is to increase the dose. In this case, increasing paroxetine to 30 mg did not have any therapeutic effect. Rather than increasing again to the maximum dose of 50 mg per day, which would have been a reasonable approach, the decision was made to try another medication, sertraline, which turned out to be effective. It has been the experience of the author that, in general, anxiety responds to antidepressants at the low end of the therapeutic dosage range, depression at low to medium range, and obsessive-compulsive symptoms at the high end of the dosage range.

The patient was tried on fluvoxamine and nefazodone to see if these agents would give better results and fewer side effects. They did not.

Antidepressants should ideally be tapered off rather than abruptly discontinued. If one antidepressant is discontinued abruptly and another started without a washout period, there can be confusion between the withdrawal symptoms from the initial antidepressant and the side effects from the medication just started.

Buspirone is sometimes used as an adjunctive medication for treatment of anxiety, obsessive-compulsive disorders, and depression. As a primary medication, buspirone is not very effective for most anxiety disorders. However, it can be used for treating mild anxiety seen in a primary care setting. Adjunctive buspirone treatment of obsessive-compulsive disorder does not have a high success rate. Fortunately in this case, it was of some benefit to the patient.

As I was reviewing the case, it was noted that clomipramine, which is a TCA possessing antidepressant and superior antiobsessional properties, was not tried with this patient, even after failure on the first two SSRIs. Clomipramine should have been tried on this patient after the second SSRI trial. If, for some reason, obsessive-compulsive symptoms reemerge in this patient, clomipramine will be chosen for a trial.

Case #35

Presenting Symptoms: The patient was a 42-year-old female with complaints of distractibility, poor concentration, anergia, decreased libido, and depressed mood. She had been doing fairly well on paroxetine 20 mg AM at the time of her first visit to me. She reported occasional crying episodes and hopelessness. She denied suicidal ideation. She also denied drug and alcohol abuse, smoking, and caffeine intake. Her medical history included gastroesophageal reflux, hypothyroidism, asthma, and fibromyalgia. Her medications consisted of levothyroxine (Synthroid), cisapride (Propulsid), and propoxyphene/acetaminophen (Darvocet N-100). She denied any acute precipitants. She had tried fluoxetine, sertraline, bupropion, and amitriptyline. The patient's mother suffered from depression, and the patient's son had attention deficit hyperactivity disorder, for which he was on pemoline.

Current Diagnosis: Dysthymia
Attention deficit disorder

Current Treatment:
1. paroxetine 45 mg with supper
2. methylphenidate 10 mg AM and 5 mg at 1 PM
3. referred for psychotherapy

Treatment Course: Paroxetine was increased to 30 mg AM, which improved depressive symptoms, but caused insomnia. The patient took it upon herself to switch the schedule and take the medication with supper. After the switch, insomnia resolved (discussed under "Comments"). Since attention deficit symptoms persisted, she was started on methylphenidate initially at 5 mg BID and eventually at 10 mg AM and 5 mg at 1 PM daily, resulting in improvement in attention deficit symptoms and, to our surprise, in her libido. Several months later, depressive symptoms such as occasional crying and anergia emerged again, secondary to several acute stressors. The dose of paroxetine was increased to 45 mg with good response within one week of the increase.

Comments: It is possible for a patient to have several coexisting conditions that may need treatment using different medications. SSRIs have insomnia and sexual dysfunction as common side effects. To minimize adverse effects on sleep, SSRIs are typically started in the morning. This patient had insomnia while taking paroxetine in the morning. When switched to an evening schedule, insomnia improved. This is unusual and was an unexpected but welcome result, demonstrating that at times medication effects are unpredictable. The inadvertent beneficial effect of methylphenidate on libido was also a welcome result. SSRIs cause sexual dysfunction in about 60 percent of patients. Stimulants partially counteract SSRI-induced sexual dysfunction. In some patients, the antidepressant dose may need to be increased periodically even after a good response for many months, due to breakthrough depression caused by additional stressors or for unknown reasons, as was the case with this patient. This is sometimes attributed to a "wearing off" effect of the antidepressant. Stimulants are sometimes used adjunctively for treatment-resistant depression.

Case #36

Presenting Symptoms: The patient was a 16-year-old male with complaints of depressed mood, irritability, mood swings, frequent fights at school, and one recent episode of shoplifting. The patient's mother described him as temperamental. He had a diagnosis of attention deficit hyperactivity disorder, for which he was on pemoline (Cylert) 75 mg AM and 37.5 mg at 2 PM. His treatment was transferred to me because of a switch of his insurance carrier. He denied suicidal ideation, intent, or plan. No other evidence of conduct disorder was present. The ADHD was well controlled on pemoline. He denied drug and alcohol abuse and smoking. The patient had previously been tried on methylphenidate, which was discontinued due to increased anxiety. The patient's father, brother, and mother had all been diagnosed with ADD. The patient's mother and grandmother suffered from depression; the mother was doing well on methylphenidate and paroxetine. Past medical history of the patient was significant for absence seizures from ages eight to ten for which he had taken phenytoin for three years. He had discontinued the anticonvulsants for the last six years and had remained seizure-free.

Current Diagnosis: Attention deficit hyperactivity disorder
Dysthymia

Current Treatment:
1. pemoline 75 mg AM and 37.5 mg at 2 PM
2. paroxetine 20 mg AM
3. referred to a therapist, but poorly compliant

Treatment Course: The patient was maintained on pemoline for a previously diagnosed ADHD. Paroxetine was started to control mood symptoms. Within a week of starting paroxetine, depressive symptoms including irritability and fighting behavior improved. Liver function tests have been within normal limits.

Comments: Various psychiatric disorders can coexist with ADHD. The most common of these are dysthymia, hypomania, anxiety disorders, cyclothymia, conduct disorder, and substance abuse. There is considerable overlap of symptoms among these disorders. Symptoms such as irritability, poor concentration, "moodiness," anxiety, oppositional behavior, distractibility, hyperactivity, impulsivity, and poor frustration tolerance can be seen in children with any of these disorders. If more than one disorder is present, each disorder is to be treated until there is a resolution of symptoms. In some cases, one medication may treat two or more conditions. For example, antidepressants such as imipramine, desipramine, venlafaxine, and bupropion can improve ADD, depression, and anxiety symptoms. Stimulants can improve ADD and depressive symptoms. However, separate medications are frequently needed for the best effect. In this case, fortunately, the first antidepressant that was tried was effective. Fluoxetine, sertraline, and venlafaxine would have been reasonable first choices for this patient. Given his history of seizure disorder, bupropion and TCAs would be relatively contraindicated. Since pemoline has been known to cause liver abnormalities in rare instances, periodic liver function tests are recommended.

If the patient's residual symptoms are judged to be secondary to hypomanic or manic conditions, or cyclothymia, additional medications such as lithium, carbamazepine, valproic acid, or clonidine may be considered. Low doses of serotonergic antidepressants are excellent for long-term treatment of anxiety disorders.

Just as there is a familial predisposition for psychiatric disorders, response to a particular medication is also shared, to some extent, among blood relatives. Since the patient's mother had been doing well on paroxetine, it was a logical first choice as an antidepressant for this particular patient. ADD, like most psychiatric disorders, tends to be familial.

Case #37

Presenting Symptoms: The patient was a 41-year-old female with complaints of depressed mood, crying episodes, anxiety, anergia, initial insomnia, poor concentration, hyperphagia, and feelings of hopelessness. She denied suicidal ideation. She also denied smoking, and drug and alcohol abuse. She reported drinking one to three cups of regular coffee daily. These symptoms had been present for about six months when she was first seen in 1991. The symptoms were worsened by marital conflicts. She denied previous psychiatric treatment. The patient's father was hospitalized for depression and was treated with alprazolam. Her medical history was unremarkable.

Current Diagnosis: Major depression, moderate, single episode
Marital conflicts

Current Treatment: 1. fluoxetine 20 mg BID
2. bupropion 100 mg AM

Treatment Course: Fluoxetine 20 mg AM was started at the first visit. When seen after two weeks, trazodone was started for insomnia. A month later, the patient reported about 40 percent improvement with no side effects. The fluoxetine dosage was increased to 40 mg AM. During a follow-up visit after four months on this dosage, the patient reported breakthrough irritability and depressed mood, prompting an increase in dose to 60 mg AM, resulting in resolution of all symptoms. Trazodone was discontinued since the patient's insomnia had resolved. Decreased libido and orgasmic dysfunction worsened following the increase in the dose of fluoxetine. After a year of being on fluoxetine, it was decided to discontinue the medication. Fluoxetine was tapered off over a period of six weeks. About two months later, depressive symptoms returned. The patient requested another less-expensive medication. She was placed on a trial of sertraline 50 mg AM for two weeks, which was then increased to 100 mg AM. Since the patient did not feel sertraline was effective, she requested trying another medication. Desipramine 50 mg gradually increased to 150 mg at bedtime for several weeks failed to improve depressive symptoms. The patient asked to be placed back on fluoxetine. Nortriptyline 25 mg PRN was added for improving premenstrual dysphoria. The patient maintained improvement on fluoxetine 60 mg AM for another year, when breakthrough symptoms of depression were again reported. It was then decided to try venlafaxine (Effexor) at 25 mg TID increased gradually to 100 mg BID. Although symptoms improved, the patient felt comparatively better on fluoxetine and requested to be switched. She was placed on fluoxetine 20 mg BID. Bupropion (Wellbutrin) 100 mg AM was added to treat anergia and sexual dysfunction. This combination proved to be effective. She has now been maintained on this combination for eight months.

Comments: Diagnostically, this patient could be considered as suffering from adjustment disorder with depressed mood instead of major depression. Further history probably would have revealed that the patient had a mild degree of depressive symptoms for years, raising the possibility of an additional diagnosis of dysthymia. The patient might then be said to have "double depression." Regardless of the precise diagnosis, it was clear that the patient had many symptoms of depression and that antidepressant medication was necessary.

Fluoxetine was well tolerated by this patient. Sertraline, desipramine, and venlafaxine were either ineffective or disliked by the patient, although higher doses of sertraline and desipramine might have produced a positive effect. The medication was changed primarily at patient request. While the physician is not obliged to change medications whenever a patient requests it, input from a cooperative and motivated patient should be seriously considered by the physician, even if the patient's suggestions do not conform to the theoretical ideals of medication trials.

Within the same class of medications, patient tolerance varies. Among SSRIs, a patient who cannot tolerate one medication may tolerate and respond to another SSRI. Medication tolerance and clinical response are highly individual matters. Antidepressants also improve premenstrual dysphoria. If SSRIs are not effective, the addition of a low dose of a TCA as needed may be helpful. Nortriptyline 25 mg or equivalent other TCA is usually sufficient.

Sexual side effects, such as decreased libido and orgasmic dysfunction, are common side effects of antidepressants and are particularly associated with SSRIs. Treatments for antidepressant-related sexual dysfunction have a low probability of success. Even when successful, they are usually only partially effective. Various interventions are listed in Chapter 3. Fortunately, for this patient, bupropion 100 mg AM was helpful. Bupropion is one of the few antidepressants that does not cause sexual dysfunction.

Case #38

Presenting Symptoms: The patient was a 23-year-old male with complaints of anger attacks, irritability, depressed mood, feelings of hopelessness, mild hyperphagia, anergia, somatic preoccupation, and poor concentration. He also reported scattered thinking and the belief that people were talking about him in a derogatory manner. The above symptoms were present for three to four years to a milder degree, but worsened over the six months prior to his first visit to me, without any identifiable precipitants. He denied suicidal or homicidal ideation. He also denied drug and alcohol abuse and smoking. He drank two cups of regular coffee daily. He denied previous psychiatric history and reported that both of his parents possibly had some degree of depression, but were not treated. The patient's medical history was unremarkable.

Current Diagnosis: Dysthymia
Consider mild ideas of reference and thinking difficulty
Schizotypal features

Current Treatment: 1. fluoxetine 40 mg AM
2. trazodone 50 mg HS

Treatment Course: The patient was first started on sertraline (Zoloft) 50 mg AM and risperidone 0.5 mg HS. Although he felt much better at his three-week appointment, he complained of dyspepsia and loose bowel movements, most likely from sertraline, which was discontinued in favor of fluoxetine 20 mg AM. His gastrointestinal symptoms subsided after switching to fluoxetine, but depressive symptoms were only moderately improved; hence, three weeks later the dose of fluoxetine was doubled to 40 mg AM, which satisfactorily resolved his depressive symptoms. The mild ideas of reference and thinking difficulty improved within three to four days of starting risperidone, a week before improvement of depressive symptoms. About two months into the treatment, risperidone was discontinued. Trazodone was added for treatment of insomnia. The patient is doing well on fluoxetine and trazodone. He is seen in the office every four months.

Comments: It is difficult to formally diagnose the very mild psychotic symptoms that some people have. Ideas of reference and thought disorder are probably too specific and too strong to describe this patient's symptoms, yet he had a mild degree of thinking abnormality. Frequently, these symptoms are easily controlled on very low doses of antipsychotic medication, which may be discontinued after several months. It has been my experience that, for some reason, these symptoms do not recur even after the discontinuation of the antipsychotic if the patient has been maintained on it for several months. Risperidone and olanzapine are excellent choices because of their low side effect profile. Other antipsychotics at very low doses used short-term are also unlikely to put the patient at risk for major side effects.

If depressive symptoms cause dysfunction, regardless of whether endogenous or reactive in origin, treatment is necessary. In this case, the patient could not identify a precipitant. However, even if the symptoms were precipitated by a stressor, the initial medication treatment strategy would have been the same. Once the patient is stabilized on an antidepressant, the length of time the patient should stay on the medication varies depending on whether or not the depression was endogenously or exogenously caused. For example, the recommendation to patients is to stay on an antidepressant for one to two years if the depression is endogenously caused, such as in dysthymia or in major depressive episodes. If the depression is precipitated by a stressor, the practical recommendation is to stay on the antidepressant for six to eight months or until the stressor is no longer present, whichever occurs later.

SSRIs and nefazodone tend to cause nausea fairly frequently. Normally, this symptom subsides within four to six days of starting the medication. Occasionally, gastrointestinal side effects persist. Although these side effects can be treated using other medications as explained in Chapter 5, it may be better to try another SSRI if the side effects are multiple and persistent.

Insomnia is commonly seen with SSRIs, especially with an activating medication such as fluoxetine. Among the various medications for insomnia, trazodone at doses of 25 to 150 mg at bedtime is an excellent choice because of advantages over benzodiazepine hypnotics. Several of my patients have reported efficacy with dosages as low as 12.5 mg at bedtime (one-fourth of a 50 mg pill, the lowest strength available). When hypnotics are used, they should be tapered off or used PRN once sleep is stabilized. As the depression resolves, the antidepressant should be slowly tapered, rather than abruptly discontinued. For unknown reasons, the chances of a relapse are lower with a slow taper over one to two months. In addition, sudden discontinuation of short half-life SSRIs can cause nausea, dizziness, headache, anxiety, and a "sick" feeling, which subside in four to six days. Because of its long half-life, fluoxetine does not cause these withdrawal symptoms. Fluoxetine's long half-life is an advantage in patients who tend to be occasionally forgetful, but a disadvantage if rapid medication change is needed, especially switching from fluoxetine to an MAOI, which requires at least a five-week interval, assuming fluoxetine had reached steady-state serum levels.

Case #39

Presenting Symptoms: The patient was a 39-year-old male with complaints of depressed mood, insomnia, obsessive worrying, mood swings, mild paranoid ideation, suspiciousness, and irritability. He denied any acute precipitants. He admitted to a ten-year history of cocaine, marijuana, and alcohol abuse. He smoked cocaine twice a week and two cigarettes of marijuana per week. He drank three to four beers, three or four days a week. The patient had reportedly abstained from abuse for two months preceding the office visit. He denied suicidal ideation. He reported smoking one pack of cigarettes per day and denied caffeine intake. The patient also denied previous psychiatric treatment. His son and daughter both suffered from depression, his mother was an alcoholic, and his brother had a substance abuse problem. The patient's medical history was unremarkable.

Current Diagnosis: Dysthymia
Polysubstance abuse
Mild paranoid ideation

Current Treatment:
1. paroxetine 30 mg AM
2. trazodone 50 mg HS
3. risperidone 0.5 mg HS
4. referred for individual and group therapy for psychiatric and substance abuse issues

Treatment Course: On the first office visit, the patient was started on paroxetine 20 mg, trazodone 50 mg, and risperidone 0.5 mg HS. On the follow-up visit after 16 days, the patient reported moderate improvement in depressive symptoms, normal sleep, and absence of paranoia and suspiciousness. The dose of paroxetine was increased to 30 mg AM with satisfactory improvement in depressive symptoms.

Comments: Patients with psychiatric problems frequently abuse drugs and alcohol, sometimes as a means of "self-treatment." On the other hand, psychiatric symptoms can be precipitated by the acute effects of substance abuse. Careful history-taking can clarify which is primary and which is secondary in most cases. If there is sufficient doubt, re-evaluation after a two-week abstinence should help.

In this patient, three different medications are used to treat various symptoms, as follows:

Symptoms	Medication
Depression	paroxetine
Insomnia	trazodone
Paranoia	risperidone

Risperidone and trazodone can probably be discontinued after several months, while the antidepressant that is the more fundamental medication may be continued for a much longer period prior to discontinuation to minimize the chances of relapse.

Other medications could have worked just as well for this patient. There are different means of achieving the ultimate goal of successful resolution of a patient's presenting symptoms.

Case #40

Presenting Symptoms: The patient was a 48-year-old female with complaints of anergia, hyperphagia, feelings of hopelessness, depressed mood, distrust of people, ideas of reference, suspiciousness, episodes of confusion, thought blocking, disorganized and slow thinking, occasional auditory hallucination with derogatory and accusatory content, irrational feelings of guilt, suicidal ideation without intent or plan, crying episodes, and anhedonia. The patient believed that the symptoms were precipitated by dental problems in 1993. She denied drug and alcohol abuse, smoking, and caffeine intake.

She denied a family history of psychiatric disorders. Her medical history was unremarkable, except for dyspepsia, for which she took over-the-counter antacids PRN.

Prior to being seen in my office, other psychiatrists and primary care physicians had tried her on various antidepressant medications. The patient reported the following side effects:

Medication	Side Effects
fluoxetine	constipation and headaches
sertraline	GI side effects
paroxetine	GI side effects
nortriptyline	hyperphagia and cramping
venlafaxine	GI side effects
desipramine	cramping and nausea
bupropion	cramping and nausea

Current Diagnosis: Major depression, severe, recurrent, with psychotic features

Current Treatment:
1. nefazodone 200 mg AM and 300 mg HS
2. risperidone 0.5 mg HS
3. zolpidem 10 mg HS PRN insomnia
4. referral to a psychotherapist for therapy

Treatment Course: The patient was started on nefazodone 100 mg BID, risperidone 1 mg HS, zolpidem 10 mg HS, and ranitidine (Zantac) 150 mg BID. She reported feeling a "little better" when seen a week later at which time nefazodone was increased to 150 mg BID. The psychotic symptoms and insomnia improved rapidly, but the depressive symptoms persisted. Two weeks later, nefazodone was increased to 200 mg AM and 300 mg HS, which led to further improvement in her depression. The dose of risperidone was decreased and maintained on 0.5 mg HS. Ranitidine was discontinued after one month.

Comments: Although one can only speculate, it is quite possible that this patient had at least mild underlying psychotic symptoms for quite some time that were not recognized by previous clinicians. The remarkable clinical improvement obtained on the above treatment after failure on seven antidepressants is attributed primarily to the addition of the antipsychotic medication. There is also the possibility that marked GI side effects prevented the patient from benefitting from the antidepressants because they were stopped prior to an adequate trial. Perhaps if she had been prescribed an H2 blocker with the other antidepressants, she would have been able to tolerate the antidepressants for longer trials. It is important for psychiatrists, as physicians, to be able to recognize and manage common medical problems that directly affect psychiatric treatment. An example is the need for H2 blockers or antacids in a patient with dyspepsia who is started on medications which are likely to be a gastrointestinal irritant, such as SSRIs, valproic acid, lithium, and others. It should also be remembered that an antidepressant without an antipsychotic in a patient with psychotic symptoms can intensify the psychosis.

It is not my belief that nefazodone was unique in its effectiveness for this patient. It is easy to miss psychotic symptoms in depressed patients unless the psychotic symptoms are florid. Yet, treating the psychosis is as important as treating the depression. Hence, my clinical attitude when approaching a patient who is severely depressed is to err on the side of caution and assume that the patient has at least mild psychotic features, unless proven otherwise. The threshold for suspecting psychotic symptoms and for starting low-dose antipsychotics for the short-term should be low when treating severe depression, because the risk of suicide and homicide is high in psychotic depression. Even if it turns out that the patient did not have psychotic features, no harm is done by exposure to low doses of an antipsychotic for one to three weeks. In most psychotic depressions, the antipsychotic can be tapered off after the acute symptoms are controlled while the patient is maintained on an antidepressant for a longer period of time, depending on individual needs.

Case #41

Presenting Symptoms: The patient was a 67-year-old male. Symptoms consisted of social withdrawal, avoidance of social contacts, seclusiveness, obsessive rumination, mild compulsive cleaning and arranging, anhedonia, severe anxiety, insomnia, depressed mood, preoccupation with punctuality, interest in solitary activities, and anergia. These symptoms, at a less severe level, had been present since early adulthood. The patient was taking thioridazine 25 mg TID, imipramine 25 mg TID, and chlordiazepoxide 10 mg TID at the time he was first seen in my office. He denied drug and alcohol abuse, smoking, and caffeine intake. This patient also denied any major medical problems.

Current Diagnosis: Dysthymia
Schizoid personality disorder with obsessive-compulsive features

Current Treatment:
1. risperidone 0.5 mg HS
2. clonazepam 0.5 mg BID
3. clomipramine 100 mg HS
4. referral for psychotherapy

Treatment Course: Thioridazine, imipramine, and chlordiazepoxide were discontinued, and the patient was started on clomipramine 25 mg HS and clonazepam 0.5 mg HS. Mild improvement was noted after two weeks. Since the patient was still symptomatic, clomipramine was gradually increased to 100 mg HS and clonazepam increased to 0.5 mg BID, which resulted in significant improvement in insomnia as well as obsessional and anxiety symptoms. However, schizoid symptoms persisted. The addition of risperidone 0.5 mg HS later in the course of treatment improved the schizoid symptoms without any identifiable side effects.

Comments: Symptoms attributed to most personality disorders are treatable. If component symptoms of a personality disorder are identified and treated using specific medications to address symptoms, treatment is usually effective. With most cases presenting to the clinician's attention, it is difficult to separate the Axis I and Axis II symptoms; hence, my approach is to focus on the most significant presenting symptoms for purposes of immediate pharmacological intervention.

Case #42

Presenting Symptoms: The patient was a 35-year-old female with complaints of severe anxiety, frequent panic attacks, depressed mood, occasional crying, irritability, anger outbursts, habitual worrying, restless sleep, anorexia, feelings of hopelessness, and anhedonia. She denied suicidal ideation. She had had these symptoms since 1989, when lymphoma was diagnosed. She had been taking alprazolam 1 mg TID for six years prior to being seen by me with the above complaints. She had been tried on various benzodiazepines, tricyclic antidepressants, and thioridazine by psychiatrists in the past. She denied drug and alcohol abuse and caffeine intake. She smoked one pack of cigarettes per day. Family psychiatric history consisted of an aunt who suffered from an anxiety disorder. The patient's medical history was significant for lymphoma and for asthma, for which she was taking metaproterenol inhaler PRN.

Current Diagnosis: Major depression, moderate
panic disorder

Current Treatment:
1. alprazolam 1 mg TID
2. fluoxetine 40 mg AM
3. doxepin 25 mg HS
4. referral for counseling

Current Treatment: The patient was kept on alprazolam 1 mg TID, which she had been taking for six years. Fluoxetine 10 mg was started. Since anorexia, nausea, and heartburn worsened, doxepin 10 mg was added. Although the patient felt better, residual symptoms of depression remained. Over the next ten months, the dose of fluoxetine was increased to the final dose of 40 mg AM, and doxepin increased to 25 mg HS, with complete remission of symptoms. Attempts at decreasing alprazolam increased anxiety; hence, the patient was maintained on alprazolam at 1 mg TID.

Comments: Alprazolam, due to its fast onset of action, potency, and relatively short duration of action, is highly addictive when used regularly at high doses for long periods of time, as are all sedatives with similar pharmacokinetics. It is very difficult to withdraw a patient from alprazolam as an outpatient once the patient becomes dependent on it. The claim by some clinicians that patients who have true anxiety disorder do not become dependent has not been substantiated by my clinical experience. My general approach to managing anxiety disorders is to use antidepressants, as described in detail in the chapter on anxiety disorders.

Various strategies are employed to decrease dependence on a short-acting sedative. Switching the patient to a long-acting sedative and then decreasing the dose gradually or giving the same medication at lower doses in shorter intervals and then decreasing the dose are effective strategies. In this case, switching to clonazepam 1 mg TID or diazepam 10 mg TID and then slowly decreasing the dose are possibilities. Alprazolam could be prescribed for this patient at 0.5 mg five to six times a day, after which it is easier to slowly decrease the dose without mobilization of significant withdrawal or rebound anxiety. The addition of an antidepressant should make it easier to decrease the dose of sedatives or to withdraw the patient from sedatives since many of the anxiety symptoms are controlled on the antidepressant. However, antidepressants do not have cross-tolerance with benzodiazepines. Whether such an approach would have actually worked for this patient is unknown.

Most patients who have a primary anxiety disorder are sensitive to antidepressants. Patients are typically started on a very low dose of an antidepressant, with small dosage increments as tolerated. This particular patient was started on fluoxetine 10 mg for this reason, but the dose had to be increased to 40 mg in order to achieve satisfactory results.

The patient did well on doxepin 25 mg HS, which treated anorexia, nausea, heartburn, and insomnia. TCAs at low doses are excellent as adjunctive medications for use with SSRIs or with antianxiety medications.

Case #43

Presenting Symptoms: The patient was a 35-year-old male with complaints of depressed mood, anergia, irritability, initial insomnia, feelings of hopelessness, anhedonia, and suicidal ideation without intent or plan. These symptoms were precipitated by marital conflicts leading to a recent separation. He denied drug and alcohol abuse. He smoked one and a half packs of cigarettes per day. He drank three cups of regular coffee daily. He denied medical problems and previous psychiatric treatment.

Current Diagnosis: Major depression, moderate, single episode
Marital problems

Current Treatment:
1. bupropion 150 mg BID
2. trazodone 25 mg HS
3. lorazepam 0.5 mg HS

Treatment Course: The patient was initially tried on fluoxetine 20 mg AM, trazodone 25 mg HS, and lorazepam 0.5 mg HS, which were ineffective except for treatment of his insomnia. After a month, fluoxetine was discontinued. Bupropion 75 mg twice a day was started, and eventually increased to 150 mg BID, with satisfactory improvement in depressive symptoms. The patient discontinued these medications after several months. Depressive symptoms relapsed after eight months. When the patient returned, he was started back on bupropion, lorazepam, and trazodone with good response.

Comments: Since bupropion requires multiple dosing, compliance is difficult, as is true with any medication that requires multiple dosing. In order to get a bupropion dose higher than 300 mg per day, at least three doses per day are required because of the single dose maximum of 150 mg. Most patients, other than the elderly and children, need 300 mg or greater per day for a satisfactory antidepressant effect. For depression primarily characterized by anergia, hypersomnia, hyperphagia, psychomotor retardation, and apathy, bupropion is an excellent choice as a first-line antidepressant. The remarkable lack of sexual side effects makes it a reasonable choice to try as a primary antidepressant at full dosage, or as an adjunctive medication at low doses, for patients with significant sexual dysfunction, either due to medication side effects or depression. A sustained-release form of bupropion expected to be introduced in December 1996 should improve compliance due to the convenience of BID dosing. The precautions regarding dosage, seizures, and specific dosing guidelines, are explained in the chapter on antidepressants. Since bupropion typically causes insomnia, adjunctive sleep medications are usually necessary, either regularly or PRN.

Case #44

Presenting Symptoms: The patient was a 55-year-old male with complaints of depressed mood, excessive worrying, irritability, initial and middle insomnia, anorexia, anergia, and anxiety. These symptoms had been present for about one and one-half years, precipitated by his daughter's chronic medical problems. The patient reported that insomnia had been a major problem for 10 to 15 years. He denied drug and alcohol abuse, smoking, and caffeine intake. He also denied previous psychiatric treatment. His medical history was significant for hypertension, hyperlipidemia, heart disease, and CHF, for which he was taking captopril (Capoten), dipyridamole (persantine), digoxin (Lanoxin), lovastatin (Mevacor), and furosemide (Lasix).

Current Diagnosis: Dysthymia

Current Treatment:
1. sertraline 100 mg BID
2. bupropion 100 mg AM and noon
3. trazodone 75 mg HS
4. lorazepam 1 mg HS
5. referral to therapist for psychotherapy

Treatment Course: The patient was initially started on sertraline 50 mg AM, which was increased over a period of four months to the maximum recommended dose of 200 mg daily, with satisfactory resolution of all depressive symptoms except anergia. Sexual dysfunction emerged as a side effect, and was more pronounced at higher doses of sertraline. Trazodone 50 mg and lorazepam 0.5 mg were also started. Insomnia improved moderately, but not completely. After trials on various dosages of trazodone and lorazepam, either alone or in different combinations, the most efficient combination with the least side effects was found to be trazodone 75 mg HS and lorazepam 1 mg HS. The patient has been on these doses now for about six months with excellent effectiveness, no noticeable side effects, and no tolerance. When nefazodone became available in early 1995, with the expectation of being an effective antidepressant without the common sexual side effects associated with SSRIs, the patient was offered a trial on nefazodone. Sertraline was tapered off over one week, and nefazodone was started at 100 mg BID, later increased to 250 mg BID. The patient was kept on this regimen for three weeks. Although sexual dysfunction improved, depressive symptoms returned, prompting the patient to request resumption of sertraline. Eventually, bupropion 100 mg AM was started in an attempt to treat anergia and sexual dysfunction. Encouraged by a mild improvement and no side effects, the bupropion was increased to 100 mg AM and at noon, which resulted in moderate improvement in anergia and sexual dysfunction without any side effects. The patient had been maintained on this combination for approximately four months at the time of this writing. The patient's digoxin level, blood pressure, and electrolytes have continued to be within acceptable levels after starting these medications.

Comments: Antidepressants are chosen based on overall efficacy, taking into consideration factors such as primary medication effects, side effects, pharmacokinetics, individual physician's experience with a particular medication, etc. The goal is to find the best medication match for the individual patient that will relieve all the symptoms without any side effects. The first choice should be the medication that will be the most effective in the shortest amount of time. Obviously, such a stroke of luck does not happen often in actual practice. Antidepressants should not be chosen based on one symptom or side effect alone. Moreover, in psychiatry, there is no one medicine that is effective for everybody. Please review Tables 2.1 and 2.2 for considerations in selecting an antidepressant for an individual patient.

Sexual side effects are not an all-or-none phenomena. Typically, the higher the dosage of an offending medication, the more marked the sexual side effects. Similarly, in general, the more severe the depression, the more pronounced the sexual dysfunction. Nefazodone does not interfere with libido or sexual performance as much as SSRIs, TCAs, or MAOIs. I have not tried it as an adjunctive medication at low doses to try to reverse the sexual dysfunction caused by other antidepressants. Bupropion, stimulants, amantadine, and others, as listed in Chapter 5, have been tried with varying success rates. If a particular medication is not effective for its primary purpose, the side effect profile is irrelevant unless used adjunctively. It is not known whether or not this patient would do well on bupropion alone, rather than on both bupropion and sertraline. An attempt to taper sertraline while increasing the dose of bupropion would be appropriate and could be tried for this patient. However, in the author's experience, symptoms such as anxiety, irritability, and obsessive worrying are not generally responsive to bupropion, whereas anergia, hypersomnia, apathy, psychomotor retardation, and decreased libido are preferentially responsive to bupropion. Unfortunately, patients' symptoms do not come in discrete "packages." Many patients are willing to accept diminished libido or some impairment in sexual functioning if more distressing presenting symptoms are satisfactorily resolved.

If insomnia is severe and chronic, as in this case, combinations of hypnotics are effective. Low doses of different medications ensure immediate results without significant side effects. See Chapter 13 for details regarding management of severe insomnia.

Although the ideal is to help resolve insomnia using sleep hygiene techniques or other nonmedication strategies, in actual practice medications are frequently needed for rapid results. Benzodiazepines alone, low-dose sedating antidepressants alone, or combinations of both are effective for treatment of most insomnias that are associated with psychiatric disorders. Specific medication guidelines are given in the chapter on insomnia. In some cases, especially when TCAs, trazodone, or nefazodone are used, separate hypnotics are not necessary. Although, as a general principle, hypnotics should be used only for short periods of time, there are patients who may need hypnotics long-term. One of the advantages of combining low doses of a sedating antidepressant along with a benzodiazepine hypnotic is that the dose of the benzodiazepine can be kept low, as demonstrated in this case of severe long-standing insomnia.

Case #45

Presenting Symptoms: The patient was a 40-year-old male with complaints of depressed mood, visual hallucinations, crying episodes, irritability, anergia, insomnia, anhedonia, and anorexia with loss of 20 pounds in the three months preceding the first visit. He denied suicidal ideation. He also denied drug and alcohol abuse, and caffeine intake. He smoked one pack of cigarettes per day. The above symptoms were precipitated by multiple medical problems. The patient was diagnosed with attention deficit disorder as a child. He took methylphenidate until age 14. He denied a family history of psychiatric problems. His medical history was significant for AIDS, chronic back pain, and hepatitis C. His medications at the time of this evaluation were fluconazole (Diflucan), acyclovir (Zovirax), fentanyl (Duragesic), cimetidine (Tagamet), and clarithromycin (Biaxin).

Current Diagnosis: Adjustment disorder with depressed mood
Mood disorder due to multiple medical problems or medications, depressive type

Current Treatment: Doxepin 10 mg BID

Treatment Course: The patient was started on doxepin 10 mg HS and lorazepam 0.5 mg HS. Significant improvement in depression and anorexia was noted when seen after two weeks. Since lorazepam 0.5 mg caused excessive sedation, this was discontinued. Doxepin was increased to 10 mg BID with satisfactory improvement in depression, insomnia, and anorexia. The patient is maintained on doxepin alone at 10 mg BID and seen once every two to three months.

Comments: Patients with serious, even terminal, medical problems often become clinically depressed. This may result from the emotional stress caused by the illness or the neurochemical effects of the medical problems and various medication effects, or both. Extremely low doses of medication are sometimes sufficient to obtain a response, particularly in patients debilitated by medical problems or in the elderly. Since this patient was emaciated, an antidepressant with weight gain as a side effect was chosen. Other TCAs could have been equally effective. In seriously medically ill patients with anergia, apathy, and depression, stimulants such as dextroamphetamine 5 to 10 mg AM, or methylphenidate 5 mg BID may be used for a short period of time. The advantages are an almost immediate response and a benign side effect profile. This patient's insomnia and severe anorexia prompted a trial on a TCA. However, it should be noted that sometimes stimulants can paradoxically improve appetite and sleep in very depressed patients. This patient's history of ADD and successful response to methylphenidate would make stimulants a reasonable option to try. If a severely depressed patient is unable to tolerate medication, ECT is an option.

An effective dose, regardless of the size of the dose, is the therapeutic dose for that particular patient. Although "therapeutic range" is a useful and commonly quoted term, it is a statistical concept applicable generically to large samples, not to specific individuals. Hence, if a patient responds to a dose that is lower than the low end of the therapeutic range, that is the therapeutic dose for this patient. Do not increase the dose only for the purpose of bringing it within the expected therapeutic range. In general, clinical response, not formulas or protocols, should primarily guide dosing adjustment.

Case #46

Presenting Symptoms: The patient was a 40-year-old female with complaints of depressed mood, anxiety, excessive worrying, anger outbursts, extreme mood swings, anergia, restlessness, obsessive somatic preoccupation, compulsive cleaning, racing thoughts, and anhedonia. She denied drug and alcohol abuse, smoking, and caffeine intake. The patient described herself as being depressed and anxious for many years, with no clear precipitants. The patient has been taking alprazolam 1 mg QID for several years when she was first seen at my office. She had previously been tried on fluoxetine, imipramine, phenelzine, nortriptyline, amitriptyline, sertraline, doxepin, buspirone, and thiothixene. All of these medications were discontinued due to the intolerable side effects or lack of effectiveness. The patient's father and sister were being treated for depression and were taking alprazolam. Her medical history was significant for mitral valve prolapse, reflux esophagitis, and temporomandibular joint dysfunction. She is currently on atenolol 50 mg daily. She reported that her father abused her physically and sexually from age 2 to age 15. This patient had been married seven times.

Current Diagnosis: Dysthymia
Generalized anxiety disorder

Current Treatment: 1. alprazolam 1 mg QID
2. referred for psychotherapy

Treatment Course: While being maintained on alprazolam 1 mg QID, the patient was subsequently tried, under my care, on clomipramine, paroxetine, lithium, carbamazepine, valproic acid, fluvoxamine, nefazodone, venlafaxine, risperidone, trifluoperazine, and thioridazine. Although she is still symptomatic on alprazolam 1 mg QID, she would be significantly more symptomatic without it.

Comments: The vast majority of patients with anxiety disorders are better treated using antidepressants as the primary medication, along with adjunctive benzodiazepines on a PRN basis. However, one rarely comes across a patient for whom antidepressants are either ineffective or not tolerated, necessitating long-term use of benzodiazepines, as illustrated in this case. All classes of antidepressants, some antipsychotics, and mood stabilizers were tried, but were unsuccessful. The main text chapter on anxiety disorders describes details of management guidelines and issues.

Case #47

Presenting Symptoms: The patient was a 27-year-old male with complaints of frequent panic attacks, depressive episodes, feelings of hopelessness, insomnia, obsessive rumination, perfectionistic tendencies, excessive preoccupation with work, anxiety, mild compulsive cleaning, and mood swings. He had been placed on imipramine, clonazepam, and sertraline in the past with no significant effect. He denied drug and alcohol abuse, smoking, and caffeine intake. The patient's father suffered from depression. The patient's medical history was significant for hypertension, and he was taking atenolol 50 mg daily.

Current Diagnosis: Panic disorder
Dysthymia
Obsessive-compulsive personality disorder

Current Treatment: 1. fluvoxamine 100 mg AM and 200 mg HS
2. alprazolam 0.25 mg QID
3. referred for counseling

Treatment Course: Various medications including fluoxetine and paroxetine were not effective. Marked improvement was seen with fluvoxamine, which was started at 100 mg HS, and gradually increased to the current dose. He is seen once every three months for medication management.

Comments: In nearly all cases, an effective medication or combination of medications can be found if the physician is determined and if the patient is cooperative. Because of the favorable side effect profile of SSRIs, my approach is to place the patient on a trial of SSRI and bupropion until most choices are exhausted. There are so many choices of SSRIs that at least one of them is likely to be effective for the majority of patients. At low- to medium-dosage range, bupropion is as safe as SSRIs. Although fluvoxamine is approved for treatment of obsessive-compulsive disorder, its actions are like other SSRIs and it is effective for all the SSRI indications.

Case #48

Presenting Symptoms: The patient was a 35-year-old female with complaints of severely depressed mood, frequent crying, anger outbursts, paranoid ideation, feelings of guilt, disorganized thinking, excessive emotional sensitivity, insomnia, feelings of hopelessness, suicidal ideation, compulsive cleaning, irritability, and anhedonia. These symptoms were precipitated by marital conflicts. She denied drug and alcohol abuse, and caffeine intake. She smoked one pack of cigarettes per day. The patient had a history of depressive episodes in the past for which she was treated by her family physician with nortriptyline, paroxetine, and sertraline. When first seen by the author, she was taking fluoxetine 40 mg AM, lorazepam 0.5 mg TID, and flurazepam 60 mg HS, as prescribed by her family physician. Her mother had a history of depression, and was doing well on nortriptyline. The patient had peptic ulcer, hiatal hernia, and irritable bowel syndrome, for which she was taking ranitidine and over-the-counter antacids.

Current Diagnosis: Major depression, severe, recurrent, with mild psychotic and obsessive-compulsive features

Current Treatment: 1. venlafaxine 50 mg TID
2. referred for psychotherapy

Treatment Course: Fluoxetine, lorazepam, and flurazepam were discontinued. The patient was started on venlafaxine 37.5 mg TID with meals, risperidone 1 mg HS, clonazepam 0.5 mg BID, and trazodone 50 mg HS. At the second visit after two weeks, she reported moderate improvement, and the dose of venlafaxine was increased to 50 mg TID with meals. A month later, she reported marked improvement, and the dose of risperidone was decreased to 0.5 mg HS. In the subsequent month, all medications except venlafaxine were discontinued. All of the symptoms, including mild psychotic and obsessive-compulsive symptoms, were resolved. This patient is seen once every three months for medication management follow-up.

Comments: Just as illnesses run in the family through shared genes, medication response also runs in the family. For this reason, it is a clinical custom to start the patient on a medication that worked for a close family member for similar symptoms. Since the patient's mother did well on nortriptyline, it was logical to try this patient on nortriptyline. A family history of medication response increases the chance that the particular medication will be effective for the patient, but does not guarantee effectiveness. Family history of medication response is only one factor that is considered in choosing a medication. The specific nature of symptoms, side effects, allergies, concurrent medical problems, concurrent medications, and previous medication history are all important factors. Since newer antidepressants have become available in the 1990s, family history of medication responsiveness to MAOIs and TCAs, which were the primary options available prior to 1990, has become somewhat irrelevant. Hence, even if a patient's mother did well on a TCA or an MAOI, I would want to place the patient on a trial of one of the newer antidepressants because of the definite advantages, the most important of which is the favorable side effect profile. Similarly, the availability of risperidone, olanzapine, and clozapine has influenced the decision-making process with regard to treatment of psychosis.

The patient was taking two benzodiazepines, lorazepam 0.5 mg TID and flurazepam 60 mg HS (twice the maximum dosage). This practice should be discouraged, unless no other intervention is effective. Full doses of two medications from the same class should be avoided, especially with benzodiazepines and antipsychotic medications, except in rare situations in which it is clinically justified. However, this does not hold true for antidepressants. More than one antidepressant is commonly used. In most of these cases, one antidepressant is given for antidepressant effects and the others for differing purposes; the reasons are usually evident by the dosages employed. The following are examples of various combinations of antidepressants that a patient could be placed on, accompanied by an explanation of their uses.

Medication and Dose	Purpose
fluoxetine 40 mg AM	treatment of depression
trazodone 50 mg HS	treatment of insomnia
bupropion 100 mg AM	treatment of anergia/ sexual dysfunction

In this hypothetical example, three antidepressants are employed for three specific purposes. If this patient had dyspepsia and anorexia, a logical addition would be doxepin 10 mg at HS with possible discontinuation of trazodone because doxepin has sedating effects that may also treat insomnia. Assume that the patient reported insomnia after stopping trazodone and after starting doxepin, and the physician does not want to subject the patient to increased TCA side effects, making it undesirable to increase the dose of doxepin. In this situation, a logical option is to resume trazodone 50 mg HS, especially for a patient who has a history of substance abuse. Because there are so many variations and adjustments that can be implemented, the physician has a variety of options. In addition, such combinations, when used in an organized, balanced, and rational manner, give a great deal of precision and control to the physician in alleviating patients' symptoms.

Clonazepam was used for this patient to control anxiety and to safely discontinue both lorazepam and flurazepam. The use of low doses of an antipsychotic for short periods of time illustrates the proper use of antipsychotics in patients who have mild psychotic symptoms associated with a primary mood disorder.

This patient also had mild obsessive-compulsive symptoms for which all SSRIs, including venlafaxine, are effective. If an antidepressant alone is not effective in controlling the major symptoms, the patient might be tried sequentially on various augmenters, as listed in Chapter 2.

Case #49

Presenting Symptoms: The patient was a 35-year-old male with complaints of depressed mood, anergia, compulsive spending, excessive worrying, hyperphagia, poor concentration, distractibility, hypersomnia, irritability, feelings of hopelessness, mood swings, and anhedonia. He denied drug and alcohol abuse. He smoked one pack of cigarettes per day, and drank two cups of regular coffee daily. The patient denied acute precipitants. He had taken imipramine and fluoxetine in the past, but they were not fully effective. The patient's grandmother had suffered from severe depression, and his mother was depressed but had not been diagnosed or treated. He denied any major medical problems.

Current Diagnosis: Major depression, moderate, with mild compulsive features
Consider mild attention deficit disorder

Current Treatment: 1. bupropion 150 mg TID
2. lorazepam 0.5 mg once daily PRN
3. referral to therapist

Treatment Course: After seizure risk and other precautions related to bupropion were explained, the patient was started on bupropion 100 mg BID, and eventually increased to 150 mg TID, with instruction to adhere to at least a six-hour interval between doses. Since anxiety and mild compulsive spending did not improve, bupropion was discontinued, and he was placed on fluoxetine 40 mg AM. Cyproheptadine 4 mg BID was tried to treat sexual dysfunction due to fluoxetine but this was not effective. Since depression persisted, the patient requested a trial of sertraline, which was tried up to 150 mg per day with only mild improvement. He was subsequently tried on clomipramine, venlafaxine, and paroxetine, all of which caused sexual dysfunction. Bethanechol, stimulants, and bupropion were added as adjunctive medications to treat SSRI-induced sexual dysfunction. None were effective. Finally, the patient requested to be switched back to bupropion, which relieved depressive symptoms moderately without causing sexual side effects. When nefazodone became available, the patient was tried on it up to 200 mg TID because of the expectation that it could improve depression and anxiety as effectively as the SSRIs, but without the sexual dysfunction. The patient reported fewer sexual side effects while on nefazodone, but depressive symptoms did not resolve satisfactorily. The patient again requested to be switched back to bupropion, which he has been taking for the last five months with moderate improvement in depression, mild improvement in anxiety, and no sexual side effects.

Comments: Bupropion is particularly effective for symptoms such as anergia, hypersomnia, apathy, psychomotor agitation, and symptoms of ADD. This patient had most of these symptoms, which resolved moderately on bupropion. This prompted the patient to request bupropion when he realized that it gave relatively better overall results compared to SSRIs and nefazodone. Although nefazodone has fewer sexual side effects compared to SSRIs, its antidepressant and sedative effects are comparable to those of trazodone, based on my experience to date. Nefazodone's antidepressant effects for treatment of severe depression have not been as robust as expected. It may be determined that nefazodone, like trazodone, may be an excellent adjunctive medication for most patients.

Bupropion has been successfully used for the treatment of certain symptoms of ADD, such as distractibility, restlessness, poor concentration, impulsivity, irritability, poor attention span, and difficulty completing tasks. However, it is not as effective as other antidepressants for anxiety disorders including obsessive-compulsive symptoms.

Case #50

Presenting Symptoms: The patient was a 32-year-old female with complaints of severe insomnia, frequent crying, depressed mood, feelings of hopelessness, anergia, excessive emotional sensitivity, irritability, temper outbursts, hyperphagia, mild ideas of reference, occasional auditory hallucinations, and anhedonia. She denied drug and alcohol abuse and caffeine intake. She admitted to smoking one pack of cigarettes per day. She denied acute precipitants. The patient had been taking paroxetine six months prior to seeing me, but it was not effective. She denied any major medical problems, except dyspepsia for which she takes over-the-counter antacids PRN.

Current Diagnosis: Major depression, severe, with mild psychotic features

Current Treatment:
1. fluoxetine 60 mg AM
2. zolpidem 10 mg HS
3. trazodone 50 mg HS
4. counseling by therapist

Treatment Course: The patient was started on fluoxetine 20 mg AM, risperidone 0.5 mg HS, lorazepam 0.5 mg HS, doxepin 10 mg HS, and ranitidine 150 mg HS. At the second visit ten days later, the patient reported only mild improvement. The dose of fluoxetine was increased to 40 mg AM, and risperidone to 1 mg HS. The patient reported marked improvement of all symptoms when seen two weeks later. Ranitidine was then discontinued. At the next visit two months later, she reported that some of the depressive symptoms were recurring, along with initial insomnia. At that visit, fluoxetine was increased to 60 mg AM, lorazepam was discontinued, and zolpidem 10 mg was started. When seen one month later, all symptoms were resolved. She was then advised to decrease risperidone to 0.5 mg HS for one week and then to stop it. She has now been maintained on fluoxetine, zolpidem, and trazodone for the last six months.

Comments: It is a prudent clinical practice to see severely depressed patients frequently in the office during the initial phase of treatment in order to monitor patients closely and to adjust medications so that the physician is confident that acute symptoms are improving. This practice is particularly important when treating patients who have severe disorders, whereas for dysthymia, anxiety disorders, and uncomplicated major depression, the usual procedure is to have patients return two to three weeks after starting an antidepressant. Since stimulants, antianxiety medications, and antipsychotics work faster than antidepressants, a two-week wait is usually not needed when these are the primary medications. In these cases, one week is sufficient to assess the acute effects of the medication. Although in most textbooks the latency period for antidepressants to show optimal response is four to six weeks, in actual practice, patients are asked to return to the physician for a follow-up appointment in two to three weeks. If no improvement at all is seen in two weeks on an antidepressant, the dose is increased, assuming that there are no side effects. In an actual practice context, patients are unlikely to return if asked to continue on the same dose for several more weeks despite lack of improvement during the first two to three weeks. With SSRIs, for which the starting doses are considered full and effective doses, the latency period is less, compared to TCAs and MAOIs whose doses have to be titrated up gradually over a period of four to seven days to get to a therapeutic range. Hence, the four- to six-week latency period is more applicable to TCAs and MAOIs than to SSRIs or bupropion. The author's extensive experience with all antidepressants suggests that, in general, most SSRIs begin to work within one to two weeks. TCAs and MAOIs begin to work after about two to three weeks. When the one week that is usually required to titrate the TCA/MAOI dose to a therapeutic range is excluded, the latency period for both SSRIs and TCA/MAOIs is comparable.

When a patient reports dyspepsia, which is usually intensified by SSRIs, the patient should be advised to take the medications with food. Additionally, it is prudent to start an H2 blocker for the first several weeks to prevent exacerbation of dyspepsia, thereby enhancing compliance. Since most SSRIs cause GI side effects during initiation of treatment, such preemptive intervention is particularly effective to assure patient satisfaction, especially with sertraline and venlafaxine, which tend to cause dyspepsia slightly more often than other SSRIs. For most mild psychotic symptoms, which are fairly common with severe mood disorders, temporary use of an antipsychotic is extremely beneficial for rapid control of acute symptoms. In most of these cases, the antipsychotic can be withdrawn in two to eight weeks.

Regarding insomnia, one hypnotic medication alone is not sufficient for some patients. The combination of a low dose of a benzodiazepine and low dose of a sedating antidepressant gives the best results. The dose of benzodiazepine hypnotic can be kept low using this approach.

The dose of fluoxetine can be increased up to 80 mg. Since the highest strength fluoxetine capsule is 20 mg, four capsules are required for a patient on 80 mg daily. This particular patient takes three capsules. The cost of a month's supply of fluoxetine 60 mg daily is approximately $150. Fortunately, this patient's insurance covers the cost of medication except for a $10 copayment per month. For most patients without third-party coverage, the expense can be exorbitant. With venlafaxine and nefazodone, and to some extent with sertraline and paroxetine, the cost impact of high dosage is relatively less, compared to fluoxetine.

Case #51

Presenting Symptoms: The patient was a 30-year-old female with complaints of trichotillomania, restless sleep, excessive worrying, depressed mood, occasional crying, irritability, anergia, and various obsessive ruminations. Compulsive hair pulling had been getting worse since age 19. She denied drug and alcohol abuse and smoking. She drank one cup of coffee daily. The patient had received counseling off and on in the past, with mild temporary relief of symptoms. She denied a family history of psychiatric disorders. She also denied any history of medical problems.

Current Diagnosis: Obsessive-compulsive disorder
Dysthymia

Current Treatment:
1. fluvoxamine 100 mg TID
2. ranitidine 150 mg HS
3. clonazepam 0.5 mg one-quarter tablet BID
4. referred to a psychotherapist

Treatment Course: The patient could not tolerate or did not benefit from the following medications: clomipramine, fluoxetine, paroxetine, sertraline, and venlafaxine. Adjunctive treatments using buspirone, trazodone, various benzodiazepines, and risperidone were tried at different times, with no improvement. When fluvoxamine became available, she was started on it initially at 50 mg BID and gradually increased to 100 mg TID, along with clonazepam 0.5 mg BID. Due to excessive sedation, the dose of clonazepam was decreased to 0.125 mg BID, an extremely low dose. The patient reported 50 percent improvement in symptoms. She has now been maintained on fluvoxamine and clonazepam for seven months. Ranitidine was started to treat nausea and dyspepsia caused by fluvoxamine.

Comments: Some obsessive-compulsive disorder symptoms are difficult to treat; hence, they require determined efforts by the physician and the patient in trying various medications sequentially and in combinations if single medication treatment is not effective. Fortunately, this patient partially responded to fluvoxamine and possibly to clonazepam. The role of clonazepam is not clear given the very low dose she is taking.

Patients with OCD nearly always have coexisting depressive symptoms, but not vice versa. Fortunately, the treatment for OCD also improves depression.

OCD patients benefit from low doses of adjunctive benzodiazepines, especially high-potency benzodiazepines such as alprazolam, clonazepam, and lorazepam.

Case #52

Presenting Symptoms: The patient was a 40-year-old male with complaints of paranoid delusions, auditory hallucinations, and insomnia. The patient was diagnosed as suffering from paranoid schizophrenia and has been fairly well stabilized on chlorpromazine 100 mg TID, benztropine 1 mg BID, and lorazepam 0.5 mg HS at the time he was first seen in my office in late 1993, having recently moved from another state. He denied drug and alcohol abuse. He smoked one pack of cigarettes and drank one cup of coffee daily. This patient had not worked for the last ten years and currently lived with his elderly mother. He had had numerous psychiatric hospitalizations in the last 15 years. The patient was a poor historian; hence, he was unable to give names of other medications tried, if any. His uncle had a "nervous breakdown" and was hospitalized several times. This patient's medical history was unremarkable.

Current Diagnosis: Schizophrenia, paranoid type

Current Treatment:
1. chlorpromazine 100 mg TID
2. lorazepam 0.5 mg HS
3. referred to psychotherapist (the patient was noncompliant with therapy)

Treatment Course: Benztropine was discontinued. The patient was strongly advised to consider clozapine, but he refused. He is currently seen once every four months for medication supervision.

Comments: Use of supplemental anticholinergics is usually unnecessary when low-potency antipsychotics that have inherent anticholinergic properties are used. Even when anticholinergic medications are beneficial along with high-potency antipsychotics, they can be gradually withdrawn after the first several months, for most patients. This approach is consistent with the general goal of treating patients using the lowest dose and the least number of medications.

Although this patient may be said to be "stabilized" from a conservative and historical perspective, it is my belief that the definition of "stabilization" as it applies to chronic psychotic patients deserves some revision with the availability of clozapine and, to some extent, risperidone and olanzapine. Chlorpromazine has helped to keep the patient's positive symptoms in fair control and thereby has stabilized him. Clozapine offers much more. The patient's overall quality of life has the potential to be further improved significantly with clozapine, thereby allowing the patient to "stabilize" at a higher level, compared to what is possible with traditional antipsychotics. Unfortunately, since this patient refused clozapine, it may take another exacerbation and resultant hospitalization for another opportunity to offer him a treatment that has the potential to significantly improve his well-being.

Assuming the patient would be willing to be switched to clozapine, hospitalization would be the appropriate venue for completing this change. The tapering off of the current antipsychotic and the upward titration of clozapine is complicated, along with the risk of exacerbation during the transition phase. The dosing strategy in switching patients to clozapine or to risperidone is discussed in Chapter 10.

Case #53

Presenting Symptoms: The patient was a 72-year-old female with complaints of anxiety, depressed mood, auditory hallucinations with persecutory content, insomnia, obsessive rumination, irritability, obsessive fear of dying, ideas of reference, and anhedonia. The patient revealed that she had been hearing voices since her late teens and avoided being home alone because of this. She stated that the voices had started again about four months prior to this office visit. Depressive symptoms emerged four months ago for the first time. The patient had been under stress due to her husband's cancer which was discovered one year ago and which worsened six months ago. She denied drug and alcohol abuse, smoking, and caffeine intake. She also denied any previous psychiatric evaluation or treatment. This patient had hypertension and arthritis. She was taking metoprolol.

Current Diagnosis: Adjustment disorder with depressed mood and anxiety
Schizotypal personality disorder with dependent features
Consider psychosis, NOS

Current Treatment:
1. risperidone 0.5 mg HS
2. clomipramine 25 mg HS
3. referral for psychotherapy

Treatment Course: Both clomipramine 25 mg HS and risperidone 0.5 mg HS were started at the first visit. When seen two weeks later, the patient reported remarkable improvement in all of the symptoms. Sustained improvement was seen two months later, with no side effects. She is now seen once every three months for medication management.

Comments: I am uncertain regarding this patient's precise diagnosis. She could be categorized as having schizophrenia, residual type; psychosis, NOS; or schizoaffective disorder, depressed. Until recently, the symptoms were of low severity, suggesting that she possibly has a schizotypal personality disorder, temporarily worsened by the stress of her husband's terminal illness.

Given her age, very low doses were prescribed. Fortunately, they worked well. Since the patient's symptoms improved to the point where she is fully satisfied with the treatment, there is no reason to increase the dose. Clomipramine was chosen to address the obsessional quality associated with her fear and anxieties.

Case # 54

Presenting Symptoms: The patient was a 49-year-old male with complaints of depressed mood, irritability, feelings of hopelessness, anger outbursts, poor self-esteem, anhedonia, anergia, middle insomnia, perfectionistic tendencies, mild obsessive preoccupation with computer games, mild ideas of reference, mild paranoia, distractibility, scattered thinking, poor concentration, and anxiety. Most of the above symptoms were present since his twenties, but had recently worsened due to the stress of family conflicts. He denied drug and alcohol abuse, smoking, and caffeine intake. This patient had had counseling off and on over the years. He denied any major medical problems.

Current Diagnosis: Major depression, mild, recurrent
Dysthymia
Consider schizotypal features
Consider adult attention deficit disorder
Consider mild obsessive-compulsive features

Current Treatment:
1. sertraline 50 mg AM
2. trazodone 50 mg HS
3. referral for psychotherapy

Treatment Course: Sertraline 50 mg AM, risperidone 0.5 mg HS, temazepam 7.5 mg HS, and trazodone 50 mg HS were started at the first visit.

The patient reported feeling much better when seen two weeks later. Temazepam was discontinued at the second visit. Risperidone was discontinued after three months. The patient has been maintained on sertraline and trazodone for the last six months.

Comments: This patient had symptoms suggestive of features of various disorders, for most of which full criteria were not met. It is common in actual practice to see patients who do not meet full criteria for *DSM-IV* diagnoses, but have dysfunctional symptoms that need treatment. It is also difficult in many cases to come up with one diagnosis that can incorporate all of the symptoms, necessitating multiple diagnoses or diagnostic possibilities. Frequently, the patient's symptoms are not sufficient to give the full diagnosis. When this occurs, it is my practice to list the diagnosis with adjectives to reflect the presence of specific symptom complexes. The following are some examples:

- Obsessive-compulsive features
- Mild paranoia
- Schizotypal features
- Mild psychotic features
- Possible mild psychotic features
- Possible attention deficit disorder

None of the above designations are diagnoses, yet they indicate the presence of symptoms that need treatment.

Antidepressants are effective for treatment of ADD symptoms, especially when depressive symptoms coexist. Among various antidepressants, norepinephrinergic antidepressants, such as bupropion and desipramine, tend to be almost as effective as stimulants in some patients, although all antidepressants can be used. Because of the safety of SSRIs, they are being used more frequently, even in children. It appears that this patient's possible ADD symptoms improved to some extent on sertraline.

Case #55

Presenting Symptoms: The patient was a 30-year-old female with depressed mood, feelings of hopelessness, anxiety, anger attacks, anergia, excessive emotional sensitivity, hyperphagia, anhedonia, and suicidal ideation without intent or plan. She admitted to binge drinking, consisting of six to eight beers on weekends. She denied drug abuse, smoking, and caffeine intake. She also denied any recent precipitants. Sertraline and fluoxetine had not been effective for these symptoms. The patient's grandmother suffered from depression. This patient denied any major medical problems.

Current Diagnosis: Major depression, moderate, single episode
Dysthymia
Alcohol abuse

Current Treatment:
1. paroxetine 60 mg AM
2. bupropion 100 mg AM
3. fenfluramine 20 mg one hour before supper
4. referral for psychotherapy
5. referral to Alcoholics Anonymous

Treatment Course: The patient was started on paroxetine 20 mg and increased to 60 mg AM over a period of three months. All presenting symptoms except anergia and hyperphagia improved satisfactorily. Bupropion 100 mg AM was added, resulting in moderate improvement in anergia. Hyperphagia persisted; hence, fenfluramine was started at a dose of 20 mg one hour before supper. Mild improvement in control of hyperphagia was reported, with slight improvement in anxiety.

Comments: Fenfluramine can be combined with nonsedating antidepressants for patients with hyperphagia, obesity, anxiety, and depression. Since it stimulates release of serotonin and has some serotonin reuptake blocking properties, it can theoretically be used as an antidepressant augmenter. The sedating effects can be of help to patients with obesity, anxiety, and insomnia. It should generally be avoided with sedating TCA because of risk of excessive sedation. Refer to Chapter 2 for precautions associated with the use of fenfluramine.

Case #56

Presenting Symptoms: The patient was a 39-year-old female with complaints of depressed mood, irritability, anxiety, crying episodes, anger episodes, feelings of hopelessness, severe anergia, decreased motivation, and suicidal ideation without intent or plan. She denied drug and alcohol abuse. She smoked one and one-half packs of cigarettes per day and drank three to five cups of coffee daily. She denied any acute precipitants. The patient had several episodes of depression for which she was hospitalized in the past. She was on amitriptyline 200 mg HS when seen at my office. The patient's sister had been diagnosed with depression. The patient denied any major medical problems.

Current Diagnosis: Major depression, severe, recurrent

Current Treatment: 1. protriptyline 20 mg AM and noon
2. buspirone 10 mg TID
3. temazepam 15 mg HS
4. referral for psychotherapy

Treatment Course: Amitriptyline was tapered off over a period of two weeks. The patient was started on temazepam 15 mg HS to relieve insomnia that emerged after the dose of amitriptyline was decreased. Bupropion, fluoxetine, and paroxetine were either ineffective or not tolerated. Protriptyline 10 mg BID, eventually increased to 20 mg AM and noon, resulted in moderate improvement in depression and anergia. Buspirone was added for treatment of chronic anxiety and for antidepressant augmentation.

Comments: Protriptyline tends to possess energizing properties, making it useful for patients who have depression with prominent anergia, apathy, and hypersomnia. Stimulating SSRIs such as fluoxetine and venlafaxine, as well as bupropion are the first-line medications for these symptoms because of their favorable side effect profile. However, there are patients for whom SSRIs and bupropion may not be effective. Among the MAOIs, tranylcypromine has excellent energizing properties.

Protriptyline at low doses is occasionally used for treatment of central sleep apnea. However, since most patients with central sleep apnea have serious multisystem illness, they are usually unable to tolerate protriptyline because of TCA side effects.

If this patient's depression worsens in the future, tranylcypromine will be considered. Buspirone is contraindicated with MAOIs.

Case #57

Presenting Symptoms: The patient was a 22-year-old female with complaints of depressed mood, frequent crying, anergia, severe insomnia, excessive worrying, irritability, anger episodes, excessive emotional sensitivity, feelings of hopelessness, and anhedonia. These symptoms worsened one and one-half years ago after the patient broke up with her boyfriend. She also drank six to seven vodka drinks daily for three months prior to her visit at the office. She denied drug abuse. She smoked one pack of cigarettes per day, and drank three to four cups of coffee daily. The patient's father suffered from depression. This patient denied any major medical problems, except for occasional dyspepsia.

Current Diagnosis: Major depression, moderate, single episode
Dysthymia
Alcohol dependence

Current Treatment:
1. fluoxetine 20 mg AM
2. doxepin 10 mg HS
3. trazodone 25 mg HS
4. complete abstention from drinking
5. coffee intake reduced to one to two cups daily
6. referral for individual psychotherapy and to Alcoholics Anonymous

Treatment Course: The patient was prescribed the following medications at the time of her first visit: (1) chlordiazepoxide 50 mg the first night, then decrease by 10 mg each night until completed (dispense 10 mg pills #15), (2) fluoxetine 20 mg AM, (3) doxepin 10 mg HS, (4) multivitamin, one tablet daily, and (5) thiamine 100 mg daily for seven days. She responded well as an outpatient and reported improvement when seen one week later. She was continued on doxepin 10 mg HS and fluoxetine 20 mg po AM. She complained of mild insomnia for which trazodone 25 mg was prescribed at the third office visit. She has done extremely well on these medications for the last six months.

Comments: For well-motivated and healthy patients, outpatient drug and alcohol detoxification is an option. My belief, based on extensive experience, is that most substance abusers have treatable underlying psychiatric symptoms that can be identified. The symptoms might be as simple as insomnia or anxiety. If the symptoms are not concurrently treated, the chances of long-term abstinence are low.

For complicated patients with severe drug and alcohol dependence, inpatient treatment is usually necessary.

Case #58

Presenting Symptoms: The patient was a 29-year-old female with complaints of depressed mood, poor concentration, scattered thinking, anergia, irritability, and anger outbursts. She denied drug and alcohol abuse and smoking. She drank two cups of coffee per day. The patient had been taking fluoxetine 20 mg AM for one year when seen at this office. Her mother had a diagnosis of schizophrenia. The patient's medical problems included back pain and headache, for which she took ibuprofen occasionally.

Current Diagnosis: Attention deficit disorder
Dysthymia

Current Treatment:
1. dextroamphetamine slow release capsule 15 mg AM
2. venlafaxine 75 mg AM and 150 mg HS
3. zolpidem 5 mg HS PRN insomnia
4. referral for psychotherapy

Treatment Course: Dramatic improvement in attention and concentration was noted after starting dextroamphetamine at 5 mg AM. The dose was eventually increased to, and stabilized on, 15 mg AM of Dexedrine spansule capsule (slow-release form of dextroamphetamine). Depressive symptoms were successfully treated using venlafaxine, starting at 25 mg po TID, and increasing gradually to the current dose. Zolpidem 5 mg is used PRN for insomnia.

Comments: Stimulants have some antidepressant properties, but they are not as potent as those of true antidepressants such as TCAs or SSRIs. Similarly, antidepressants have some beneficial effect on ADD, but stimulants generally give the best results. When distinct ADD symptoms and depressive symptoms coexist, often both stimulants and antidepressants are needed for optimal outcome. The combination of SSRIs and stimulants have been tolerated well by patients, in the author's experience. Since venlafaxine has some norepinephrinergic activity, it is probably more suitable for ADD and depression than other SSRIs. (Venlafaxine is technically not an SSRI, but for ease of discussion, I have included venlafaxine in the SSRI group.) However, the norepinephrinergic potency of venlafaxine is probably not sufficient to adequately treat the full spectrum of ADD symptoms.

Case #59

Presenting Symptoms: The patient was a 35-year-old male with complaints of depressed mood, anxiety attacks, excessive worrying, irritability, crying episodes, feelings of hopelessness, anergia, and anhedonia. The patient had a history of suicidal ideation and had overdosed eight months before the initial visit. He admitted to a history of cocaine abuse in the past, but had abstained from it for the past year. He denied alcohol abuse. He smoked one and one-half packs of cigarettes per day, and drank two cups of coffee daily. At the time of his first visit to the office, he was taking fluoxetine 40 mg AM, methylphenidate 5 mg TID (for ADD), and trazodone 50 mg HS, started by the patient's previous psychiatrist in another city. The patient's brother had a diagnosis of panic disorder. This patient denied any major medical problems.

Current Diagnosis: Major depression, severe, recurrent
Attention deficit disorder (by history)
History of cocaine abuse

Current Treatment:
1. fluoxetine 60 mg AM
2. methylphenidate slow release 20 mg AM
3. trazodone 50 mg HS
4. bupropion 100 mg AM

Treatment Course: Fluoxetine was increased to 60 mg AM at the first visit to control depressive symptoms. After calling the previous psychiatrist's office to verify prescription and dose of methylphenidate, the patient was given a prescription. At the second visit about four weeks later, the patient reported improvement in all depressive symptoms except anergia, which persisted; hence, bupropion 100 mg AM was added with moderate but satisfactory improvement in anergia. The patient has been functioning well on this regimen.

Comments: When patients present with a request for continuation of controlled drugs, it is important to verify the prescription and dose with the previous physician, regardless of history of substance abuse. If immediate verification is not possible, a prescription for several days may be given, pending verification. For medications that are not commonly abused, such verification is not usually necessary, unless there are questions regarding exact dosing.

Because of bupropion's seizure risk, it is used at low doses when employed as part of a combination regimen, as in this patient. If this patient's depression reemerges, a reasonable option will be to discontinue fluoxetine and bupropion, and to try venlafaxine, which has serotonergic and norepinephrinergic properties.

Case #60

Presenting Symptoms: The patient was a 49-year-old female with complaints of anxiety attacks, depressed mood, anergia, and anxiety, for which she had been taking two tablets of Triavil 2/10 at bedtime for ten years, and paroxetine 10 mg HS for two years. She recently moved from another state, and was seen at my office. She denied drug and alcohol abuse and smoking. She drank three cups of coffee daily.

Current Diagnosis: Dysthymia
Paranoid features (as reported by the patient's previous psychiatrist)

Current Treatment: 1. paroxetine 30 mg HS
2. risperidone 0.5 mg HS
3. amitriptyline 25 mg HS
4. referral for psychotherapy

Treatment Course: Triavil is a mixture of perphenazine and amitriptyline. Triavil was discontinued; instead, the patient was started on risperidone 0.5 mg HS and amitriptyline 25 HS, and the dose of paroxetine was increased to 20 mg HS. The patient's previous psychiatrist was contacted to ascertain the need for the low dose of antipsychotic that she had taken for about ten years. It was revealed that the patient had paranoid symptoms that improved on Triavil. The patient was not able to identify paranoia as a problem she had had in the past. Her presenting symptoms improved satisfactorily on her current medications.

Comments: If a patient has been on an antipsychotic–even at low doses–the decision to discontinue the antipsychotic should not generally be made without obtaining information regarding the circumstances that led the previous psychiatrist to start the antipsychotic. The reason is that, in most cases, antipsychotic medication is started and maintained for long periods of time because of the presence of psychotic symptoms. It is sometimes tempting to discontinue an antipsychotic, especially if the patient is on a low dose and has no current psychotic symptoms or presenting complaints that are suggestive of a psychotic process. The reason why the patient is not symptomatic is most likely because the patient has been taking the antipsychotic. If it is decided to take the patient off of the antipsychotic, it is preferable to taper off the medication very slowly, so that if psychotic symptoms emerge, the dose can be rapidly reinstituted.

Because risperidone and olanzapine both have a better side effect profile with a low incidence and severity of extrapyramidal symptoms and possible decreased risk of tardive dyskinesia, my practice has been to switch patients to risperidone or olanzapine if possible. The effectiveness and improved side effect profile of risperidone and olanzapine should make them the first-line general purpose antipsychotics, whereas clozapine is superior in the treatment of chronic forms of major psychotic disorders, including schizoaffective disorder and schizophrenia with predominantly "negative" symptoms.

Case #61

Presenting Symptoms: The patient was a 21-year-old male with complaints of depressed mood, difficulty focusing, disorganized thinking, poor concentration, distractibility, anergia, social withdrawal, seclusiveness, dislike of close interaction with people, excessive worrying, and anhedonia. These symptoms had been present since early adolescence. He denied drug and alcohol abuse and caffeine intake. The patient was prescribed thioridazine for a brief period at age 13, for unknown reasons. The patient denied any major medical problems.

Current Diagnosis: Dysthymia
Attention deficit disorder
Schizoid personality disorder

Current Treatment:
1. bupropion 100 mg TID
2. risperidone 0.5 mg HS
3. fluoxetine 20 mg AM
4. referral for psychotherapy

Treatment Course: Bupropion was started at 100 mg BID and gradually increased to 100 mg TID. Depression and attention deficit symptoms improved moderately. Since fear of people, scattered thinking, and social withdrawal persisted, risperidone 0.5 mg and fluoxetine 20 mg were added, resulting in some improvement in these symptoms.

Comments: Bupropion is effective in depression characterized by anergia and for treatment of ADD. For schizoid personality features, a combination of a low dose of an antipsychotic and an antidepressant is sometimes beneficial.

Case #62

Presenting Symptoms: The patient was a 22-year-old female with complaints of extreme anger outbursts with minimal provocation; frequent assaultiveness, including punching walls and doors and destroying property; anxiety; excessive emotional sensitivity; and initial insomnia. She denied drug and alcohol abuse, and caffeine intake. She smoked one pack of cigarettes per day. These symptoms had been present for many years. Regarding family psychiatric history, the patient described her father as moody.

Current Diagnosis: Intermittent explosive disorder

Current Treatment:
1. paroxetine 45 mg AM
2. lorazepam 1 mg HS PRN
3. trazodone 100 mg HS
4. referral for psychotherapy

Treatment Course: The patient was initially started on paroxetine 20 mg AM and was gradually increased over a period of two months to 45 mg

AM with satisfactory control of explosive episodes. Trazodone and lorazepam were added to treat insomnia.

Comments: SSRIs and other antidepressants are usually effective for impulse control disorders, but SSRIs seem to be particularly effective. If SSRIs are not effective, other medication options are mood stabilizers, beta-blockers, clonidine, or antipsychotics. Combination treatment may be necessary if one medication by itself is not sufficient to control behavior. Severe impulse control disorders have serious consequences for the individual and others, and should be aggressively managed. If immediate control is necessary, antipsychotics are the best choice. Some of the severe, chronic, and refractory cases involving violent behavior may respond to clozapine. Combination short-term treatment using antipsychotics has the advantage of bringing the behavior rapidly under control while the antidepressants and/or mood stabilizers have time to become effective, at which time the antipsychotic can be slowly tapered off. The availability of risperidone and olanzapine has made the risk of neuroleptic side effects less of a concern, especially for short-term use at low doses.

Case #63

Presenting Symptoms: The patient was a 57-year-old female with complaints of somnambulism at a frequency of one to two episodes per week since 1985, excessive worrying, agoraphobia, perfectionistic tendencies, anxiety, and mild compulsive arranging. The obsessive-compulsive characteristics had been present for as long as the patient could remember. She admitted to a habit of drinking four glasses of wine daily since 1983. She smoked two packs of cigarettes per day, and drank three cups of coffee daily. She denied any acute precipitants. Her medical history was unremarkable.

Current Diagnosis: Sleepwalking disorder
Obsessive-compulsive personality disorder
Alcohol dependence, mild

Current Treatment: 1. clomipramine 50 mg HS
2. psychotherapy

Treatment Course: Alcohol was safely discontinued using tapering doses of chlordiazepoxide at a rate of 40 mg on the first day, 30 mg on the second day, 20 mg on the third day, and 10 mg on the fourth day. Clomipramine 25 mg HS was started on the day of her first office visit and increased to 50 mg starting the second week, with excellent results. She has been maintained on this medication for one year. She reported no further episodes of sleepwalking and satisfactory improvement in all other symptoms.

Comments: Somnambulism is a phenomenon that typically occurs in sleep stages 3 and 4. Alcohol can worsen almost all parasomnias, including sleepwalking. TCAs and sedatives, which decrease the intensity of slow-wave sleep improve sleepwalking. Given this patient's obsessive-compulsive personality features, the choice of clomipramine is readily apparent. Since her alcohol consumption preceded the onset of sleepwalking, it is possible that alcohol has etiological significance. In fact, the suppression of sleepwalking may have been due to abstention from alcohol rather than due to the effect of clomipramine. Given her obsessive-compulsive personality disorder symptoms, she could benefit from maintenance on clomipramine for several years.

Case #64

Presenting Symptoms: The patient was a 49-year-old female with complaints of anxiety, excessive worrying, obsessive fear of losing close friends or relatives, excessive somatic preoccupation, restless sleep, vague fears, perfectionistic tendencies, depressed mood, and anhedonia. These symptoms had been present since early adulthood, but had worsened during the last two to three years with no acute precipitants. She denied drug and alcohol abuse, smoking, and caffeine intake. The patient had been taking alprazolam 0.5 mg BID, prescribed by her primary care physician. She had taken chlordiazepoxide many years ago. The patient's mother suffered from depression. The patient was on atenolol 50 mg daily for mitral valve prolapse and on ranitidine 150 mg BID for peptic ulcer.

Current Diagnosis: Obsessive-compulsive features
Obsessive-compulsive personality
Depressive features

Current Treatment: 1. paroxetine 20 mg AM
2. alprazolam 0.25 mg PRN for anxiety

Treatment Course: The patient was started on paroxetine 20 mg AM, which improved all of the presenting symptoms. Alprazolam was decreased to 0.25 mg BID for several weeks, and then changed to infrequent PRN use. Since paroxetine caused mild sedation during the daytime, the schedule was switched to bedtime with further improvement in sleep and optimal daytime alertness. The patient has been on paroxetine for three years and wants to continue the medication indefinitely.

Comments: Obsessive-compulsive symptoms respond to antiobsessional medications, even if the patient does not meet the criteria for a formal diagnosis of obsessive-compulsive disorder. Obsessive-compulsive symptoms rarely exist without depressive and anxiety symptoms. Fortunately, antiobsessional medications such as clomipramine and SSRIs nicely control obsessive-compulsive symptoms, depression, and anxiety.

Case #65

Presenting Symptoms: The patient was a 40-year-old male with complaints of depressed mood, anergia, anhedonia, poor concentration, distractibility, hyperphagia, irritability, feelings of hopelessness, and initial insomnia. He denied drug and alcohol abuse. He smoked one pack of cigarettes per day and drank two cups of coffee daily. He had been taking long-acting nifedipine 30 mg daily for hypertension.

Current Diagnosis: Major depression, moderate, single episode
Mild attention deficit disorder symptoms

Current Treatment: 1. venlafaxine 75 mg BID
2. dextroamphetamine 10 mg AM

Treatment Course: The patient was first tried on bupropion 100 mg BID, then gradually increased to 150 mg TID, on which he did well for about one year. Since depressed mood and anergia reemerged, he was switched to venlafaxine 25 mg TID, and eventually increased to 100 mg TID. Depression improved but anergia persisted; hence, dextroamphetamine was added as an adjunctive medication after decreasing the dosage of venlafaxine to 75 mg BID, with excellent results. Results have been sustained for five months so far.

Comments: Stimulants are excellent adjunctive medications for treating refractory depression, particularly in patients with anergia, hypersomnia, apathy, and attention deficit disorder symptoms if energizing antidepressants such as fluoxetine, bupropion, and venlafaxine are only partially effective. Tranylcypromine is an antidepressant with stimulant effects but, being a MAOI, it is generally used as a last resort in current clinical practice.

Case #66

Presenting Symptoms: The patient was a 28-year-old female with complaints of difficulty organizing and focusing thoughts, vague thinking, feelings of having "close contacts" (as described by the patient) with people, introversion, social withdrawal, apathy, avoidance of social situations, obsessive worrying, and seclusiveness. These symptoms had been present since her early teens. She was brought to the office by her parents, with whom she lives. She denied drug and alcohol abuse, smoking, and caffeine intake. She also denied any history of major medical problems.

Current Diagnosis: Schizotypal personality disorder with schizoid, obsessional, and dependent features

Current Treatment: 1. risperidone 1 mg HS
2. fluoxetine 20 mg AM

Treatment Course: The patient was initially started on risperidone 0.5 mg, which was increased to her current dose of 1 mg. The increased dose improved thought disorganization and unnatural feelings. Fluoxetine was later added, initially at 10 mg AM, and eventually at 20 mg, which significantly improved apathy, worrying, and social withdrawal.

Comments: Personality disorders are treatable if constituent symptoms are identified and treated using specific medications. Usually, low doses are sufficient for treating personality disorders, with borderline personality disorder being an exception.

Chapter 17

Complex Cases

CASES 67 TO 100

Case #67

Presenting Symptoms: The patient was a 35-year-old male with complaints of depressed mood, anxiety, initial insomnia, restless sleep, irritability, increased emotional sensitivity, anger outbursts, anergia, seclusiveness, fear of leaving the house, belief that people were staring at him and degrading him, and anhedonia. His girlfriend had left him four months earlier because of his suspiciousness and distrust of her–symptoms that the patient reported had been present for many years. Depressive symptoms were precipitated by the breakup with his girlfriend. He denied auditory and visual hallucinations. He also denied suicidal or homicidal ideation, intent, or plan; drug and alcohol abuse; and caffeine intake. He smoked two packs of cigarettes per day. He denied any previous psychiatric treatments and any family psychiatric history. He denied medical problems.

Current Diagnosis: Adjustment disorder with depressed mood and paranoid symptoms
Paranoid personality disorder

Current Treatment:
1. paroxetine 20 mg AM
2. risperidone 0.5 mg HS
3. trazodone 50 mg HS
4. clonazepam 1 mg HS
5. continued counseling
6. requested to return in three months

Treatment Course: The patient was started on paroxetine 20 mg AM, risperidone 1 mg HS, and lorazepam 0.5 mg HS. Two weeks later, the patient reported no improvement in his anxiety, fears, or insomnia, and requested a change of medications. Paroxetine and lorazepam were discontinued, and he was started on clomipramine 25 mg HS and clonazepam 1 mg HS, with increase of risperidone to 2 mg HS. When seen after two weeks, he complained of feeling tired and drained. At this visit, risperidone was decreased to 1 mg HS, clomipramine discontinued, clonazepam decreased to 0.5 mg HS, trazodone started at 50 mg HS, and fluoxetine started at 20 mg AM. Two weeks later, the patient complained of anxiety attacks and insomnia. He felt that of all the antidepressants tried, paroxetine improved his symptoms the most; hence, fluoxetine was discontinued, clonazepam increased back to 1 mg HS, and paroxetine resumed at 20 mg AM. The patient reported significant improvement two weeks later. Risperidone was decreased to 0.5 mg HS. The patient has been fully functional with no residual symptoms or side effects on his current medications. He is seen in the office once every three months.

Comments: In clinical practice, it is rare to see a patient with a personality disorder and no overlapping Axis I symptoms. It is difficult to distinguish whether depressive symptoms or paranoid symptoms are primary in this patient, although his primary presenting complaints were depressive symptoms precipitated by the breakup with his girlfriend who probably felt alienated and frustrated by the patient's paranoid attitude. The patient does not meet the full *DSM-IV* criteria for paranoid personality disorder. In psychiatric practice, it is the presence of symptoms that defines treatment. Thus, if a patient presents with depressive and paranoid symptoms that are causing distress, treatment is warranted, regardless of whether or not the patient meets the full criteria for one or more specific diagnoses. Alternatively, one could describe this patient as suffering from major depression, moderate, with mild psychotic features, although this is not a *DSM-IV* diagnosis. Regardless of the diagnostic terms used, treatment is the same. Insomnia frequently needs to be treated as a separate problem as is done with this patient using trazodone and clonazepam. Several other treatment options are possible: one could conceivably use amoxapine at bedtime for this patient to possibly treat depression, paranoia, and insomnia all at once; another TCA could be used to treat the depression and insomnia; and a low-potency antipsychotic could be used at bedtime to treat both mild paranoia and insomnia. All of these approaches are reasonable. However, in my view, SSRIs are preferable to TCAs and MAOIs, and risperidone or olanzapine is preferable to traditional antipsychotics. The various advantages are described in the respective chapters on individual medications in this text. Individual medications for insomnia treat the problem without major side effects, thereby increasing patient comfort and compliance. Although this patient is on four different medications, the dosages are low and carefully balanced to achieve an excellent response with no side effects. The dose of clonazepam can be slowly tapered off. If insomnia returns, trazodone can be increased to 100 mg HS. Most patients are eventually able to discontinue benzodiazepines. This patient will probably be kept on paroxetine 20 mg AM and risperidone 0.5 mg HS for one to two years before an attempt will be made to withdraw these medications.

Case #68

Presenting Symptoms: The patient was a 50-year-old male with complaints of panic attacks once a day, severe insomnia, racing thoughts, inability to function at work, extreme irritability, crying episodes, anger, manic episodes rapidly alternating with depressed mood, scattered thinking, and compulsive behavior. He denied suicidal or homicidal ideation, drug and alcohol abuse, smoking, and caffeine intake. He had three psychiatric hospitalizations with a diagnosis of manic-depression. He had tried numerous antidepressants, mood stabilizers, and antipsychotics in the past. His father had a diagnosis of manic depression. The patient's medical problems included borderline hypertension and dyspepsia for which he was not on any medications.

Current Diagnosis: Bipolar disorder, depressed, with rapid-cycling
panic disorder
Obsessive-compulsive features

Current Treatment:
1. paroxetine 20 mg HS
2. risperidone 0.5 mg HS
3. Depakote sprinkle capsule 250 mg BID and HS
4. trazodone 50 mg HS
5. lorazepam 1 mg HS
6. return in two months

Treatment Course: The patient was pressured by coworkers and his wife into coming to the office. He refused to be hospitalized or take one week off from work despite the presence of severe symptoms. He was extremely reluctant to take medications because of possible side effects. With considerable persuasion from everyone, he agreed to take the medications. He was started on Depakote sprinkle capsules 125 mg TID and 250 mg HS, ranitidine 150 mg BID, risperidone 0.5 mg HS, and lorazepam 1 mg HS. When seen a week later, he reported feeling better overall, but still complained of depressive symptoms, mood swings, and insomnia. The dose of Depakote sprinkle capsules was increased to 250 mg TID, paroxetine started at 20 mg AM, and trazodone started at 50 mg

HS. He was continued on risperidone 0.5 mg HS and lorazepam 1 mg HS. Significant improvement, with no major side effects, in all of the presenting symptoms was reported when the patient was seen after two weeks. This surprised the patient because previous episodes had been controlled only by fairly long hospitalizations. Since the patient reported yawning during the daytime, probably from paroxetine, he was instructed to switch paroxetine to bedtime. The valproic acid serum level was 38 ng/ml. Liver function tests and TSH were within normal limits.

Comments: This patient could be diagnosed with bipolar I disorder, mixed features, and the treatment would be identical. The Depakote sprinkle capsule was chosen because it is less irritating to the stomach, which is important in this patient because of a preexisting dyspepsia. Ranitidine 150 mg was given for several weeks for additional protection against gastric irritation. Other mood stabilizers, such as carbamazepine, lithium, verapamil, and clonazepam had been tried in the past with no effect on mood. Because of the antihypertensive and antimanic properties of calcium channel blockers, verapamil might have been a consideration. However, verapamil does not possess antimanic properties significant enough to impact on this patient. This patient had been tried on valproic acid in the past, which was discontinued because of nausea and heartburn. Although therapeutic serum level of valproic acid for the treatment of a seizure disorder is between 50 and 100 ng/ml, the patient responded well at a lower serum level and there was no reason to increase the dose. This reinforces the general principle that clinical response should be the primary criterion in determining dosage in psychiatric applications, as long as guidelines regarding blood levels and dosages are not exceeded. Paroxetine seems to have improved depressive, compulsive, and panic symptoms. Risperidone at low doses, along with Depakote, improved scattered thinking and racing thoughts. Trazodone and lorazepam effectively treated insomnia with no daytime sedation. The patient did not miss any time from work. He has reported that on his current medications he has felt the most "level" he has been in the last 20 years. The patient was referred to a psychotherapist, but he refused this, saying that he did not need it.

Bipolar disorders, especially with manic, hypomanic, or mixed episodes, are psychiatric emergencies because these patients can become irrational, impulsive, destructive, and labile without warning. Bipolar disorder with mixed or rapid-cycling features is considered a severe form of bipolar disorder. A combination regimen involving one or more mood stabilizers, an antidepressant, and an atypical antipsychotic may be necessary in some cases. Clozapine should be considered for severe treatment-resistant patients. Ideally, hospitalization is the best intervention. If this is not possible, the next best alternative is to initiate immediate treatment in the office, which was the only option in this case. A common dilemma that physicians encounter when dealing with severely symptomatic bipolar patients is whether or not to commit patients involuntarily if the patient refuses treatment. Manic behavior frequently results in considerable financial, occupational, and interpersonal consequences, which may not be sufficient to meet the criteria for involuntary commitment in most states. Yet, the patient's thinking and behavior are irrational. Being irrational or "crazy" is not a sufficient reason to force a patient to receive treatment. This can be frustrating to clinicians because they know that the patient and family members suffer when the patient refuses voluntary treatment, which is typical with manic episodes. Unfortunately, in most cases the legal requirements to fulfill the criteria for involuntary treatment will not be met until too much disruption and damage have taken place in patients' lives.

Case #69

Presenting Symptoms: The patient was a 60-year-old male. He was involuntarily brought by police and admitted to the inpatient psychiatric unit after he became assaultive toward his wife, destructive to property, hostile, and agitated. Several months prior to his psychiatric hospitalization, he suffered a cerebrovascular accident that damaged the speech center and caused expressive aphasia. Since the stroke, he had been exhibiting violent rages, paranoid ideation, crying episodes, and extreme mood swings. He also suffered from anorexia and insomnia. His wife reported that he had had an irritable and angry temperament for all of his adult years and that the stroke made his anger and moodiness even worse. However, rage attacks, assaultive behavior, and paranoia were never observed prior to his stroke. He had been in the habit of drinking two to three beers daily. Alcohol worsened the mood lability. He denied drug abuse. He smoked one pack of cigarettes daily, and drank one to two cups of regular coffee daily. The patient's medical history was unremarkable, except as described above. He denied previous psychiatric treatment and denied a family history of psychiatric disorders, except that the patient's father was described as "hot tempered."

Current Diagnosis: Personality change due to CVA, combined type
Other possible diagnoses:
Alcohol abuse
Dysthymia
Bipolar disorder, NOS

Current Treatment: 1. fluoxetine 60 mg AM
2. carbamazepine 200 mg TID
3. Triavil 4/10 HS (Triavil is a brand name for a fixed-ratio tablet containing perphenazine and amitriptyline.)

Treatment Course: The patient's agitation was controlled using haloperidol 5 mg IM and lorazepam 1 mg IM in the hospital. After the first dose of IM medication, he became cooperative and was started on fluoxetine 20 mg AM, carbamazepine 200 mg BID, lorazepam 0.5 mg TID, and Triavil 2/10 HS. The dose of fluoxetine was increased to 40 mg AM after seven days. The dose of carbamazepine was increased to 200 mg TID to achieve a therapeutic serum level. Lorazepam was tapered off prior to discharge. The patient was discharged after nine days and before optimal results were achieved because he refused to stay any longer. It was only with considerable persuasion and threats of separation by his wife that he stayed for the nine days. When seen in the office after three weeks, his wife reported continuing mood disturbance, although not as severe as prior to his hospitalization. The fluoxetine dose was increased to 60 mg in the morning. At the next follow-up appointment, his wife reported improvement in the patient's irritability and anger outbursts, but complained of suspiciousness. The dose of Triavil was increased to 4/10 at bedtime. A month later, the patient's symptoms had improved to the point that family members were able to tolerate him. He is now seen in the office every six months. According to his wife, he drinks one to two beers a day, despite the recommendation to abstain. Psychiatric treatment has also made it possible for him to cooperate with his speech therapist without becoming frustrated and hostile.

Comments: Prior to his stroke, this patient may have had dysthymia, cyclothymia, or a personality disorder, and probably mild alcohol abuse. His family barely tolerated his temperament. The CVA significantly worsened the existing symptoms to the point that he was out of control. The mechanism of exacerbation may be related to the disinhibitory effects of the stroke or to the extreme helplessness and frustration related to the motor sequelae of the stroke, or both. Regardless of the etiology, symptom control was necessary. From his wife's description of his premorbid personality, it is likely that he would have benefitted from an antidepressant even before the stroke, particularly one of the SSRIs. Paranoia was a feature that appeared to have emerged after the stroke. Assaultiveness and rage attacks may be considered a quantitatively more severe form of hostility, anger outbursts, and irritability, which were preexisting features. The patient's wife had considered divorce many years earlier because of difficulty coping with his temper but continued in the marriage for the sake of their children. There were four overlapping symptoms that were thought to respond optimally to four separate medications in this patient.

Main Target Symptoms	Medication
Mood–anger, irritability, crying	fluoxetine
Extreme mood swings	carbamazepine
Paranoia, assaultiveness	perphenazine
Anorexia, insomnia	amitriptyline

Some of the medications have overlapping effects on symptoms. It would have been ideal to have been able to place this patient on systematic and sequential medication trials in the safe setting of a hospital. Given the increasingly constraining limitations of hospitalization and length of treatment, such an approach is no longer realistic. Third-party payers do not approve lengthy hospital stays, and patients may not be able to afford long hospitalizations. The longer the hospitalization, the more the patients' lives are disrupted. It is common knowledge that antidepressants take from 7 to 21 days for optimal effect. In most cases, the number of days in the hospital is not sufficient for making a definitive determination as to whether or not the antidepressant is truly effective at the starting dose. Out of practical necessity, the clinician has to make a judgment and provide a treatment that will control symptoms rapidly. Although all physicians make judgments, the task is more subjective in the specialty of psychiatry, hence more dependent on the particular psychiatric clinician's understanding of the patient's problems. This is in significant contrast to most other medical specialties, where radiographs and laboratory tests such as blood tests, and cultures provide more objective and definitive information, enabling the physician to institute specific treatment with a very high degree of confidence and prognostic certainty. The use of combinations of medications is necessary for rapid symptom control. It is my view that the judicious use of combinations, based on an understanding of which medications improve which target symptoms, improves treatment outcome and maximizes the patient's overall functioning, without making the patient overmedicated or "drugged up." It is possible, but unlikely, that the patient could have done as well on a single medication. When I suggested to the family that we taper off one or more medications sequentially to see if fewer medications would sustain the improvement, the family ardently requested that we not change what was "working." Amitriptyline is probably not necessary at this point. Perphenazine could also be discontinued or the dose decreased without adverse consequence. Fluoxetine is the primary medication required in this patient at this time, with carbamazepine helping adjunctively. If an antipsychotic is needed, risperidone, which was not available at the time the patient was hospitalized, would have been the first-line antipsychotic. Olanzapine, a recently introduced antipsychotic, would also be an excellent choice. Any of the SSRIs would have done an equally good job; I happened to choose fluoxetine. Paroxetine, nefazodone, mirtazapine, venlafaxine, and fluvoxamine were not available at the time. Similarly, valproic acid would have been a reasonable choice. The important concept is that medications from different classes were chosen to address different target symptoms. The specific medication under each class is not as important. The dosages should also reflect the purpose. For example, amitriptyline at low doses can provide appetite stimulation, improved sleep, and mild anticholinergic effects (which are beneficial to patients on high-potency antipsychotics) but is without antidepressant effects. At high doses, amitriptyline acts as an antidepressant with perhaps excessive side effects. Both the choice of medication and the dosage are important for achieving the right "balance," whereby all the symptoms are under satisfactory control without side effects.

Case #70

Presenting Symptoms: The patient was a 59-year-old male admitted involuntarily to the psychiatric unit after he voiced homicidal threats. Symptoms consisted of paranoid delusions, extreme agitation, hostility, insomnia, labile affect, and uncooperativeness. He had a history of seizure disorder for which he underwent a left temporal lobectomy in the late 1950s, resulting in better seizure control. He had been noncompliant with haloperidol, which he has taken intermittently for many years. It is not certain what precipitated the recent relapse. Possible reasons include noncompliance with haloperidol or breakthrough partial complex (temporal lobe) seizure. He has excellent seizure control on primidone (Mysoline) 750 mg per day and phenytoin (Dilantin) 400 mg per day. To the best of my knowledge, he had been compliant with his antiseizure medications. Anticonvulsant levels were therapeutic at the time of admission. He denied any recent history of drug and alcohol abuse, smoking, and caffeine intake. Reportedly, he has an irritable temperament. He has a mild right hemiparesis secondary to craniotomy. He was alert and oriented. The patient's family history was positive for seizure disorder, but not for psychiatric disorders.

Current Diagnosis: Psychotic disorder due to a brain lesion and seizure disorder, (previously known as organic psychosis)

Current Treatment: 1. risperidone 2 mg HS
2. paroxetine 20 mg HS
3. lorazepam 1 mg HS

Treatment Course: Several doses of haloperidol 5 mg IM and lorazepam 1 mg IM given concurrently in the hospital improved the patient's agitation and made him sufficiently cooperative so that he accepted medications orally. During the first three days of his hospital stay, he refused to be examined by the neurologist and internist who were consulted for management of his nonpsychiatric medical problem. His anti-seizure medications were not changed. He was started on risperidone 0.5 mg QID, paroxetine 20 mg AM, and lorazepam 1 mg HS. After three days, he became much more cooperative and less hostile. The CT scan showed changes consistent with left temporal lobectomy. The EEG showed left anterior temporal slowing with rare sharp activity. All other labs, including chemistries, thyroid, B12 and folate levels and erythrocyte sedimentation rate were within normal limits. His psychosis and temperament improved significantly, and he was discharged after about seven days of inpatient treatment.

Comments: This patient's psychiatric symptoms appeared after the craniotomy, but it is unclear as to how many years later. Temporal lobe epilepsy, also known as complex partial seizure, is sometimes associated with psychosis. Unless there is a clear temporal association, it is difficult to determine whether or not the psychosis is primary or secondary. This distinction is clinically important, because if medical causes of psychosis can be identified and corrected, resolution of the psychosis is expected. Steroid-induced psychosis or mania and psychosis due to anticholinergic toxicity are examples. Since the patient's seizures were fairly well controlled on phenytoin and primidone for many years, it was decided not to switch the patient to carbamazepine or valproic acid, both of which could have "psychiatric" benefits in addition to seizure treatment.

Acute psychosis, characterized by agitation, homicidal thoughts, and delusions, is an emergency and should be treated rapidly using antipsychotics, regardless of the cause. The combination of haloperidol and lorazepam IM, as used in this case, is an effective combination to rapidly decrease agitation. It can be given every hour as needed. In most cases, one to two doses are sufficient. The causative factor, such as a medical condition or drug intoxication, should be managed concurrently, until the psychotic symptoms subside. Some medical conditions, such as a seizure disorder, are chronic. Appropriate treatment of the seizure may not control the psychosis, which then is seen as a separate disorder requiring long-term treatment, as in this case. Risperidone at a fairly low dose was effective in controlling the psychosis.

SSRIs are excellent for improving irritability, anger, and moodiness even if it is part of one's characteristic temperament. Paroxetine was successfully used in this case to control the irritable temperament, which may have been exacerbated by the brain lesion. Other SSRIs could have been chosen. SSRIs and MAOIs tend not to lower seizure threshold as much as TCAs and bupropion, which would be relatively contraindicated in this patient.

The elderly and patients with brain lesions are highly sensitive to antipsychotics. Therefore, the starting dose should be low, with slower and smaller dosage increments. Once symptom control is achieved, the dose of the antipsychotic can be gradually decreased to a maintenance level, which usually is about 50 to 75 percent of the dose that was needed to control the acute symptoms. Use of low doses of adjunctive benzodiazepines enable the patient to maintain control on lower doses of antipsychotics.

Case #71

Presenting Symptoms: The patient was a 30-year-old female with complaints of depressed mood, insomnia, anorexia, paranoid ideation, ideas of reference, anergia, and anhedonia. She denied suicidal ideation. She also denied drug and alcohol abuse, smoking, and caffeine intake. The symptoms were precipitated by the loss of her job. The patient had no history of psychiatric treatments and no family history of psychiatric disorders. She had no medical problems.

Current Diagnosis: Schizophrenia, chronic paranoid type
Diagnosis at the time of the initial evaluation: Major depression with mild psychotic features

Current Treatment:
1. clozapine 100 mg TID and 300 mg HS
2. clonazepam 0.25 mg HS
3. Part-time volunteer work
4. Return in three months

Treatment Course: The patient was first treated with nortriptyline 100 mg HS, haloperidol 5 mg HS, and benztropine 1 mg BID, with satisfactory improvement. Several months later, the patient became suicidal and acutely agitated, and was hospitalized. The dose of haloperidol was increased to 5 mg BID and she was discharged after a week of hospital treatment. She took an overdose while visiting relatives in another state and was subsequently hospitalized for ten days. No medication changes were made. About three months later, she had yet another exacerbation, necessitating hospitalization. During this hospitalization, medications were changed to thiothixene 5 mg AM and 10 mg HS, lithobid 300 mg TID, fluoxetine 20 mg AM, and lorazepam 1 mg HS. She was discharged after about ten days. During the third hospitalization, she revealed that she had been experiencing auditory hallucinations and paranoid delusions. Between the second and the third hospitalizations, various medications including clomipramine, fluphenazine, and imipramine were tried with no significant advantage. There was no evidence of noncompliance. Signs of tardive dyskinesia became visible about six months after the third hospitalization. The patient was still complaining of psychotic symptoms but reported that they were at a tolerable level. At this time, the patient was hospitalized to initiate clozapine, which controlled her psychosis at a total daily dose of 600 mg. Divalproex sodium (Depakote) 250 mg TID was started for seizure prophylaxis. Depakote was tapered off after a year. Clonazepam 0.25 mg was given for insomnia. After switching to clozapine, signs of tardive dyskinesia completely disappeared. The patient has remained free of psychotic and depressive symptoms since clozapine was started three years ago. She is now seen once every three months. Leukocytosis with a WBC in the range of 15,000 to 19,000/mcl, normal neutrophil fraction, and high neutrophilia have persisted since starting clozapine. Hematology and infectious disease consultations were obtained to rule out hematological or infectious disorders. Her CBC is monitored weekly as per clozapine protocol.

Comments: This patient initially presented with primarily depressive symptoms precipitated by the loss of her job. The depressive symptoms were moderate in severity and the psychotic symptoms were mild. The patient had no obvious delusions or hallucinations. Based on these, the initial diagnosis could very well have been adjustment disorder with depressed mood. The mild ideas of reference could be considered an understandable reaction to the stress of losing her job. As the illness evolved, more severe psychotic symptoms consisting of well-formed ideas of reference, paranoid persecutory delusions, and hallucinations emerged to the extent that the intensity of psychotic symptoms were in excess of her depressive symptoms. Another explanation is that this patient had been psychotic all along, but the symptoms were not identified either because the patient was very guarded or because the clinician did not recognize the symptoms. My view is that the stress of losing her job lead to the manifestation of prodromal psychotic symptoms along with predominant depressive symptoms. Psychotic patients or patients who have latent psychosis frequently present with depression or anxiety. In fact, as noted in other sections of this book, most patients' presenting complaints include depression, anxiety, insomnia, hypersomnia, and anorexia, regardless of the definitive ultimate diagnosis. Psychiatric diagnosis is frequently an evolving process. For example, what was diagnosed as a major depression or generalized anxiety disorder could turn out to be bipolar disorder or one of the psychotic disorders, although the reverse is less likely. Since normalcy and psychosis are on a continuum, there can be quantitative differences in the degree of psychosis, with some patients having mild psychotic symptoms and others with severe symptoms. Mild psychotic symptoms can be prodromal presentations of more malignant but latent psychopathology. Regardless of the eventual significance, clinical prudence dictates that even mild psychotic symptoms should be identified and treated. Since symptoms can evolve or change over time, the clinician should be vigilant so that appropriate treatment revisions are instituted. In hindsight, the most effective medication for this patient would have been clozapine at the initial presentation if it were known that the patient would have a deteriorating course with increasing severity of psychosis. It should be noted that, although the manufacturer's recommendation is that clozapine should be used only for treatment of refractory schizophrenia, my view is that if clinical evaluation suggests that the psychotic disorder is likely to be chronic, there is no clinical reason to put the patient through less effective treatment when clozapine is available, as long as other clozapine treatment and monitoring protocols are followed. In this patient's case, three hospitalizations, several suicide attempts, considerable personal anguish for the patient and her family, and approximately two years of distress were endured before the patient was started on clozapine, which was available when the patient was first seen by me. To complicate matters, the managed care company reviewers felt that the patient was an "acting-out borderline" and initially refused to cover her second hospitalization after a suicide attempt with a drug overdose. Unfortunately, "borderline" has become a psychiatric "four-letter word." This issue is discussed in detail in my companion book *Personality Disorders: New Symptom-Focused Drug Therapy* (The Haworth Press, 1997).

This patient fit the criteria for various diagnoses such as major depression with psychotic features; Bipolar disorder, depressed; schizoaffective disorder, depressed; paranoid schizophrenia; and paranoid disorder. The prominence of florid paranoid symptoms during the year immediately prior to her starting clozapine, lack of adequate response to the antidepressant, significant functional deterioration, and complete resolution of symptoms on clozapine alone (for three years so far) suggest a diagnosis of paranoid schizophrenia. However, as is common with complex psychiatric disorders, if this patient presents with predominant depressive symptoms in the future, which is possible, the diagnosis could change to schizoaffective disorder, depressed. An antidepressant may possibly be added to her drug regimen.

Treatment with clozapine has restored the patient's functional skills at least partially, whereas prior to clozapine treatment, she was living a dysfunctional and unproductive life plagued by various symptoms. Since her WBC is now chronically elevated, it is necessary to rely on other indicators to evaluate the presence of infection or other conditions in which the WBC is one of the useful markers. The patient and the family have to be made aware of this and of the need to contact her primary care physician should symptoms or signs of infection occur.

The dose of clozapine will be gradually decreased to 300 to 400 mg per day if symptoms do not reemerge. Because of the setback to the patient's life should a relapse occur, I do not have the courage to recommend that this patient discontinue clozapine, despite patient inquiries regarding this issue. My rationale is that since the patient has a chronic illness, the treatment is also expected to be chronic, similar to the length of treatment for essential hypertension or diabetes. Attempts to maintain her on 300 mg per day will be made cautiously while her mental status is more frequently monitored. However, completely tapering off of the medication is very risky for a patient with a chronic diagnosis.

Case #72

Presenting Symptoms: The patient was a 40-year-old female. She was first seen in the hospital, where she was admitted involuntarily, status post suicide attempt by an overdose of carbamazepine that had been prescribed by her previous psychiatrist for bipolar disorder. The symptoms were suicidal ideation, depressed mood, irritability, anger outbursts, moodiness, frequent panic attacks, crying episodes, anorexia, anhedonia, and extreme emotional sensitivity. The suicide attempt was precipitated by marital conflicts. She denied drug and alcohol abuse. She smoked one-half pack of cigarettes per day and drank one to two cups of coffee per day. She had had a previous psychiatric hospitalization for suicidal ideation two months prior to this hospitalization, at which time she was diagnosed with bipolar disorder, started on carbamazepine, and followed as an outpatient. She denied a family history of psychiatric disorders. Her medical history was significant for dyspepsia and migraine headaches.

Current Diagnosis: Major depression, severe, recurrent
Panic disorder
Dysthymia
Histrionic features

Current Treatment: 1. paroxetine 30 mg AM and at noon
2. zolpidem 10 mg HS PRN insomnia
3. nortriptyline 25 mg HS

Treatment Course: The patient was discharged in improved condition on paroxetine 20 mg AM, doxepin 10 mg HS, risperidone 0.5 mg HS, and ranitidine 150 mg HS. Since she was still depressed, paroxetine was increased to 30 mg AM. Dizziness prompted discontinuation of doxepin. Instead, nortriptyline 10 mg was started to stimulate her appetite and assist weight gain as the patient weighed only 102 pounds, for a height of 5 feet 4 inches. She continued complaining of depressive symptoms; hence, the dose of paroxetine was increased to 30 mg AM and 15 mg at noon. Since she did not have any side effects and continued to have some depressive symptoms, the dose was again increased to a final dose of 30 mg BID. An increase of nortriptyline to 25 mg improved the appetite to the patient's satisfaction, without dizziness. Zolpidem 10 mg was prescribed PRN for insomnia. Risperidone was discontinued after four weeks. The depressive symptoms, panic attacks, insomnia, and anorexia resolved almost completely on the current medication on which the patient has now been maintained for about four months. The patient reported that she now feels more emotionally stable than she has in the last ten years, an observation supported by her husband.

Comments: When patients present with considerable emotional turmoil manifested by severe anxiety, depression, moodiness, and histrionic tendencies, it is tempting to give a diagnosis of cyclothymia or bipolar disorder. Some patients volunteer that they have "extreme mood swings." The exact nature of the mood swings should be understood, specifically: Do the mood swings consist of clear manic or hypomanic episodes? What is the duration? What were the behaviors or thoughts during those episodes?, etc. In many cases, what patients describe as mood swings are changes from an irritable or depressed mood to feeling normally happy or euthymic. If the patient had had the chance to be treated by her previous psychiatrist during her second hospitalization when she overdosed, this would probably have been recognized and medication changed to include an antidepressant. Any acute presentation can involve diagnostic uncertainty; I, as a physician, am not immune to such diagnostic perplexity. In many situations, psychiatric diagnosis and treatment are evolving processes, with changes in diagnosis and treatment made as the patient is better understood. The ideal goal, obviously, is to make the correct diagnosis and to choose all of the right medications the first time.

The effective use of a TCA for appetite stimulation is again illustrated. Although the maximum recommended dose of paroxetine is 50 mg per day, some patients tolerate and need higher doses, as in this case. Similarly, the relative safety of SSRIs afford the physician the option of increasing the dose above the recommended range if the individual clinical situation dictates it. Recently, the drug manufacturer raised the maximum dose of paroxetine to 60 mg per day.

Panic disorders respond well to antidepressants, especially to SSRIs. In this patient, severe depression and frequent panic attacks were controlled on paroxetine. Other SSRIs could have been equally effective. Adjunctive PRN use of benzodiazepines is beneficial, although in this case it was not necessary.

This patient probably had histrionic personality features. The author believes that at least the emotional reactivity and lability associated with a histrionic personality disorder could respond to SSRIs, as it probably did in this case. Medication treatment is logical when personality disorder characteristics are understood in terms of treatable symptoms. Such an approach and specific treatment guidelines are described in my companion book *Personality Disorders: New Symptom-Focused Drug Therapy* (The Haworth Press, 1997).

Case #73

Presenting Symptoms: The patient was a 40-year-old female with complaints of chronically depressed mood, anxiety, insomnia, racing thoughts, episodes of confusion and thought disorganization, memory loss for discrete periods of time, irritability, impulsivity, panic attacks, a history of several suicidal attempts by cutting her wrist, feelings of hopelessness, compulsive counting, an obsessive preoccupation with self-mutilation, episodes of vague auditory hallucinations, extreme mood swings, a history of prescription benzodiazepine abuse, and anhedonia. She denied any recent drug and alcohol abuse. She smoked one-half pack of cigarettes per day. She denied caffeine intake.

Her past psychiatric history was significant for approximately ten psychiatric hospitalizations. She had been tried on nearly all antipsychotics, antidepressants, benzodiazepines, lithium, carbamazepine, and valproic acid.

Previous psychiatric diagnoses by different psychiatrists were as follows:

- Borderline personality disorder
- Multiple personality disorder
- Bipolar disorder
- Temporal lobe epilepsy
- Cyclothymia

- Schizoaffective disorder
- Acute psychotic episode
- Schizophrenia, chronic undifferentiated type
- Major depression, severe, with psychotic features
- Adjustment disorder with depressed mood
- Panic disorder
- Personality disorder, NOS

She had a history of being severely physically and emotionally abused as a child. She was a college graduate and had a teacher's certificate. She lived in a halfway house at the time of the initial evaluation.

The patient's father had been diagnosed with depression. Her medical history is significant for reflux esophagitis and migraine headaches. Hyperventilation EEG showed intermittent activity from frontal regions, suggesting a suspicion of a partial complex seizure disorder. She was given carbamazepine for three months in 1989, but had stopped because of an exacerbation of her headaches. Valproic acid was tried in 1993, and was discontinued due to abdominal pain, nausea, and vomiting. She did not feel that either carbamazepine or valproic acid was of any help. Nonpsychiatric medications included omeprazole 20 mg AM, metoclopramide 5 mg QID, conjugated estrogen 1.25 mg days 1 to 25, and medroxyprogesterone 10 mg days 16 to 25.

Current Diagnosis: Schizoaffective disorder, depressed
Obsessive-compulsive disorder
Personality disorder, NOS
Borderline personality disorder
Consider multiple personality disorder

Current Treatment:
1. clomipramine 75 mg HS
2. chlorpromazine 25 mg QID
3. risperidone 2 mg HS
4. benztropine 0.5 mg BID
5. temazepam 15 mg HS
6. trazodone 100 mg HS
7. weekly psychotherapy by a psychologist

Treatment Course: Various medications, including carbamazepine, valproic acid, and all available SSRIs were tried under my care, with no success. Propranolol LA 80 mg was tried intermittently to treat migraine headaches and akathisia. Buspirone was started adjunctively, but was not helpful. Urecholine 25 mg had to be occasionally used for urinary hesitation caused by the anticholinergic effects of the medications. Chlorpromazine and risperidone were tried alone and in various dosage combinations until the most effective doses were found. She has been able to stay out of the hospital now for one and one-half years, which is the longest hospitalization-free interval since her psychiatric illness began in her late twenties. She is seen in the office once every four months. She sees a psychologist once every week.

Comments: Complicated, chronic, and severely ill patients with mood symptoms typically have multiple psychiatric diagnoses. A patient's major problem can be described in one or two words using a standardized diagnosis. As emphasized in this text, the clinician needs to focus on the specific symptoms of the individual patient, in order to choose medications and other treatments. This principle is even more true when dealing with patients having complex psychiatric problems. Diagnoses, including the various personality disorders, have to be translated and understood in terms of component symptoms for effective treatment to begin. All of the diagnoses for this patient, given by other psychiatrists, are probably justified at the time they were made. By the same token, another psychiatrist could justifiably arrive at a diagnosis different from my current diagnosis. Such diagnostic variability is common when dealing with patients as complex as this one.

Borderline personality disorder is often used as a derogatory and hostile term for patients who are not responding to treatment and who have difficult temperaments. Many patients with manic, hypomanic, psychotic, and depressive characteristics are agitated, hostile, needy, angry, impulsive, intrusive, labile, ambivalent, self-destructive, impatient, hyperactive, manipulative, defiant, threatening, and accusatory during the acute phases of their illness and when their symptoms are not properly controlled. These symptoms can be easily interpreted as indicative of a personality disorder, usually that of a borderline personality disorder. There are many instances that I can remember when successful medication treatment of the patient completely resolved the so-called "personality disorder." It is important to resist the tendency to label any difficult or complex patient with a diagnosis of personality disorder. This tendency is often seen in the nursing staff in an inpatient setting, probably a result of their frustration with having to deal with these patients around the clock, day in and day out.

For purposes of pharmacological treatment, dissociative symptoms probably should be considered a form of a mini-psychotic episode, and as such can effectively be treated using low doses of antipsychotic medication. Fortunately, the psychopharmacologist only has to deal with one body, regardless of the number of personalities, all of which are affected by the same medication. However, for the psychotherapist, the number and prominence of various personalities are important considerations while conducting therapy. Symptoms, if they are dysfunctional and treatable, should be treated irrespective of which personality manifested the symptoms. Careful and thorough evaluation of patients diagnosed as suffering from multiple personality disorder will usually reveal varying numbers of symptoms from the mood and psychotic spectrum of disorders.

The need for a combination of two or more antipsychotics on a fairly long-term schedule is extremely rare. In the acute treatment period, it is fairly common to use two antipsychotics. For example, when switching from a traditional antipsychotic to clozapine or risperidone, the old antipsychotic is tapered off while the dose of the new antipsychotic is increased gradually. Another example is that of the patient who becomes acutely agitated while being introduced to an antipsychotic which does not have a parenteral form. In the latter case, another antipsychotic that is available in parenteral form is used on a PRN basis. Another situation occurs when a patient responds exceptionally well to a low-potency antipsychotic in some respects, such as control of agitation or insomnia, but cannot tolerate a higher dose to control delusions or hallucinations. Another antipsychotic, usually a high-potency antipsychotic that is better tolerated and effective for the latter symptoms would be appropriate to add. There are other rare clinical situations when a combination of two antipsychotics is reasonable. I can remember only one other case among more than 800 patients on antipsychotics who needed two antipsychotics for optimal maintenance treatment, except for combinations involving clozapine and risperidone.

It is usually unnecessary to give anticholinergic medication while the patient is on low-potency antipsychotic or sedating TCAs, which have inherent anticholinergic effects. There is a risk of anticholinergic excess, leading to central anticholinergic syndrome when one or more highly anticholinergic medications are used, particularly when high doses are used in elderly patients. However, there are some patients who benefit from additional anticholinergic medication, despite being on low-potency antipsychotics.

If this patient has another relapse necessitating hospitalization, consideration will be given to a trial of clozapine, which, if effective, can probably supplant the need for all of her current psychotropic medications.*

---

*Subsequent to the preparation of the final pages of this book, the patient suffered another relapse and had to be hospitalized. She is now functioning well on just two medications, clozapine 200 mg HS and fluoxetine 40 mg AM.

Case #74

Presenting Symptoms: The patient was a 55-year-old female with complaints of depressed mood, frequent crying episodes, feelings of hopelessness, suicidal ideation, middle insomnia and early morning awakening, auditory hallucinations with persecutory content, irritability, anhedonia, and a history of several suicide attempts by overdose. She admitted to drinking three to four beers and two to three glasses of wine daily for the past several months. She denied drug abuse and smoking. She drank two to three cups of regular coffee daily. The patient had had four previous psychiatric hospitalizations. She had a course of electroconvulsive therapy during one of those admissions. Various antipsychotics, including haloperidol and fluphenazine, were tried in the past. At the time of her first visit, she was on nortriptyline 50 mg HS, buspirone 10 mg BID, and temazepam 30 mg HS. She denied a family history of psychiatric disorders. This patient's medical history was significant for insulin-dependent diabetes mellitus, and hyperlipidemia for which she was taking insulin and lovastatin (Mevacor).

Current Diagnosis: Schizoaffective disorder, depressed
Alcohol dependence (resolved)

Diagnosis at First Visit (1993): Major depression with psychotic features

Current Treatment:
1. venlafaxine 75 mg TID
2. risperidone 2 mg BID
3. temazepam 30 mg HS
4. referred for psychotherapy

Treatment Course: The patient was hospitalized voluntarily from the office. She was medicated with chlordiazepoxide 75 mg the first day, 50 mg the second day, and 25 mg the third day for alcohol detoxification. She was discharged after a ten-day stay on the following medications: perphenazine 12 mg HS, paroxetine 20 mg AM, propranolol 10 mg TID (for akathisia), and trazodone 50 mg HS. After a month, she stopped the medications against medical advice because she felt that she was doing well on temazepam 30 mg HS and lorazepam 0.5 mg BID, which she was taking from a supply she had at home. Since she reported behavior suggestive of hypomanic episodes, she was tried on lithium, and then on carbamazepine, both unsuccessfully. She was also started on clomipramine, trifluoperazine, and chlorpromazine at various times with some improvement. In March of 1994, she had to be hospitalized when she presented with auditory hallucinations, ideas of reference, paranoia, and suicidal ideation. She was successfully treated with risperidone 3 mg BID, clomipramine 50 mg HS, and lorazepam 0.5 mg HS. Because of significant weight gain, clomipramine was discontinued, and the patient was instead started on venlafaxine 25 mg TID, which was eventually increased to 75 mg TID. After discontinuation of clomipramine, she reported muscle rigidity for which benztropine 1 mg TID was effective. This was tapered off after two months without recurrence of muscle rigidity. She was placed back on temazepam 30 mg because she felt that lorazepam was less effective. The dose of risperidone was decreased to 2 mg BID after about four months. She still experiences occasional auditory hallucinations for which she is instructed to take an extra tablet of risperidone PRN.

Comments: The patient was initially thought to have a major depression with psychotic features, but more information about the patient's symptoms, gained over a one-year period, revealed that the patient probably had periods during which psychotic symptoms were predominant compared to depressive symptoms. The diagnosis, therefore, was changed to schizoaffective disorder, depressed, although this change had no practical bearing on treatment. Hypomanic symptoms were transient and could have been due to the disinhibiting effects of benzodiazepines or from the abrupt stopping of antipsychotics. For a while, her episodic shopping binges had a compulsive quality for which clomipramine was tried but was not unequivocally effective. Neither this behavior nor alcohol abuse have recurred to date. Although medication response or nonresponse is neither necessary nor sufficient for diagnostic confirmation, such information is one piece of data among many to help clarify a diagnosis. In this particular case, a lack of response to adequate trials on lithium and carbamazepine makes it less likely that the patient has bipolar characteristics.

Frequently, the need for separate antiparkinsonian, anticholinergic, or dopaminergic medications can be avoided if a patient on high-potency antipsychotic medication is also on TCAs, which have varying degrees of anticholinergic effects. For instance, this patient developed pseudoparkinsonian symptoms while on risperidone after clomipramine was withdrawn, necessitating temporary addition of benztropine. On the other hand, additive anticholinergic effects from different medications can lead to anticholinergic toxicity. In many patients, anticholinergic medications can be slowly tapered off after two to three months.

If breakthrough psychotic symptoms occur infrequently and are recognized as such by the patient, an extra dose of antipsychotic on a PRN basis usually controls these symptoms. In addition, such a strategy gives the patient a greater sense of control and responsibility and rewards the "observing ego."

If this patient experiences a relapse of the depression and/or psychosis in the future, consideration will be given to a trial on clozapine, which has the potential to eliminate the need for antidepressants and temazepam, especially if depressive symptoms are secondary to psychosis. It is very difficult to determine whether or not depression is primary or secondary when both depression and psychosis coexist. Clozapine can also effectively treat "negative" symptoms, many of which overlap with depressive symptoms.

Case #75

Presenting Symptoms: The patient was a 35-year-old male with complaints of severe chronic anxiety, panic attacks at a frequency of three to four per week, depressed mood, irritability, anger outbursts, anergia, middle insomnia, history of compulsive checking behavior, anorexia, crying, feelings of hopelessness, episodic auditory hallucinations, difficulty focusing thoughts, and anhedonia. He admitted consuming seven to eight drinks of vodka daily for six months. He smoked two and one-half packs of cigarettes per day. He denied caffeine intake. He also denied suicidal or homicidal ideation. His symptoms emerged six months ago, precipitated by marital conflicts. He denied a previous psychiatric history. The patient's mother was doing well on fluoxetine for depression. His medical history is significant for borderline hypertension for which he is not on any medications.

Current Diagnosis: Major depression with possible mild psychotic features
Generalized anxiety disorder
Panic disorder without agoraphobia
Marital problems
Alcohol dependence (resolved)

Current Treatment:
1. fluoxetine 40 mg AM
2. alprazolam 0.5 mg PRN (the patient takes three alprazolam a week on average)
3. referred for psychotherapy
4. referral to Alcoholics Anonymous

Treatment Course: The patient was prescribed chlordiazepoxide 10 mg pills with instruction to take 50 mg the first night, 40 mg the second night, 30 mg the third night, 20 mg the fourth night, and 10 mg the fifth night, along with a high potency multivitamin, to safely withdraw from alcohol. His liver function tests are normal. Concurrently, he was started on fluoxetine 20 mg AM and risperidone 0.5 mg at HS. Depressive and anxiety symptoms were moderately improved after four weeks. Symptoms improved to a satisfactory level after fluoxetine was increased to 40 mg AM. Risperidone was discontinued after two months. The patient has been able to abstain from alcohol for one year so far. He is seen in the office once every three to four months.

Comments: Reliable and compliant patients without major medical problems who have a mild to moderate alcohol dependence are good candidates for outpatient detoxification when done under close outpatient supervision. These patients are encouraged to call the physician in between office visits for a telephone check regarding withdrawal symptoms and vital signs, which the patients can monitor themselves. Of course, reliable and compliant alcoholics are not very common. Fortunately, this outpatient detoxification was successful. As a minimum, liver function tests and CBC are recommended prior to initiating outpatient alcohol detoxification.

Many severely depressed patients have psychotic symptoms that are usually mild (and transient when treated). Psychotic symptoms, even if mild, should not be ignored, because the combination of depression and psychotic symptoms has the potential to be very dangerous. Once the depression has lifted, the antipsychotic can be withdrawn, usually in three to four weeks. In most cases, low doses of the antipsychotic drug are sufficient. However, it is critical for the physician to be alert to recognizing the presence of psychotic symptoms.

It is typical to choose the same medication for a patient if a close relative did well on that medication for similar indications. Just as some disorders tend to run in families, medication responses also tend to run in families. However, the recent availability of several new antidepressants with more favorable side effect profiles compared to TCAs and MAOIs have altered this practice to some extent. For example, the fact that a close relative did well on phenelzine or doxepin six years ago when SSRIs were not available would not be sufficient reason to start the patient on one of those medications without giving the patient the benefit of a trial on one of the newer antidepressants, such as SSRIs or bupropion. If however, a TCA or MAOI has to be chosen, then it is desirable to choose the particular TCA or MAOI with which the relative was treated.

Case #76

Presenting Symptoms: The patient was a 37-year-old male with a history of bipolar disorder for which he was stabilized on lithium (Lithobid) 300 mg BID, hydroxyzine (Vistaril) 25 mg TID, amitriptyline 10 mg HS, and thiothixene 2 mg TID at the time he was first seen. During manic episodes, he had racing thoughts, grandiose delusions, pressured speech, extreme hostility, labile affect, insomnia, and hyperactivity, accompanied by alcohol abuse. He had had several previous psychiatric hospitalizations. His brother was on lithium for bipolar disorder. The patient smoked one pack of cigarettes per day, and drank two to three cups of coffee daily. He denied any medical problems.

Current Diagnosis: Bipolar disorder, manic
Alcohol abuse

Current Treatment:
1. lithium carbonate 600 mg BID
2. risperidone 3 mg HS
3. clonazepam 0.25 mg AM and 0.5 mg HS
4. paroxetine 20 mg AM
5. propranolol 20 mg AM
6. gabapentin 300 mg TID
7. referred for psychotherapy and Alcoholics Anonymous

Treatment Course: The patient was kept on the same combination of medications that he had been on when first seen. After three months, he stopped the medications and started drinking, resulting in a relapse necessitating an involuntary hospitalization. He was discharged on divalproex sodium 250 mg TID, bupropion 100 mg BID, lithium carbonate 300 mg TID, and thiothixene 5 mg HS. He did well on this combination for about ten months, when he had another relapse after decreasing medications on his own. Again, he was involuntarily committed by the police to the psychiatric unit where he was treated for 16 days. He was discharged on risperidone 2 mg TID, lithium carbonate 600 mg AM and 900 mg HS, and clonazepam 1 mg HS. He was also tried on carbamazepine, which had to be discontinued due to a skin rash. His lithium level on the above dose was 0.8 mEq/L. A greater lithium dosage to obtain a higher plasma level caused typical lithium side effects, which were intolerable. He eventually refused to take divalproex sodium and instead was placed on gabapentin, which he has been taking faithfully. He has been able to avoid inpatient hospitalization and to hold part-time jobs for the last two years.

Comments: Bipolar disorder patients present with varying levels of severity. Some patients can be maintained on mood stabilizers alone, either on a single mood stabilizer or a combination. Most patients with bipolar disorder need a combination of one or more mood stabilizers as the primary medication and low doses of antipsychotics as well as antidepressants. Acutely manic and agitated patients are initially managed in the same manner as acutely psychotic patients. Severely manic patients are typically admitted involuntarily and managed in the inpatient unit. Detailed guidelines in managing manic patients are given in Chapter 9. Any severe mental illness requiring hospitalization or intensive outpatient treatment interferes with occupational functioning and can cause significant disability. This patient was terminated from a job that he had held for about five years, despite supportive letters and telephone assurances given to his employer by the author in an effort to save his job. His wife nearly divorced him. There were disastrous financial consequences. Eventually, he became dependent on Social Security Disability income. Given the major psychological, occupational, and social losses associated with each episode, and the general tendency for each subsequent episode to be more severe than the previous one, patients who have bipolar disorder must be considered for long-term maintenance on medications. The clinical significance of manic episodes in psychiatry may be compared to the significance of an uncontrolled seizure disorder in neurology or unstable angina in cardiology, except that with bipolar disorder, the benefit of objective diagnostic tests is not available, making medication prophylaxis even more important.

Most patients and their significant others can be educated to recognize worsening of their symptoms and to adjust their medication temporarily to control breakthrough symptoms. Since mood stabilizers have a latency period after initiation or dosage adjustment, other fast-acting medications such as benzodiazepines and antipsychotics are more suitable for this purpose. A useful analogy to which patients can relate is to compare the functions of different medications to that of cruise control and the brakes in a car. A mood stabilizer functions like cruise control in keeping the car going at an even speed, whereas antipsychotics and benzodiazepines act like a brake that is applied intermittently to slow the car down when the "speed" is excessive. Such analogies serve to educate patients and prompt their interest and curiosity. Furthermore, patients feel that they have control over their illnesses, which makes them more responsible for their own well-being. Obviously such analogies are best described to patients during the maintenance period, when patients are in emotional and behavioral control.

The majority of patients suffering from bipolar disorder tend to abuse alcohol and/or illicit drugs. The presenting complaint might be substance abuse. Concurrent treatment of substance abuse and the underlying psychiatric disorder is crucial in stabilizing the patient. The prevalence of substance abuse among patients with psychiatric disorders is so high that the clinician is prudent to search for occult substance abuse problems in every patient who presents with psychiatric complaints.

Case #77

Presenting Symptoms: The patient was a 36-year-old female who presented with symptoms such as depressed mood, severe anxiety, various obsessive preoccupations, initial and middle insomnia, social withdrawal, anhedonia, rapid mood swings consisting of dysphoria and hyperthymia, frequent suicidal ideation, paranoid ideation, episodic auditory hallucinations with a persecutory content, and ideas of reference. These symptoms at varying severity had been present for at least ten years. She was taking risperidone 3 mg BID, sertraline 50 mg AM, and lorazepam 0.5 mg TID, prescribed by her inpatient psychiatrist during her recent psychiatric hospitalization. Although her symptoms improved on the medications, she was still symptomatic. She was previously tried on various traditional antipsychotics and antidepressants with unsatisfactory results. She had had two previous psychiatric hospitalizations. She denied drug and alcohol abuse except binge drinking during brief manic episodes. She denied smoking and caffeine intake. She has been unable to hold a job despite having several years of college education. The patient's aunt suffered from schizophrenia. She denied any major medical problems.

Current Diagnosis: Schizoaffective disorder, bipolar type (with obsessive features)
Alcohol abuse (associated with manic episodes)

Current Treatment:
1. olanzapine 10 mg HS
2. lamotrigine 50 mg HS
3. clomipramine 50 mg HS
4. lorazepam 0.5 mg BID PRN for anxiety
5. continue psychotherapy by the referring psychologist

Treatment Course: Since the patient remained symptomatic while taking the medications she was prescribed at the time of discharge from her most recent hospitalization, it was decided to change her medications. Risperidone was tapered off over a period of four days. She was simultaneously started on olanzapine 5 mg HS on the first two days and then increased to 10 mg HS. Sertraline was discontinued and she was given clomipramine 50 mg HS. In addition, she was placed on lamotrigine initially at 25 mg HS and eventually at 50 mg HS. She was instructed to change the lorazepam schedule to 0.5 mg BID PRN for anxiety. The medication changes were made on the same day that she was seen in my office. She has reported a dramatic improvement in all of her symptoms. Although it is too early to conclude that these medications will maintain the remarkable improvement, I feel that, given the superior response to these medications, she is likely to be significantly more functional than she had been with other medication regimens in the past.

Comments: The patient did not respond satisfactorily to various traditional antipsychotics as well as risperidone. Although risperidone is considered an excellent medication for the treatment of psychotic symptoms, it is not effective in some patients. Olanzapine is another SDA antipsychotic recently introduced in the United States. It appears that olanzapine was uniquely effective for this patient's symptoms. She presented with other disparate symptoms that were not expected to respond to olanzapine and required adjunctive medications as listed below.

Target Symptoms Cluster	Medication Class	Medication
psychotic symptoms	antipsychotic	olanzapine
mood swings	mood stabilizer	lamotrigine
obsessive features	antiobsessional	clomipramine
dysphoria	antidepressant	clomipramine
anxiety	anxiolytic	lorazepam (PRN)
insomnia	hypnotic	lorazepam (PRN)

Clomipramine has antiobsessional, antidepressant and anxiolytic properties, all of which were of benefit to this patient. Although the dose of clomipramine may appear subtherapeutic at 50 mg HS, there is no compelling clinical reason to increase the dose because the patient has reported nearly complete resolution of these symptoms. In addition to its primary antipsychotic effects, olanzapine has antianxiety effects. Perhaps olanzapine alone might have improved all the symptoms the patient had. A sequential medication trial could have clarified this possibility. However, my clinical experience indicates that different medications are frequently necessary for optimal resolution of distinct symptom clusters. Olanzapine is tolerated well by most patients. Olanzapine seems to have slightly better anxiolytic effects (probably due to decreased incidence and severity of akathisia) compared to risperidone although both are excellent as first-line antipsychotic medications. The patient reported that she is now able to benefit more from psychotherapy due to her improved ability to think rationally and be in control of her emotions. Refer to Chapter 11 for a detailed clinical profile of olanzapine.

Case #78

Presenting Symptoms: The patient was a 52-year-old male with complaints of alcohol dependence consisting of a habit of drinking 18 beers daily for several years, withdrawal symptoms, severely depressed mood, crying episodes, irritability, feelings of hopelessness, and suicidal ideation. The patient had been abusing alprazolam by taking more than the prescribed doses. He denied other drug abuse and caffeine intake. He smoked two packs of cigarettes daily. The patient was started on alprazolam 0.5 mg TID for anxiety several months ago by his family physician. He denied any other psychiatric history. This patient had been taking captopril for hypertension.

Current Diagnosis: Alcohol dependence (in remission)
Major depression, severe

Current Treatment:
1. paroxetine 30 mg AM
2. risperidone 1 mg HS
3. doxepin 10 mg HS
4. trazodone 50 mg HS
5. naltrexone 50 mg HS
6. referral to Alcoholics Anonymous and counseling

Treatment Course: Alcohol withdrawal was treated using tapering doses of chlordiazepoxide. He received routine medications for patients with a history of alcohol abuse such as thiamine, folic acid, and multivitamins during the first week of hospitalization. He was not given any medications at the time of discharge. When seen in the office two weeks after discharge, he complained of depressive symptoms, severe insomnia, anorexia, and a mild craving for alcohol. Thus, he was started on sertraline 50 mg AM, trazodone 50 mg HS, and doxepin 10 mg HS. He did well for about six months; then, depressive symptoms reemerged. The dose of sertraline was increased to 100 mg AM. There was no improvement after three weeks; hence, the dose of sertraline was increased to 100 mg AM and noon. Since the patient also reported mild paranoid ideation, he was started on risperidone 1 mg HS while continuing on doxepin, naltrexone, and trazodone. Naltrexone was started in early 1995 when it was approved for use in alcoholics. The patient's depressive and paranoid symptoms improved significantly. He is currently maintained on these medications, has been abstinent for one year so far, and has been compliant with participation in Alcoholics Anonymous.

Comments: Sedatives with long half-lives are typically used for treatment of alcohol withdrawal. My medications of choice for this purpose are phenobarbital, chlordiazepoxide, and diazepam. All of these medications can be given orally, intramuscularly, or intravenously. If a patient has hepatic dysfunction, one third of the usual dose of the above medications can be given. Another option in patients with hepatic dysfunction is to use benzodiazepines, such as lorazepam and oxazepam which have no active metabolites. The approximate dose can be calculated from the amount of alcohol consumed daily. One beer, one glass of wine, or one ounce of hard liquor is considered one drink. The formula for calculating the approximate dose follows. Dosing must be individualized because there is considerable variation in drug tolerance among individuals.

Using Table 17.1, it can be calculated that a patient in the habit of drinking ten drinks will need an initial dose of 150 mg of phenobarbital, 80 mg of chlordiazepoxide, 50 mg of diazepam, 6 mg of lorazepam, and 150 mg of oxazepam. Of these medications, lorazepam and oxazepam must be in divided doses, although it is preferred that all of them be given in divided doses. The long half-life medications may be completely tapered off in three to five days, whereas lorazepam and oxazepam may be gradually tapered off over five to seven days. Half of the dose should be used if given parenterally. In general, medication should be administered by IM or IV route only if the patient cannot tolerate medications orally. Manufacturers' guidelines may be consulted for precise dosing and rate of administration, since they vary for different medications. If patients need extra doses for control of breakthrough withdrawal symptoms, additional doses can be given on a PRN basis during the tapering period. Patients who consume three or fewer drinks daily may not experience significant withdrawal symptoms and hence may not need pharmacological intervention for treating alcohol withdrawal symptoms.

TABLE 17.1. Alcohol Withdrawal: Approximate Initial Dose of Sedatives Based on Number of Drinks

Medication*	Route	Oral Dose per Drink**
phenobarbital	PO, IM, IV	15 mg
chlordiazepoxide	PO, IM, IV	8 mg
diazepam	PO, IM, IV	5 mg
lorazepam	PO, IM, IV	0.5 mg to 0.75 mg (in divided doses)
oxazepam	PO	15 mg (in divided doses)

Notes: *Refer to Chapter 8 for a detailed discussion of administration instructions.
**Dose should be reduced by half and be given in three to four divided doses if IM or IV route is employed.

Most alcoholics and drug abusers have underlying psychiatric symptoms that can be discovered under careful scrutiny. Unfortunately, many substance abuse treatment programs have a fairly concrete and extreme approach that devalues the usefulness of medications. Some programs equate all psychotropic medications to "drugs." The inadvertent effect of such an attitude is that patients become conflicted regarding the use of beneficial medications, and eventually are at a greater risk of relapse because of suboptimal outcome related to unresolved underlying symptoms.

It is important to avoid medications having addictive, dependence, or abuse potential in patients who have a history of substance abuse. Fortunately, SSRIs, various TCAs, diphenhydramine, hydroxyzine, buspirone, trazodone, and nefazodone are available for effective treatment of anxiety and insomnia, which are particularly common among drug and alcohol abusers.

Case #79

Presenting Symptoms: The patient was a 49-year-old female with complaints of depressed mood, scattered thinking, difficulty organizing thoughts, anxiety, crying episodes, mild paranoia, apathy, social withdrawal, forgetfulness, feelings of hopelessness, anhedonia, and poor work performance. These symptoms were intensified by conflicts with her supervisor at work. She denied drug and alcohol abuse and caffeine intake. She smoked one-half pack of cigarettes daily. She was seen by a psychiatrist one time four years ago, and was diagnosed as dysthymic. No medication treatment was recommended at that time. Her son has a diagnosis of paranoid schizophrenia. She denied any major medical problems.

Current Diagnosis: Major depression, moderate, with mild psychotic features
Dysthymia
Consider simple schizophrenia (not a current *DSM-IV* diagnosis)

Current Treatment:
1. fluoxetine 40 mg AM
2. trazodone 50 mg HS
3. risperidone 0.5 mg HS
4. referral for psychotherapy

Treatment Course: Various other diagnoses, such as attention deficit disorder, generalized anxiety disorder, and presenile dementia were considered during the course of treatment. The patient was tried at various times on bupropion and stimulants with no effect. She experienced increased agitation when risperidone was increased; yet, when risperidone was discontinued, symptoms such as scattered thinking and poor concentration returned. The current combination of drugs has improved her symptoms about 40 percent, according to the patient's estimate. However, she has not improved to the point that she is capable of functioning at work.

Comments: There are many patients in whom psychotic symptoms are not prominent, yet extremely dysfunctional symptoms such as apathy, scattered thinking, poor concentration, mild suspiciousness, excessive interpersonal sensitivity, mild ideas of reference, frequent errors at work due to apparent cognitive dysfunction, dysphoria and lack of drive make them unable to function in the workplace. They are able to function at home and to lead simple lives, as long as they are not stressed by the demands of work or other social responsibilities. Such nonflorid symptoms initially present diagnostic uncertainty because various easily treatable diagnoses that can present with similar symptoms must be ruled out, such as adult attention deficit disorder, depression, and anxiety disorders. Since treatment of each of these disorders must be tried sequentially and may need trials on various medications prior to moving on to consider another diagnostic possibility, considerable time is required to obtain a better diagnostic understanding. For example, in the case of depression, a medication ideally must be tried at the maximum tolerable dose within the approved dosage range with an estimated two- to three-week wait after dosage initiation and after each dosage increment in order to conclude that the medication is ineffective. With so many distinct classes of antidepressants, even if the physician tries the patient on only one medication from each class, five to six medication trials are necessary. In most cases, a trial of more than one medication from the same class may be required to conclude that the patient is not responsive to antidepressants. Within the SSRI category, it is frequently observed that patients who do not respond at all to one SSRI, respond to another. Adding the time it takes to try the various augmenters, it is obvious that the time period to conclude that a particular patient is treatment-resistant can well exceed one year. In most cases of chronic mild depressive symptoms associated with a mild thought disorder and mild cognitive dysfunction, electroconvulsive therapy is not effective. A low dose of clozapine is theoretically appealing, but hard to justify given the absence of prominent positive symptoms.

This patient has been out of work now for ten months. Long-term disability is anticipated. It took considerable explanation to convince the disability insurance carrier that the work dysfunction is real. Since there are no florid symptoms, and since the patient is fairly functional at home, it is understandably difficult for those who are not experts in the field to realize that nonflorid symptoms can also cause severe dysfunction.

Chronic treatment-resistant depression is one of the most disabling conditions. With treatment, some improvement is to be expected, but complete resolution of symptoms is rare. A small number of patients will remain dysfunctional and depressed all of their lives. Treatment will prevent further deterioration and severe complications, such as suicide or inability to care for one's self. It is possible that some of the treatment-resistant chronic depressions represent negative symptoms of schizophrenia, which is resistant to treatment with antidepressants, whereas a medication such as clozapine, olanzapine, and risperidone which have comparatively superior effects on negative symptoms, could improve these symptoms.

Case #80

Presenting Symptoms: The patient was a 59-year-old female with complaints of severely depressed mood, suicidal thoughts, frequent crying, a history of a suicidal attempt 15 years ago by an overdose of amitriptyline, early morning awakening, obsessive rumination, psychomotor agitation, feelings of guilt, anhedonia, and melancholia. She denied any acute precipitants. She denied drug and alcohol abuse and smoking. The patient had had several previous psychiatric hospitalizations for severe depression. She was on bupropion, perphenazine, lorazepam, and trihexyphenidyl at the time of admission. She had tried various medications in the past, including fluoxetine, lithium, various tricyclics, and antipsychotics. Two of her sisters had been diagnosed with depression and another with bipolar disorder. A brother suffered from obsessive-compulsive disorder. Medical history is significant for hypertension, for which she had been taking guanfacine (Tenex).

Current Diagnosis: Major depression, severe, recurrent, melancholic type

Current Treatment:
1. Status post nine ECT treatments
2. venlafaxine 75 mg BID
3. hydroxyzine 25 mg HS
4. referral for psychotherapy

Treatment Course: Brief trials of clomipramine, venlafaxine, imipramine, and paroxetine at various times in conjunction with lithium and risperidone, were ineffective in the hospital. Hence, the patient was given nine ECT treatments, which resulted in remarkable improvement. She was discharged on venlafaxine 37.5 mg po BID and hydroxyzine 25 mg HS. During the course of outpatient treatment, the dose of venlafaxine was gradually increased to 75 mg po BID to treat mild worsening of depressive symptoms. She has been doing well for the last year.

Comments: For reasons unknown to date, some patients with severe depression respond dramatically to ECT, whereas others do not respond satisfactorily. Those who respond still need to be on a maintenance antidepressant to sustain the improvement, unless periodic maintenance ECT is instituted. Although the idea of outpatient maintenance ECT is theoretically appealing, it has very limited application in practice for a number of reasons. Patients dislike it. The logistics involved in administering ECT on an outpatient basis can at times be unwieldy. It has been observed on several occasions that an antidepressant that was ineffective for the patient prior to ECT seemed to work better after ECT, as seemed to be the case with this patient. Whether this is a true medication maintenance effect or continued response to ECT for this patient can only be answered in time. However, it is a fairly common observation that most patients who are not treated with antidepressants after ECT will have a relapse in 6 to 12 months.

The advent of new antidepressants has given more medication options to the physician. Appropriate use of augmenters along with the use of new antipsychotics such as risperidone and clozapine has dramatically increased the chances of successfully treating complicated and severe depressions using combinations of medications, when managed appropriately. Hence, the use of ECT is expected to be less frequent, even in severe depressions. The psychiatrist must be aggressive in using the newer medications in a combination format in most cases in order to enable the patient to benefit from the advantages offered by them. Various medication strategies of a complex nature are described in Chapter 2. Also, review Chapter 6 for clinical and practical aspects of ECT.

Case #81

Presenting Symptoms: The patient was a 40-year-old female with complaints of racing thoughts, pressured speech, irritability, mood swings, episodes of depressed mood, anger attacks, violent episodes, hypomanic episodes, hyperphagia, anxiety, insomnia, and a past history of alcohol and cocaine abuse, which reportedly ended three years ago. She had a history of several suicidal gestures and attempts by overdose and self-mutilation. She denied current drug and alcohol abuse and smoking. She drank one to two cups of coffee daily. The patient had had two psychiatric hospitalizations previously, the last hospitalization being three years ago. She was on clonazepam 0.5 mg QID, carbamazepine 400 mg po BID, and sertraline 50 mg AM when seen at my office. The patient reported that her father had fits of anger. Her medical history is significant for motor vehicle accidents in 1987 and 1989 in which she had a closed head injury resulting in concussion. Most of her psychiatric problems apparently predated her head injury.

Current Diagnosis: Bipolar disorder, NOS
Consider mood disorder due to head injury
Borderline personality disorder

Current Treatment:
1. divalproex sodium 250 mg BID
2. Eskalith CR 450 mg HS
3. clonazepam 0.5 mg TID
4. risperidone 1 mg HS
5. trazodone 200 mg HS
6. referral for psychotherapy

Treatment Course: Since the patient was still symptomatic on the medications she was taking at the time of her first visit to my office, medications were changed to divalproex sodium, lithium, and trazodone while maintaining the patient on clonazepam 0.5 mg QID. Her lithium level on the above dose was found to be 0.4 mEq/L, and valproic acid level was 32 ng/ml. Mood swings, racing thoughts, and pressured speech have been well controlled on divalproex sodium and lithium. During the course of treatment, it was discovered that she had had paranoid ideation for many years. Risperidone 0.5 mg improved the paranoia somewhat but an increase to 1 mg almost completely treated the paranoia. The patient has been functioning well on the present combination of medications for more than a year.

Comments: One of the goals of pharmacologic treatment is to use the lowest dose of medication that will control discrete symptoms. One of the advantages of combination treatment is that low doses of multiple drugs control a variety of symptoms with minimal side effects. Another goal of treatment is to use the least number of medications to treat the symptoms. However, in treating disparate symptoms, different medications are both desirable and necessary. The dosages of divalproex sodium and lithium are kept low as indicated by low serum levels. Clinical response is much more important than rigid adherence to obtaining predetermined target serum levels in most cases. Generally, in maintenance treatment, low dosages can be used successfully, thereby minimizing side effects. Most patients with a chronic bipolar disorder require lithium and/or valproic acid, carbamazepine, gabapentin, or lamotrigine for effective control of mood swings. Since there is an overlap between symptoms of bipolar disorder and borderline personality disorder, mood stabilizers can be used for the treatment of borderline personality disorder with predominant mood symptoms. This patient is currently on the greatest number of medications that she has ever been at one time, but she is also the most functional and the most stable that she has ever been in her adult life. Balanced, disciplined, rational, and symptom-focused combination treatment is not only safe and effective, but also enables patients to function at their highest potential.

Case #82

Presenting Symptoms: The patient was a 30-year-old female with complaints of depressed mood, chronic feeling of emptiness, anger attacks, extreme mood swings, irritability, insomnia, feelings of hopelessness, excessive dependency on her boyfriend and her mother, scattered thinking, crying episodes, impulsivity, frequent suicidal ideation without intent or plan, episodes of hypomania, and anhedonia. She had a history of several suicidal gestures by cutting her wrists. The patient reported that she had been moody and depressed since age 15. Recent stressors include conflicts with her family and her boyfriend. She had a past history of alcohol dependence, but denied any current drug or alcohol abuse. She smoked one pack of cigarettes per day. She denied caffeine intake. The patient was on alprazolam 0.5 mg TID when first seen in my office. She had had one hospitalization at which time she was started on lithium, which she discontinued soon after discharge. Her mother and sister have a history of depression.

Current Diagnosis: Bipolar disorder, NOS
Consider cyclothymia
Borderline personality disorder with histrionic and dependent features

Current Treatment:
1. Eskalith CR 225 mg AM and 450 mg HS
2. sertraline 50 mg AM
3. trazodone 50 mg HS
4. risperidone 1 mg HS
5. propranolol long-acting 60 mg AM
6. levothyroxine 0.075 mg AM
7. referral for psychotherapy

Treatment Course: The patient was started on Eskalith CR 450 mg BID, fluoxetine 20 mg AM, and trazodone 50 mg HS, while alprazolam was gradually tapered off over a period of three weeks. The patient complained of restlessness and agitation after about ten days of starting fluoxetine, which was then discontinued. She was switched to sertraline, which was well tolerated. The patient revealed that she has had thoughts of harming people and extreme hostility toward people. She also had attacked her boyfriend on several occasions and had episodes of depersonalization. She was tried on carbamazepine, which was not effective. Perphenazine 4 mg HS controlled the above symptoms effectively. When risperidone became available, she was switched to risperidone 2 mg HS, which was eventually decreased to her current dose of 1 mg HS. Lithium caused hypothyroidism, which was treated using levothyroxine 0.075 mg AM. She complained of fine tremors of her fingers, thought to be induced by lithium. Propranolol improved the tremors. TSH has been within normal limits at 1.91 mciu/ml. The patient is seen once every four months for medication management.

Comments: It is difficult to sort out the precise diagnosis among mild forms of bipolar disorder, cyclothymia, and personality disorder with borderline, narcissistic, and histrionic features. Fortunately for the practicing physician, the precise diagnosis is not as important as eliciting or identifying symptoms that help to choose the effective medications. For this particular patient, the author is still not certain of the diagnosis, despite treating the patient for more than three years. Regardless of the true diagnosis, it is clear that the current medications are extremely effective, as evidenced by the patient's emotional stability, which, according to her, is currently at its best in the last 10 to 15 years.

Case #83

Presenting Symptoms: The patient was a 15-year-old female with complaints of behavior problems, distractibility, restlessness, extreme mood swings, promiscuity, running away, alcohol and drug abuse, impulsivity, anger outbursts, racing thoughts, depressed mood, insomnia, disorganized thoughts, anorexia, anhedonia, a history of suicidal gestures, and suicidal ideation without intent or plan. She denied any acute precipitants. She smoked one-half pack of cigarettes per day. Prior to being seen at my office, this patient was tried on fluoxetine, hydroxyzine, sertraline, risperidone, stimulants, desipramine, trazodone, divalproex sodium, various antipsychotics, lithium, and carbamazepine. She had had several psychiatric hospitalizations and had been expelled from school for behavior problems. The patient's mother had severe mental illness; the patient was being raised by her grandmother. Her aunt has a diagnosis of schizophrenia. The patient denied any major medical problems.

Current Diagnosis: Bipolar disorder, NOS
Conduct disorder
Polysubstance abuse
Consider attention deficit disorder
Consider schizoaffective disorder, bipolar type
Borderline personality disorder

Current Treatment:
1. Depakote sprinkle capsule 250 mg BID and 500 mg HS
2. fluoxetine 20 mg AM
3. Triavil 2/25 HS
4. clonidine 0.1 mg BID
5. ranitidine 150 mg HS
6. referral for psychotherapy

Treatment Course: Various medications, including methylphenidate, bupropion, paroxetine, and imipramine were ineffective. The addition of Triavil and clonidine significantly improved restlessness, distractibility and impulsivity. Ranitidine was added to control treatment-emergent dyspepsia. The patient has shown marked improvement compared to her baseline, but is still emotionally fragile. If this combination is not effective in the future, a trial on clozapine will be considered.

Comments: Without aggressive outpatient medication management, this patient's behavior and emotional functioning would be likely to deteriorate to the point of needing long-term hospitalization.

Behavioral symptoms in an adolescent are likely to be attributed to conduct disorder or a personality disorder. However, symptoms of bipolar disorder in an adolescent are not well formed or "mature." Therefore, typical symptoms of mania or depression seen in adults are not always applicable to adolescents. Psychiatric manifestations of mood disorders in adolescents consist of behavioral symptoms for the most part. Aggressive outpatient medication treatment should be pursued for adolescents presenting with what appears to be conduct disorders, personality disorders, or other behavioral problems. Inpatient hospitalization can be prevented or the frequency reduced when symptom-focused medication treatment is provided, just as in adults.

The addition of clonidine significantly improved concentration, distractibility, and restlessness in this patient, whereas stimulants and bupropion were not effective. Even for a complex, seemingly treatment-resistant case, diligent efforts by the physician in trying different medications and combinations, as well as cooperation by the patient, will result in the eventual identification of medications that are helpful to the patient.

Case #84

Presenting Symptoms: The patient was a 40-year-old female with complaints of multiple obsessive and compulsive symptoms and depressed mood, which were satisfactorily treated on sertraline 100 mg QID (total 400 mg daily), lithium carbonate 300 mg TID, trazodone 50 mg HS, and diazepam 5 mg HS. The patient was stabilized on these medications by her psychiatrist. She recently moved from another state and wanted to continue these medications. Her medical history was unremarkable. Her previous psychiatrist had tried her on other medications, including fluoxetine and clomipramine, without success. Lower doses of sertraline were not effective. The patient denied drug and alcohol abuse, smoking, and caffeine intake. The patient's mother had compulsive symptoms (cleaning rituals) according to the patient, but had not been treated.

Current Diagnosis: Obsessive-compulsive disorder (severe)

Current Treatment:
1. Continue sertraline 100 mg QID.
2. Continue lithium 300 mg TID.
3. Continue diazepam 5 mg HS.
4. Continue trazodone 50 mg HS.
5. referral for psychotherapy

Treatment Course: Since this patient has been doing well on the above medications, she is maintained on them.

Comments: Patients with OCD tend to need antiobsessional medication at the higher end of the dosage range. This particular patient is on double the maximum recommended dose of 200 mg of sertraline, yet is reporting no side effects. In fact, she has shown an excellent response to the high dose of sertraline. Laboratory studies including liver function tests were normal. The considerable safety margin of SSRIs enables trial on higher than the recommended doses for treatment-resistant cases, whereas with non-SSRI antidepressants, one has to be much more cautious.

Even if a meaningful plasma level of sertraline is available, a plasma level is not necessary in this case because the patient is tolerating the medication well with excellent results.

Lithium, trazodone, and benzodiazepines are employed in this case as adjunctive medications. The patient's lithium level was 0.7 mEq/L.

There is no severity level classification for OCD, according to *DSM-IV*. However, clinical experience shows that OCD can occur in quite a range of severity levels. I have found it helpful to use specifiers, such as mild, moderate, and severe to describe and to convey the severity level more accurately.

Case #85

Presenting Symptoms: The patient was a 58-year-old male with complaints of anxiety, vague fears, insomnia, anxiety attacks, excessive meticulousness and punctuality, excessive worrying, obsessive preoccupation with a fear of dying, depressed mood, and compulsive arranging. He reported that the obsessive-compulsive tendencies had been present for more than 30 years. He was previously tried on doxepin, clomipramine, and alprazolam, which were not quite effective. He denied drug and alcohol abuse and smoking. He drank one cup of coffee daily. The patient denied a family history of psychiatric disorders. He also denied any major medical problems.

Current Diagnosis: Generalized anxiety disorder
Consider panic disorder
Obsessive-compulsive personality disorder

Current Treatment:
1. paroxetine 45 mg AM
2. clonazepam 0.25 mg BID
3. Triavil 2/10 HS
4. referral for psychotherapy

Treatment Course: Other medications tried at various times in my office were buspirone, fluoxetine, diazepam, risperidone, venlafaxine, amitriptyline, and fluvoxamine. None of these were fully effective. Eventually, the patient responded well to the present combination of medications, which he has been taking for the last six months.

Comments: The doses of clonazepam and Triavil are extremely low; yet, the addition of these medications to the primary medication (paroxetine) had a noticeably beneficial effect and resulted in overall improvement. Antipsychotics are generally not indicated for anxiety disorders or for nonpsychotic symptoms. However, there are some patients whose anxiety symptoms respond nicely to low doses of antipsychotics, but not to benzodiazepines, for unknown reasons. A possibility exists that these patients could have a mild alteration in the balance of the dopamine neurotransmitter system, which manifests clinically as anxiety rather than psychosis. Generally, very low doses of antipsychotics can be tried in these patients as a last resort, after trying various antidepressants, antianxiety medications, and buspirone. If a patient is to be maintained on the antipsychotic for more than three to four months, it is important to inform the patient of the risk of tardive dyskinesia. In the case of elderly patients, tardive dyskinesia can be a risk after one to two months if the dose of the antipsychotic is fairly high. Risperidone, olanzapine, and sertindole probably have a low risk of causing tardive dyskinesia compared to traditional antipsychotics. Clozapine is not known to cause tardive dyskinesia.

Case #86

Presenting Symptoms: The patient was a 27-year-old female with complaints of paranoia, racing thoughts, pressured speech, hostility when frustrated, reckless spending, labile affect, ideas of reference, and insomnia. She denied suicidal or homicidal ideation. The patient suffered marked deterioration in personal and occupational functioning over the last seven years, despite having a college degree. History from family members revealed that the patient had always been somewhat suspicious, secretive, emotionally sensitive, and distrustful. She had been noncompliant with taking antipsychotics and lithium, which were prescribed by other psychiatrists in the past. She denied drug and alcohol abuse and caffeine intake. She smoked one pack of cigarettes per day. The patient's uncle had several "nervous breakdowns."

Current Diagnosis: Schizoaffective disorder, bipolar type
Consider bipolar disorder
Consider schizophrenia, paranoid type
Paranoid personality disorder
Consider delusional disorder, persecutory type

Current Treatment:
1. recommendation of voluntary hospitalization at the first visit, refused
2. risperidone and lithium prescribed as an outpatient treatment option; the patient never returned after the first visit

Treatment Course: The patient's family brought the patient to the office, requesting that she be hospitalized. Since she refused voluntary hospitalization and since she did not meet the clinical criteria for involuntary hospitalization at the time, she was offered outpatient treatment. The patient's family members, which included a physician, were upset that the author did not initiate involuntary commitment. The patient failed to show up for her next appointment.

Comments: Mental health professionals occasionally encounter cases like this. The patient is chronically and severely mentally ill and absolutely needs intensive inpatient treatment. This patient probably would have done well on clozapine or risperidone, along with a mood stabilizer. The family's frustration and reaction are entirely justified and understandable; yet all patients, including severely and chronically ill, have the right to refuse treatment. All states provide for evaluating and treating a psychiatric patient involuntarily under certain strict conditions, which vary from state to state. However, most states allow involuntary commitment and treatment only if one of the following criteria is met:

1. The patient has threatened to harm himself or herself, others, or property, due to mental illness.
2. The patient has attempted to or did harm himself or herself, others, or property, due to mental illness.
3. The patient has been or will be imminently incapable of caring for himself or herself, risking serious harm to himself or herself, due to mental illness.

Most states do not allow for involuntary commitment even if extreme and overwhelming negative consequences have occurred or are imminently likely to occur due to mental illness. Examples include giving away one's belongings and money in a manic state, or resigning from a stable job based on paranoid beliefs, or other extremely irrational acts.

In the absence of meeting such strict criteria, as required by individual states, the physician has no legal basis to commit a patient involuntarily, even if the physician feels that the patient needs inpatient treatment and the family demands it. The presence of severe mental illness alone is not sufficient for initiating involuntary commitment. Similarly, harming oneself or others is not sufficient to commit someone involuntarily to a psychiatric facility. For instance, a terminal patient expected to live for several months would not be psychiatrically hospitalized involuntarily in the absence of severe depression or psychosis, despite suicidal ideation or attempts. Also, people who assault others or commit murder are usually placed in jail rather than committed to a psychiatric hospital.

The clinician's duty is to apply clinical criteria and clinical judgment in individual cases to decide whether or not the patient meets the particular state's legal guidelines for involuntary commitment. Determination at a later time as to whether or not the patient met the legal criteria for involuntary commitment is the responsibility of the court system.

Although the physician's ultimate goal of making people well is noble, the means to achieving the goal must follow the state's legal guidelines, taking into consideration the patient's right to refuse psychiatric evaluation and/or treatment, even if such refusal is based on irrational beliefs and lack of insight and not in the best interest of the patient.

There is no question that this patient will suffer further deterioration and possible serious adverse consequences in the future, and, therefore, is expected to meet clinical criteria for involuntary commitment at a later date. However, most states require the risk of imminent and serious consequences to justify commitment.

Case #87

Presenting Symptoms: The patient was a 77-year-old female with complaints of pressured speech, insomnia, confusion, flight of ideation, racing thoughts, paranoia, anxiety, agitation, and labile affect. The patient was hospitalized for this condition. She had a long history of bipolar disorder, for which she had been taking lithium and thioridazine. She had had several hospitalizations in the past. She denied drug and alcohol abuse, smoking, and caffeine intake. The patient's medical history was positive for transient ischemic attacks, arthritis, cataracts, and headache. EKG showed first degree AV (atrioventricular) block.

Current Diagnosis: Bipolar disorder, manic

Current Treatment:
1. divalproex sodium 250 mg BID
2. risperidone 0.5 mg HS
3. lorazepam 0.5 mg HS PRN for insomnia

Treatment Course: Because of the patient's EKG abnormalities and diminished responsiveness to lithium, she was switched to divalproex sodium 250 mg BID while in the hospital. Thioridazine was discontinued in favor of risperidone 1 mg BID. She was also given lorazepam 0.5 mg AM and HS while in the hospital. Her condition improved significantly within a week of these medication changes. She was discharged after about eight days of hospitalization and continued to improve as an outpatient. The dose of risperidone was gradually decreased to the current dose of 0.5 mg HS. Lorazepam 0.5 mg is taken only PRN. The patient's son reported that her current functioning on these medications is the best it has been in ten years. An attempt will be made to discontinue risperidone at the next visit and to keep the patient only on divalproex sodium.

Comments: Some patients fail to respond to lithium after doing well on it for many years for unknown reasons. In these patients, the addition of, or switch to, carbamazepine, gabapentin, lamotrigine, or valproic acid is usually effective. Lithium is best avoided in elderly patients with cardiac problems. Thioridazine can also lead to EKG abnormalities and should be cautiously used in the elderly. Fortunately, this patient's mania responded well to the combination of divalproex sodium, risperidone, and lorazepam with no significant side effects. Her liver function tests have been normal.

Case #88

Presenting Symptoms: The patient was a 63-year-old female who presented with symptoms such as depressed mood, anxiety, anhedonia, middle insomnia, frequent crying episodes, feelings of hopelessness, frequent suicidal ideation without intent or plan, irritability, agitation, and constant anger. She reported that she has had a depressive tendency all of her life. She had one psychiatric hospitalization two years earlier with a diagnosis of major depression, severe. She had tried fluoxetine, sertraline, and nefazodone prior to seeing me. She denied drug and alcohol abuse, smoking, and caffeine intake. The patient's son had bipolar disorder. Her father had depression and attempted to commit suicide. The patient's medical history was positive for gastroesophageal reflux, hypertension, arthritis, and asthma for which she had been taking omeprazole, cisapride, conjugated estrogen, nabumetone, hydrochlorothiazide, and diltiazem, and using an albuterol inhaler.

Current Diagnosis: Major depression, severe, recurrent with probable psychotic features
Dysthymia

Current Treatment:
1. olanzapine 10 mg HS
2. fluoxetine 40 mg AM
3. temazepam 15 mg HS
4. trazodone 50 mg HS
5. referral for psychotherapy

Treatment Course: The diagnoses when this patient was first seen in my office were major depression, severe, recurrent, and dysthymia. During the course of treatment, the primary diagnosis was changed to that of major depression, severe, recurrent, with probable psychotic features. Other medications tried in my office were paroxetine, venlafaxine, clomipramine, bupropion, mirtazapine, dextroamphetamine, and a low dose of risperidone. None of these were effective. Prior to her psychiatric hospitalization under my care, she experienced a severe exacerbation with symptoms such as extreme hopelessness, increased agitation, suicidal ideation with a plan of overdosing on multiple medications, and increased anger. She was immediately referred to consult a psychiatrist who provides ECT for consideration for urgent hospitalization for ECT, which the patient was willing to try. However, the consulting psychiatrist could not schedule the patient for several weeks. Meanwhile, the patient became more acutely suicidal and was seen in the emergency room which again failed to get her into the ECT program despite the author's efforts. She was subsequently hospitalized under my care and out of desperation was placed on clozapine, which significantly improved the anger, agitation, suicidal ideation, and hopelessness. The addition of fluoxetine resolved her depressed mood. She was discharged from the hospital after five days on clozapine 100 mg HS, fluoxetine 40 mg AM, and temazepam 15 mg HS. Although there was remarkable improvement in all of the severe symptoms, the patient complained of apathy and anergia despite trials on methylphenidate and bupropion adjunctively. When olanzapine became available, she was switched to olanzapine on an outpatient basis according to the following crossover schedule.

	Clozapine	Olanzapine
Day 1	75 mg HS	5 mg HS
Day 2	50 mg HS	10 mg HS
Day 3	50 mg HS	10 mg HS
Day 4	25 mg HS	10 mg HS
Day 5	25 mg HS	10 mg HS
Day 6	12.5 mg HS	10 mg HS
Day 7	12.5 mg HS	10 mg HS
Day 8	discontinue	continue 10 mg HS

The patient tolerated the crossover to olanzapine well and reported improvement in symptoms matching that obtained with clozapine, but without the anergia and apathy. The patient's energy level and affect were visibly improved. She was maintained on fluoxetine 40 mg AM. Trazodone 50 mg HS satisfactorily treated insomnia, which worsened after clozapine was discontinued. The current regimen of medication has been maintained for two months without any loss of efficacy.

Comments: This patient did not manifest any of the typical psychotic symptoms that would have prompted the choice of an antipsychotic as the primary medication early in the course of treatment. The only symptoms that could share psychotic symptomatology were persistent and seething anger, and mental agitation. Without clozapine treatment, the patient was at high risk for a serious and imminent suicide attempt. I believe clozapine might have saved her life. Olanzapine fortunately eliminated the anergia and apathy while nearly completely treating the depressive symptoms. The patient had taken fluoxetine up to 60 mg in the past with no significant improvement. Therefore, it is my belief that the antipsychotic is responsible for the remarkable improvement in this patient. Clozapine and olanzapine are antipsychotic medications indicated for the treatment of psychoses, not for the treatment of depression. Purists, particularly in the academia, might disagree with the use of an antipsychotic as the primary medication in this patient because of the absence of obvious symptoms of psychosis. There is a possibility that I failed to detect the presence of psychotic symptoms, that the patient intentionally or unintentionally concealed typical psychotic symptoms, or that the patient presents a yet-to-be recognized condition that is responsive to atypical antipsychotics. Risperidone was tried up to 2 mg along with various antidepressants. Whether or not the patient would have responded to risperidone at the optimal dose of 4 to 6 mg per day is unknown. At the time risperidone was tried, there was the belief that the primary medication would be an antidepressant. It is also possible that if I had persisted and tried the patient on complex combinations of antidepressants and antidepressant augmenters as described in Chapter 2, the patient might have responded. However, based on my clinical experience, I seriously doubt that antidepressant medication combinations would produce such dramatic improvement as was observed in this patient. If olanzapine was not effective, the options would have been a trial on risperidone at its optimal dose of 4 to 6 mg per day or reintroduction of clozapine. Patients who respond well to clozapine tend to do poorly when switched to other antipsychotics. Therefore, a medication switch may not be prudent unless there is clinical justification. Although the clozapine trial was implemented almost by default due to the inability to initiate ECT in a timely manner, the patient and I are happy that the course of events fortunately culminated with a surprisingly positive outcome for the patient. In a clinical practice setting, treatment must be adapted for the benefit of the individual patient. The use of specific *DSM-IV* criteria and FDA drug indications should be as general guidelines rather than as rigid canons. This idea is particularly applicable in the field of psychiatry where clinical evaluation, patient monitoring of progress, and assessment of the effectiveness of treatment are more subjective than in almost all other medical specialties in which objective tests are routinely employed.

Case #89

Presenting Symptoms: The patient was a 40-year-old female with complaints of severely depressed mood, suicidal ideation, crying episodes, feelings of hopelessness, persecutory delusions, guilt feelings, episodic auditory hallucinations with persecutory messages, anhedonia, and insomnia. The patient had had several suicide attempts and about four previous psychiatric hospitalizations. Her previous psychiatrist had treated her with fluoxetine, imipramine, amitriptyline, thiothixene, haloperidol, trifluoperazine, diazepam, and alprazolam. She denied drug or alcohol abuse and caffeine intake. She smoked one pack of cigarettes per day. The patient's mother had a diagnosis of depression. This patient's medical history is positive for back pain.

Current Diagnosis: Schizoaffective disorder, depressed
Consider major depression, severe, recurrent, with psychotic features

Current Treatment:
1. clozapine 50 mg BID and 200 mg HS
2. paroxetine 30 mg HS
3. referral for psychotherapy

Treatment Course: The patient was hospitalized and was discharged on risperidone 3 mg BID, trazodone 400 mg HS, and diazepam 5 mg HS. The patient continued to complain of anxiety, insomnia, auditory hallucinations, and depression. When she required another hospitalization for severe depression, all medications were discontinued and the patient was started on clozapine, to which she responded well. Moderate depression and anxiety remained, for which paroxetine 30 mg was prescribed. She has done well on this regimen for two years. Auditory hallucinations, paranoia, and feelings of guilt are well controlled.

Comments: Depression and suicides are common among chronically ill patients, whether it is due to psychosis or some other illness. Although risperidone is superior to traditional antipsychotics and hence is the current drug of choice among the antipsychotics, it is my opinion that for severe chronic psychotic conditions, clozapine is the best medication available today.

Case #90

Presenting Symptoms: The patient was a 29-year-old female with complaints of severely depressed mood, suicidal ideation, frequent crying, severe insomnia, racing thoughts, compulsive checking, agitation, feelings of hopelessness, excessive anger, extreme mood swings, guardedness, and impatience. These symptoms had been present for many years. She denied drug and alcohol abuse and smoking. She drank eight cups of coffee daily. The patient's mother and sister suffered from depression. The patient had been taking ranitidine for a peptic ulcer.

Current Diagnosis: Bipolar disorder, NOS
Consider major depression, severe, single episode, with mild compulsions

Current Treatment:
1. fluoxetine 40 mg HS
2. carbamazepine 200 mg BID
3. risperidone 1 mg BID
4. clonazepam 1 mg HS
5. decreased coffee intake to two cups per day
6. referral for psychotherapy

Treatment Course: The patient was started on fluoxetine 20 mg AM and zolpidem 10 mg HS. She reported some improvement for two months, but then complained of anxiety and insomnia. She was switched to paroxetine 20 mg AM, trazodone 50 mg HS, and lorazepam 0.5 mg HS, which improved the symptoms. After about two months, she become abruptly suicidal and was involuntarily hospitalized and discharged on venlafaxine 75 mg BID. However, the patient requested to be switched back to fluoxetine because she felt comparatively better on it. Carbamazepine, clonazepam, and risperidone were sequentially added to treat specific symptoms. She is currently doing well on these medications. Carbamazepine level is 4.8 ng/ml. White blood count is within normal limits.

Comments: It is sometimes difficult to distinguish between a bipolar disorder and severe depression. Although treatment is based on specific symptoms, diagnosis gives a general idea about a patient's problems, and hence should be as specific as possible. When suicidal ideation or an attempt is a symptom, the presentation is complicated and therefore needs aggressive and intensive intervention.

Suicidality does not always indicate a primary diagnosis of depression. Patients with schizophrenia, bipolar disorder, paranoid disorder, obsessive-compulsive disorder, and other disorders may become suicidal at times. Aggressive management of fundamental symptoms can literally save their lives by treating the illness, thereby preventing suicides.

Case #91

Presenting Symptoms: The patient was a 39-year-old female with complaints of severely depressed mood, insomnia, suicidal ideation, frequent panic attacks, excessive worrying, agoraphobia, seclusiveness, social withdrawal, fear of driving, crying episodes, anger outbursts, counting and checking rituals, racing thoughts, extreme fear of being alone, suspiciousness, anergia, mood swings, and anhedonia. She denied drug and alcohol abuse and caffeine intake. She smoked one-half pack of cigarettes daily. The medications used by previous psychiatrists were fluoxetine, buspirone, bupropion, alprazolam, clonazepam, nortriptyline, imipramine, trifluoperazine, haloperidol, and thioridazine at various times, with mild to moderate improvement, which was never sustained. The patient's mother suffered from depression. The patient denied major medical problems.

Current Diagnosis: Major depression, severe, recurrent, with psychotic features
Obsessive-compulsive disorder
Panic disorder

Current Treatment:
1. tranylcypromine 20 mg AM and 10 mg at noon
2. trazodone 100 mg HS
3. clonazepam 0.5 mg HS
4. risperidone 0.5 mg BID
5. referral for psychotherapy

Treatment Course: At my office, this patient was tried on other medications such as sertraline, paroxetine, venlafaxine, fluvoxamine, nefazodone, clomipramine, methylphenidate, Triavil, and amoxapine during the course of one year with no lasting improvement. Her anergia, depression, and anxiety persisted. She was offered electroconvulsive therapy, but she refused. The current combination of medications has shown moderate improvement for the last three months, but it remains to be seen whether or not the improvement will be sustained. Her anergia, anxiety, and depression are better, but she is still afraid of leaving her home alone or of driving.

Comments: MAOIs are very useful and uniquely effective in treatment-resistant depressions. Some patients who have shown superior response on an MAOI fail to respond to other antidepressants, including TCAs and SSRIs. Among MAOIs, tranylcypromine has energizing properties compared to phenelzine. Production of isocarboxazid (Marplan) was discontinued several years ago, probably because of a lack of sufficient demand. The availability of SSRIs and bupropion has further decreased the use of MAOIs, which still offer important options for selected patients.

Despite aggressive management, there are some patients whose depression does not respond fully to available treatment methods. If this patient suffers another relapse on tranylcypromine, a trial on clozapine will be considered.

Case #92

Presenting Symptoms: The patient was a 20-year-old male with complaints of depressed mood, irritability, feelings of hopelessness, crying episodes, compulsive washing and cleaning rituals, social withdrawal, dislike of social situations, obsessive preoccupation with fear of getting sick, compulsive tapping, avoidance of intimate relationships, ideas of reference, guilt feelings, belief that he should be punished, and paranoia. He denied suicidal ideation. He also denied drug and alcohol abuse, smoking, and caffeine intake. These symptoms had been present for several years, causing the patient to drop out of college. No acute precipitants were reported. He had been taking paroxetine 40 mg AM and clonazepam 0.5 mg BID for six months prior to seeing me. The patient reported mild improvement on these medications. His medical history is significant for spastic colon.

Current Diagnosis: Obsessive-compulsive disorder
Schizoaffective disorder, depressed
Schizoid personality disorder with schizotypal and avoidant features

Current Treatment:
1. risperidone 3 mg HS
2. clomipramine 75 mg AM and 150 mg HS
3. clonidine 0.1 mg TID
4. referral to a psychotherapist

Treatment Course: The patient was initially started on clomipramine 25 mg, with a gradual increase in dose over a period of two months to 75 mg AM and 150 mg HS. He was also placed on perphenazine 2 mg HS and temazepam 15 mg HS. He improved progressively from the first week of treatment. When risperidone became available, perphenazine was discontinued and risperidone 2 mg HS was started. The dosage of risperidone was gradually increased to 1.5 mg BID and 3 mg HS. Temazepam was discontinued after about six weeks. All symptoms improved to the point that he resumed his college studies and was doing well. He complained of excessive sweating even at night, for which propranolol LA 80 mg was tried, but was unsuccessful. A trial on clonidine 0.1 mg TID was moderately effective in decreasing sweating. He is now maintained on clonidine. After about six months of stabilization and progress, an attempt was made to slowly taper off risperidone. A decrease to risperidone 3 mg was tolerated well. When the dosage was decreased to 1.5 mg HS, the psychotic symptoms gradually returned to the degree that he could not complete the courses he was taking at the time. The dosage of risperidone was increased back to 3 mg HS, with complete suppression of symptoms. The patient was able to resume his studies on his current regimen of medications.

Comments: Diagnostically, this patient presents with symptoms characteristic of various diagnoses. Even though there is some diagnostic uncertainty, treatment so far has been very effective because all of the symptoms are being treated. Clomipramine at high doses significantly decreases seizure threshold. Therefore, a ceiling of 250 mg per day in divided doses has been established. If there is any concern regarding increased seizure risk for a particular patient for any reason, the addition of an anticonvulsant such as valproic acid, gabapentin, carbamazepine, or lamotrigine along with clomipramine should be considered for prophylactic purposes.

Since antipsychotic medication can cause tardive dyskinesia, it is advisable to try to wean a patient off an antipsychotic if possible, especially when psychotic symptoms are not prominent. Risperidone is a new antipsychotic that is claimed to have less risk of tardive dyskinesia, based on theoretical expectations, when compared to traditional antipsychotics. However, there is still some risk with its use, as opposed to clozapine, which has very little risk of causing tardive dyskinesia. Noteworthy is the fact that risperidone has not been in use long enough to accurately assess the actual risk of developing tardive dyskinesia, which typically is a side effect that emerges only after chronic use. In this patient, slowly decreasing risperidone appeared desirable. The observation that his psychotic symptoms returned at a dose of 1.5 mg not only indicated that he needed a higher dose for adequate control of symptoms, but also suggested that the patient had more prominent psychotic symptoms than had been initially suspected. Although response or lack of response to a medication should not routinely be relied on to make, confirm, or refute a diagnosis, there are certain limited clinical situations in which medication response can be one of the factors in clarifying a diagnosis. For example, a dramatic response to a medication usually bolsters the clinician's confidence in the diagnosis that dictated the choice of the particular medication. Certain conditions, such as attention deficit disorder or mild psychosis, that present with vague symptoms that are common to a variety of disorders, give an opportunity to cautiously try a medication. For instance, although stimulants have a nonspecific invigorating effect in most people, the effects on patients who have ADD are usually dramatic, sometimes likened to "turning on a light." In this particular patient, increase of risperidone to 3 mg promptly suppressed the psychotic symptoms, enabling the patient to resume college studies.

Excessive sweating is seen with various antidepressants, especially SSRIs. A number of medications may be employed to reduce or eliminate this symptom. Propranolol 10 to 20 mg TID or long-acting propranolol

60 to 120 daily, clonidine 0.1 mg BID-TID, clonidine transdermal patch, guanfacine (Tenex) 1 to 2 mg HS, or benzodiazepines are sometimes effective. Since clomipramine lowers the seizure threshold, patients may be instructed to avoid activities that might increase the risk of seizures, such as alcohol abuse, sleep deprivation, and excessive caffeine intake. Valproic acid, gabapentin, lamotrigine, carbamazepine, or phenytoin may be considered for seizure prophylaxis for patients whose seizures might be exceptionally hazardous. For example, a professional truck driver who has to be on clomipramine at the high dosage range may benefit from seizure prophylaxis, whereas a sedentary worker may not need such protection.

Case #93

Presenting Symptoms: The patient was a 40-year-old female. She was first seen in the hospital where she was admitted involuntarily with the following symptoms: suicidal ideation, intent and plan of overdosing on medication, severely depressed mood, agitation, restlessness, increased anger, racing thoughts, extreme mood swings, anxiety attacks, paranoid ideation, ideas of reference, persecutory delusions, severe insomnia, frequent sobbing, and feelings of hopelessness. She denied drug and alcohol abuse. She smoked one pack of cigarettes and drank two cups of coffee daily. The patient had had several psychiatric hospitalizations in the past, and had been treated on various TCAs. History also revealed that she had mood symptoms and conduct disturbance of mild severity since adolescence. Her daughter was diagnosed with bipolar disorder. The patient is on tamoxifen for a breast tumor.

Current Diagnosis: Schizoaffective disorder, depressed
Consider bipolar disorder, NOS
Personality disorder, NOS

Current Treatment:
1. carbamazepine 200 mg BID
2. paroxetine 30 mg AM
3. perphenazine 16 mg HS
4. clonazepam 0.5 mg HS
5. propranolol LA 120 mg AM
6. benztropine 0.5 mg BID
7. referral for psychotherapy

Treatment Course: The patient was stabilized on perphenazine, paroxetine, and clonazepam while in the hospital and discharged after seven days. The remaining medications were added during outpatient follow-up. The patient has been functioning fairly well on these medications for about two years.

Comments: The patient had several distinct symptoms, each of which needed treatment using different medications as follows:

Symptoms	Medication(s)
Depression, anxiety	paroxetine, clonazepam
Psychotic features	perphenazine
Mood instability	carbamazepine, paroxetine
Insomnia	clonazepam
Akathisia	benztropine, propranolol, clonazepam

Some medications have overlapping effects. Common examples are given below:

Medication	Possible Overlapping Indications
Benzodiazepines	anxiety, insomnia, akathisia, acute dystonia, agitation, alcohol withdrawal symptoms
Mood stabilizers	mood instability, depression, anxiety, rage, etc.
Antidepressants	depression, anxiety, anger, attention deficit disorder
Antipsychotics	psychosis, hostility, agitation, anxiety

Although medications have overlapping effects, different medications may be necessary to obtain an optimal effect. For example, although akathisia is improved with benzodiazepines, the preferable primary medications are usually beta-blockers or anticholinergics. A medication may have beneficial effects for a variety of symptoms but may be a poor choice as a primary medication for treating certain symptoms. For instance, although antipsychotics have some antianxiety effects, they are generally avoided for treatment of anxiety in favor of other medications such as antidepressants and benzodiazepines.

My speculation is that with a switch to risperidone, this patient could probably discontinue propranolol and benztropine. Switching to clozapine might enable discontinuation of propranolol, benztropine, clonazepam, carbamazepine, and even paroxetine. These options could not be tried in this patient because of her financial limitations and unwillingness to alter a treatment protocol that has been fairly effective.

Case #94

Presenting Symptoms: The patient was a 49-year-old female with complaints of chronic severe depression, vague fears, chronic anger and hostility, excessive somatic preoccupation, social withdrawal, anergia, anxiety attacks, chronic anxiety, multiple suicidal attempts by overdose, frequent crying, emotional neediness, severe insomnia, hopelessness, and anhedonia. She denied active psychotic symptoms or paranoia. She also denied drug and alcohol abuse. She smoked one pack of cigarettes per day and drank one to two cups of coffee daily. The patient reported that she had been treated for depression since her early twenties. Doxepin had helped for about five years, but stopped working spontaneously. She was tried on various TCAs and some antipsychotics in the past. She had had about five inpatient hospitalizations prior to beginning treatment at my office. The patient's mother had a history of depression. The patient was taking levothyroxine for hypothyroidism, and estrogen supplements.

Current Diagnosis: Major depression, severe, recurrent
Consider "negative" schizophrenia (not a *DSM-IV* diagnosis)

Current Treatment:
1. clozapine 200 mg HS
2. paroxetine 10 mg AM
3. atenolol 50 mg AM (for clozapine-induced tachycardia)

Treatment Course: The patient was initially seen in the hospital where she was admitted after yet another suicide attempt. She was discharged on paroxetine 30 mg AM, perphenazine 8 mg HS, and lorazepam 0.5 mg TID. There have been many exacerbations and she has had several inpatient psychiatric hospitalizations during the last two years. Medications unsuccessfully tried under my care are listed below. Full trials were given unless side effects interfered.

Antidepressants	Antipsychotics	Other Adjunctive Medications
imipramine	perphenazine	clonazepam
clomipramine	thioridazine	lithium
nortriptyline	thiothixene	carbamazepine
protriptyline	risperidone	trazodone
fluoxetine		buspirone
paroxetine		valproate
sertraline		
venlafaxine		
fluvoxamine		
nefazodone		
phenelzine		
bupropion		

She was referred for electroconvulsive therapy, which was discontinued after ten treatments for lack of improvement. As a desperate attempt, she was subsequently hospitalized under my care and started on clozapine, which produced a moderate response within two weeks. Atenolol was added to control tachycardia caused by clozapine. Paroxetine 10 mg was started on an outpatient basis for mild depressive symptoms. The patient has shown slow but steady improvement since she was started on clozapine three months ago.

Comments: Some chronic, severe, and refractory depressions may represent the "negative" or "deficit" symptoms of schizophrenia and deserve a trial on clozapine, if other standard medication treatments and ECT fail. Since clozapine has the best effects on negative symptoms among the medications currently available in the United States, including risperidone and olanzapine, it is my opinion that clozapine has the best probability of successfully treating the "negative" symptoms. Hence, it is important for the psychiatrist to think of clozapine when presented with severe depression or bipolar disorder that is refractory to aggressive management using standard approaches.

A point of interest is that this patient was described by the psychiatric nursing staff as a "borderline personality." During several of her hospitalizations, the staff had conveyed their sense of hopelessness and frustration both indirectly and directly by suggesting that, having a personality disorder, the patient would not be likely to benefit from treatment. The patient's hopelessness, anger, hostility, anxiety, neediness, impatience, and irritable mood when not responding to treatment made her an ongoing challenge to the staff. It is very satisfying to see the so-called personality disorders fade with effective treatment. The important point is to not give up on patients with personality disorders or chronic depression. With so many new medications now available, symptoms and conditions that were refractory to treatment several years ago are now more likely to respond to appropriate treatment.

Case #95

Presenting Symptoms: The patient was a 40-year-old female with complaints of depressed mood, extreme mood swings, insomnia, racing thoughts, auditory hallucinations, episodic compulsive spending, episodic grandiose delusions, paranoid delusions, thought broadcasting, thought insertion, intermittent binge drinking, and labile affect. She denied drug abuse. She smoked one pack of cigarettes per day, and drank one to two cups of coffee daily. Her past psychiatric history was significant for multiple hospitalizations including a three year, long-term residential treatment in a psychodynamically oriented facility. She was on fluoxetine 20 mg AM and mesoridazine 50 mg HS at the time she was first seen by me as a follow-up referral after her discharge from the three-year private hospitalization. She denied any major medical problems.

Current Diagnosis: Schizoaffective disorder, bipolar type

Current Treatment:
1. Eskalith CR 450 mg BID
2. carbamazepine 200 mg TID
3. risperidone 3 mg BID and 4.5 mg HS
4. clonazepam 1 mg HS
5. paroxetine 45 mg AM
6. trazodone 50 mg HS
7. referral for psychotherapy

Treatment Course: This patient experienced a very complicated treatment course while under my care, including four brief hospitalizations and multiple medication trials in a four-year period. The medication trials included clomipramine, nefazodone, naltrexone, perphenazine, fluphenazine, haloperidol, valproate and clozapine. She has been the most functional on her current combination of medications. As far as can be determined, she has abstained from drinking for the last eight months.

Comments: Complicated patients require complex treatment using multiple medications. Unfortunately, clozapine, which was tried in 1992 and 1994, was not effective. Her current global assessment of functioning (GAF) score is estimated at 50. Without treatment using medications, her GAF score is usually in the 20 to 30 range. It is unlikely that even with continued compliance and treatment, her GAF score would exceed 70. (GAF score is an estimate of the patient's overall level of functioning ranging from 1, suggesting the most extreme dysfunction, to 100, representing the most superior functioning. The GAF score is recorded on Axis V. Although there is no normal limit, a score above 70 usually indicates adequate functioning. Since technical details on multiaxial diagnosis and GAF scoring are beyond the scope of this text, please refer to the *DSM-IV* for further information.)

Case #96

Presenting Symptoms: The patient was a 39-year-old female with complaints of depressed mood, frequent crying, obsessive rumination related to her ex-husband, anergia, feelings of hopelessness, frequent suicidal thoughts without intent or plan, anxiety attacks, and anhedonia. The patient had a history of several episodes of severe depression from which she recovered ten years ago. Her current episode was precipitated by her divorce. She had had several previous hospitalizations. Most recently, she was tried on fluoxetine and trazodone, which were not effective. She denied drug and alcohol abuse, smoking, and caffeine intake. The patient's mother is doing well on paroxetine for depression.

Current Diagnosis: Major depression, severe, recurrent

Current Treatment:
1. perphenazine 2 mg TID
2. amitriptyline 25 mg TID
3. alprazolam 0.25 mg QID
4. referral for psychotherapy

Treatment Course: This patient was tried on paroxetine, sertraline, venlafaxine, fluvoxamine, nefazodone, clomipramine, amitriptyline, imipramine, bupropion, phenelzine, and tranylcypromine. Adjunctive medications tried were lithium, thyroid supplements, risperidone, buspirone, and dextroamphetamine. The only medication that was effective was phenelzine, which unfortunately stopped working after about four months. The patient revealed that many years ago she did well on Etrafon (perphenazine and amitriptyline); hence, she was placed on Etrafon with dramatic improvement. Alprazolam was prescribed for panic anxiety, which was not controlled on Etrafon.

Comments: Etrafon, also known by the brand name Triavil, is a fixed-ratio mixture of perphenazine and amitriptyline, available in 2/10, 2/25, 4/10, 4/25, and 4/50 strengths in brand and generic versions. This patient had no obvious psychotic symptoms. It is still puzzling as to why this patient responded so well to Etrafon when she failed to respond to numerous antidepressants, including amitriptyline. Apparently the antipsychotic, perphenazine, was critical in converting her to a responder, yet she did not respond to adjunctive risperidone at low doses.

It is possible that the patient could have had a thought disorder or cognitive dysfunction so mild and latent that it was clinically evident neither to the author nor to the patient. The perphenazine was uniquely effective for this problem.

Projective psychological testing might possibly have uncovered a latent thought disorder, but cost considerations and practical irrelevance of test results related to clinical management in this particular case would have made testing difficult to justify. In other words, medication management is unlikely to change, regardless of test result findings, as far as this patient is concerned.

Case #97

Presenting Symptoms: The patient was a 45-year-old female with extreme mood swings, racing thoughts, pressured speech, episodes of depression and anergia, insomnia, scattered thinking, episodes of confusion, suicidal ideation, and obsessive preoccupation with chronic fatigue syndrome and health-food-related issues. She attempted suicide by overdose six years ago. She denied drug and alcohol abuse and smoking. She drank two cups of coffee daily. She had been taking fluoxetine 20 mg, doxepin 150 mg HS, and clonazepam 2 mg HS, prescribed by an out-of-state chronic fatigue syndrome specialist. She had had one psychiatric hospitalization subsequent to the overdose episode. Her medical history is positive for fibromyalgia, chronic fatigue syndrome (CFS), and back pain.

Current Diagnosis: Bipolar disorder, depressed
Obsessive-compulsive features
Schizotypal features

Current Treatment:
1. fluoxetine 40 mg AM
2. risperidone 0.5 mg BID
3. Eskalith CR 450 mg BID
4. clonazepam 2 mg HS
5. hydroxyzine 50 mg HS
6. referral for psychotherapy

Treatment Course: Sequential addition of lithium and risperidone improved mood swings, depression, and disorganized thinking. Hydroxyzine was added as an adjunctive medication for insomnia, which was a complaint despite being on clonazepam 2 mg HS. With the increase in the dose of fluoxetine to 40 mg, there was a decrease in the intensity of her preoccupation with chronic fatigue syndrome. Her lithium level was 0.7 mEq/L.

Comments: Most patients diagnosed with CFS improve on antidepressants, particularly energizing antidepressants such as bupropion, fluoxetine, venlafaxine, desipramine, and tranylcypromine. Some patients with the diagnosis of CFS approach their illness with incredible zeal and are offended by any suggestion that they might be depressed. In order to persuade CFS patients to comply with treatment, an approach that has worked well for me so far is to tell CFS patients that depression and anxiety usually accompany CFS. Their identification with CFS is such that if the treatment is in some way connected to CFS, they readily accept treatment, whereas if they are told that their symptoms might possibly be explained as due to depression, they are likely to be resistant to further intervention and may seek another physician.

It is possible that at least some patients diagnosed as having CFS may actually be suffering from an atypical form of depression with somatization, obsessive-compulsive, or psychotic features.

Case #98

Presenting Symptoms: The patient was a 40-year-old male with complaints of severely depressed mood, crying episodes, frequent suicidal ideation, increased anger, feelings of hopelessness and worthlessness, anger outbursts, ideas of reference, difficulty trusting people, confused thinking, anergia, anorexia, initial insomnia, restless sleep, irritability, and anhedonia. These symptoms were recently precipitated by a marital breakup. He denied drug and alcohol abuse, and smoking. He drank two to three cups of coffee daily. He took ibuprofen occasionally for back pain. No formal treatment was being pursued for dyspepsia.

Current Diagnosis: Major depression, severe, single episode, with mild psychotic features
Marital problems

Current Treatment:
1. sertraline 50 mg AM
2. doxepin 10 mg HS
3. risperidone 0.5 mg HS
4. temazepam 7.5 mg HS
5. referral for psychotherapy

Treatment Course: The patient was started on all of the above-listed medications at the time of his first visit. He reported marked improvement in anxiety, paranoia, suicidality, insomnia, and anorexia when seen five days later. He was continued on the same medications and doses. When seen two weeks after the second visit, depressive symptoms were moderately improved. He has been doing well on these medications now for two months. Risperidone will be discontinued in the near future.

Comments: This is an example of a hospitalizable patient who improved satisfactorily and rapidly with aggressive outpatient treatment, using four different medications which were started simultaneously at the first visit, all at low doses, to address various symptoms as follows:

– sertraline	depression, anxiety, anger
– risperidone	ideas of reference, guardedness, anger
– doxepin	anorexia, dyspepsia, insomnia
– temazepam	insomnia

Some overlap is beneficial in keeping the dosages low. For example, since doxepin has some sleep-inducing effects, it was possible to keep the dose of temazepam extremely low at 7.5 mg, whereas without doxepin the dose of temazepam would have been 15 or 30 mg. Aggressive medication management that comprehensively treats all discrete symptoms enables many severely ill patients to be treated in the office setting, making it possible to reduce hospitalizations. Similarly, effective, comprehensive, and aggressive management of patients who require hospitalization reduces the number of days that the patient needs to stay in the hospital.

Case #99

Presenting Symptoms: The patient was a 49-year-old male with complaints of homicidal ideation and threats toward his ex-wife, stalking his ex-wife despite a restraining order, frequent suicidal ideation, deep-seated anger, hostility, distrust of people, extreme selfishness, bitterness, anergia, hypersomnia, lack of remorse for violent behavior toward his ex-wife, threats to commit suicide if sentenced to jail, and obsessive-compulsive personality characteristics. These symptoms, at less severity, had been present for many years. His history also suggested the presence of conduct problems during his teenage years. He denied drug and alcohol abuse and caffeine intake. He smoked one pack of cigarettes daily. The patient had been taking sertraline 150 mg daily for six months when first seen at my office.

Current Diagnosis: Schizoaffective disorder, depressed
Antisocial personality disorder with paranoid, obsessional, and narcissistic features

Current Treatment:
1. risperidone 2 mg AM and 4 mg HS
2. fluoxetine 40 mg AM
3. referral for psychotherapy

Treatment Course: The patient was hospitalized and started on the above medications. He was discharged after a ten-day hospitalization that resulted in significant improvement in suicidal and homicidal ideation and anger. He reported that he no longer felt obsessed with the idea of killing his ex-wife or with suicidal thoughts.

Comments: The combination of hostility, externalization of blame, obsessive hatred, and antisocial features can be deadly. Those symptoms require intensive treatment. Antipsychotic medication is immediately the most important medication for the presence of anger and externalization. SSRIs are particularly effective in the long-term management of anger, as well as in the control of any emotion that has obsessional features, including obsessive love or hatred. Extreme anger and hostility are symptoms sufficient to cause consideration of starting an antipsychotic even in the absence of typical psychotic symptoms. If SSRIs or mood stabilizers eventually control these symptoms, the antipsychotic may be completely tapered off.

Case #100

Presenting Symptoms: The patient was a 34-year-old female with complaints of depressed mood, suicidal ideation, history of numerous suicidal attempts by overdosing and cutting her wrists, paranoia, anger, hostility, social withdrawal, extreme ambivalence, severe insomnia (a total sleep duration of less than two hours per day, according to the patient's estimate, verified by her husband), physical violence toward her husband, anger outbursts, and labile affect.

The patient has a long psychiatric history, beginning in 1980 when she was first hospitalized for depression. Since then, she has had approximately 65 (sixty-five) psychiatric hospitalizations, many of which were involuntary. Most voluntary hospitalizations were of one to three days duration because typically the patient left against medical advice several days after signing herself in. Since psychiatrists and psychiatric hospitals in her city refused to treat the patient, her husband had to bring her to another city (a two-hour drive) to find psychiatrists and psychiatric hospitals that, unaware of her history, would agree to treat her. Finally, the new psychiatric hospital staff refused to readmit her for treatment because of their frustration in dealing with her (despite her having adequate private insurance coverage). Her local psychiatrist also refused to continue treating her after she became violent in his office. She has had various diagnoses in the past, including borderline personality disorder, schizoaffective disorder, personality disorder, NOS, and depression. Some of her previous psychiatrists and most nursing staff describe her simply as "borderline." She has been tried on nearly all psychiatric medications, including lithium, valproate, carbamazepine, desipramine, amitriptyline, nortriptyline, imipramine, doxepin, amoxapine, trazodone, bupropion, fluoxetine, sertraline, venlafaxine, phenelzine, tranylcypromine, isocarboxazid (no longer available), haloperidol, fluphenazine, chlorpromazine, thioridazine, thiothixene, trifluoperazine, loxapine, chlordiazepoxide, diazepam, clonazepam, alprazolam, triazolam, and zolpidem. At the time she was first seen in my office, her medications and dosages as prescribed by her previous psychiatrist were the following:

- phenelzine 45 mg AM, 45 mg noon, 30 mg PM (120 mg daily)
- loxapine 75 mg daily
- benztropine 2 mg TID
- alprazolam 2 mg QID

She denied drug and alcohol abuse, smoking, and caffeine intake. The patient's father and brother reportedly suffered from nervous breakdowns and alcoholism. Her medical history was significant for hypertension, migraine headaches, and peptic ulcer. She had been taking enalapril, atenolol, ranitidine, and sumatriptan SC.

Current Diagnosis: Schizoaffective disorder, depressed
Borderline personality disorder

Current Treatment:
1. clozapine 100 mg BID and 400 mg HS
2. paroxetine 20 mg AM
3. diazepam 10 mg HS
4. Depakote sprinkle capsule 250 mg TID
5. Risperidone 2 mg HS
6. continue psychotherapy

Treatment Course: The patient was first seen in my office with her husband. Her complete history was reviewed in detail, and the patient was evaluated. They were advised that I would provide psychiatric services as long as she was compliant with treatment recommendations and that noncompliance of a significant nature would result in immediate termination. The first recommendation was to electively and voluntarily hospitalize the patient with a specific plan of trying clozapine. The risks and benefits of clozapine treatment were discussed. They were told to think about the recommendations and to call me when she was ready for hospitalization to start clozapine. She was advised to seek the services of another psychiatrist if she decided not to be hospitalized for a trial of clozapine. The patient's husband called within a week, consenting to hospitalization, which was arranged the same day. All psychiatric medications that she had been on were discontinued. Clozapine was started in accordance with Sandoz protocol, as reproduced in Chapter 11. Supplemental haloperidol was given during the first seven days to control agitation. Phenobarbital on a tapering schedule was given for ten days to treat alprazolam withdrawal. The first seven days of hospitalization were very stormy, with frequent use of seclusion and restraints, use of IM haloperidol and lorazepam on many occasions, and frequent threats by the patient to leave against medical advice. Divalproex sodium was added for seizure prophylaxis. Paroxetine improved depressive symptoms. Supplemental risperidone at 2 mg HS controlled breakthrough "positive" symptoms not controlled by clozapine. A long-acting sedative such as diazepam was chosen to treat insomnia and to provide possible additional seizure protection. The clozapine level was 532 ng/ml. Her GAF score during the past year and at admission was estimated at 35. At the time of discharge it was 55. If treatment continues to go well, it is expected that she will show further slow and gradual improvement.

Comments: Difficult and complex patients are often labeled "borderline" by mental health professionals. Even when the patient actually has borderline personality disorder, there are nearly always Axis I diagnoses that are treatable. It is frequently found that when the Axis I disorder is effectively managed, the personality disorder symptoms subside to a degree that they become dormant. I believe such is the case with this patient. She has not had a hospitalization in the last two years, which is remarkable, given her history of a hospitalization every one to two months. It is too early to be sure that her recovery is long-term, but the preliminary indications from reports by her and her husband are that she is functioning better now than she has been in the last 15 years.

In general, a warning by the clinician that the patient will be terminated for noncompliance should not routinely be given to patients unless noncompliance becomes a problem in the course of treatment. It is understood and expected that patients will be compliant. In fact, a preemptive warning of termination for noncompliance with no provocation can suggest hostility or an antagonistic attitude on the part of the clinician. However, for certain patients with severe personality disorders and/or substance abuse in whom noncompliance has been a problem in the past, an initial warning may be necessary and therapeutic. Such an approach gives the clinician better control over the management of the patient. If the patient becomes noncompliant with significant aspects of treatment, the clinician will have no choice but to terminate treatment of the patient, because continuation of treatment in the face of noncompliance leads to further loss of control of the treatment process. When the threat is promptly carried out, the patient is more likely to be compliant with the next clinician. If noncompliance is a major concern based on the patient's past psychiatric history, it may even be beneficial to the patient to be told that noncompliance is expected and that the patient will be terminated so that hopefully there will be improved compliance with the next clinician. This could have a paradoxical effect, in that it can serve much like a psychological "vaccination" and possibly forestall noncompliance. There are many variations of this technique, depending upon the unique clinical situation. Such techniques are part of the general clinical skills necessary to be an effective clinician, and hence are beyond the scope of this text.

MAOIs should not be abruptly discontinued unless the clinician is prepared to treat the withdrawal symptoms, consisting of anxiety, insomnia, nightmares, vivid dreams, and agitation. In rare cases, even transient psychosis and delirium can result. MAOIs may be tapered off over a period of seven days to minimize any withdrawal symptoms. This patient was taking phenelzine 120 mg, which is significantly higher than the maximum recommended dose of 90 mg per day; hence, withdrawal symptoms were expected in this patient. However, for various clinical reasons, it was decided to stop phenelzine abruptly and to manage the withdrawal symptoms. These symptomes were controlled on phenobarbital, haloperidol, and clozapine, which the patient was taking for other purposes.

The seizure risk on clozapine above 500 mg daily is estimated at 5 to 6 percent, which is substantial. Therefore, seizure prophylaxis using valproate, gabapentin, or lamotrigine should be considered in patients receiving clozapine at or above 500 mg daily. Of all valproate preparations, depakote sprinkle capsule is the least irritating to the gastrointestinal tract. Since this patient had peptic ulcer, it was crucial to choose a medication form that was unlikely to exacerbate the gastrointestinal problem.

If clozapine must be discontinued for some reason, other options that may be considered for this patient are risperidone, olanzapine, sertindole, clomipramine, nefazodone, or electroconvulsive therapy, which have never been tried, assuming the patient remains compliant. Occasionally, it is necessary to add high-potency antipsychotics such as risperidone, haloperidol, or thiothixene for control of breakthrough "positive" symptoms in a patient receiving clozapine.

This patient presents a chronic suicidal risk. It is critical not to minimize the risk simply because she has not been successful, despite numerous attempts over a period of 15 years. It is emotionally stressful for a clinician to work with a chronically suicidal patient unless the clinician is able to assume a professional attitude and is able to use a mild level of defenses such as intellectualization, rationalization, and isolation of affect when a patient is successful in committing suicide. The clinician must accept the reality that determined patients will attempt to commit suicide or homicide, or engage in other acts of violence to themselves or others, despite the best efforts of the clinician. Long-term commitment in psychiatric units, 24-hour observations, and no-suicide contracts are neither practical nor effective if a patient is sufficiently determined. Most institutions do not keep patients long-term, even if the clinician is successful in getting the patient admitted on a court order. I have had the experience over the years of sending some of the most self-destructive and dangerous patients to state psychiatric hospitals to discover that some of them were discharged to their communities after several weeks or months. The reality, therefore, is that there is no such thing as permanent hospitalization even for the most chronically suicidal patient. Ongoing 24-hour observation and supervision is obviously impossible. No-suicide contracts will not prevent a truly suicidal or homicidal patient from acting on thoughts or impulses. The clinician's approach should be to help the patient overcome those thoughts and prolong life. Any physician or therapist working with severely emotionally disordered patients will, sooner or later, have to deal with a patient suicide or suicide attempts, and will, on rare occasions, deal with a patient who has attempted or committed a homicide. Suicide and homicide, or attempts thereof, are risks associated with severe mental disorders, just as sudden death is a risk associated with severe cardiovascular disease. The clinician's task is to recognize the risk, if recognizable, and to manage the patient in order to reduce the risk, using available and practical clinical techniques. Just as prolonging the life of a patient with severe cardiovascular disease is considered a medical success, in psychiatry it should be considered a success if, due to treatment, the patient lives longer or commits–or attempts to commit–suicide or homicide later than would be the case without treatment. In dealing with such patients, my approach, in addition to providing aggressive treatment in the office or hospital, has been to advise the patient and significant others of chronic risks, practical options, absence of any guarantee of success, and of my plan to do what is practical to attempt to help the patient. With some severely disordered patients, the expectation should be that of palliative rather than curative treatment, because the risk of suicide or destructive behavior is so high and chronic that the question is more appropriately *when,* rather than *if,* the behavior will be manifested. When patients drink alcohol or abuse drugs, such behaviors become even less predictable. To make matters worse, the mental health clinician has very little control over the behavior of a suicidal or homicidal psychiatric patient, whereas in most other medical specialties (1) patients are generally more motivated and compliant; (2) the risks are more predictable; (3) substance abuse, which can disrupt any inhibition patients might have, is usually not a complicating factor; and (4) legal considerations related to patients' rights, involuntary treatment, confidentiality, and competency are generally less controversial.

Despite the true lack of control over patients' behavior, the clinician must not be indifferent when treating a dangerous patient. The clinician has the responsibility to do a reasonable clinical evaluation, recognize any risks if suggested by the clinical evaluation, and to offer treatment, if indicated. To give an extreme illustration, if a patient reports suicidal thoughts, the clinician should not say or do anything that might aggravate the condition and should not dismiss the serious nature of such a report. On the contrary, if the patient denies any suicidal or homicidal ideation during the clinical evaluation but then commits suicide on the way home from the clinician's office, there is simply nothing that the clinician could have done. Another scenario exists when a patient admits to suicidal or homicidal thoughts but denies any intent or plan, agrees to seek help if intent or plan develops, assures the clinician that he or she will not act on the thoughts, and agrees to follow treatment recommendations. Should this patient commit suicide in the near future, there again is nothing the clinician could have done to intervene. If a clinician insists on hospitalizing or involuntarily committing every patient with suicidal or homicidal thoughts, nearly 75 percent of the patients in every mental health clinician's practice would be in the hospital. All clinicians will agree that patients having suicidal or homicidal intent or plan need inpatient treatment or some other immediate intervention to protect themselves or others. Patients experiencing suicidal or homicidal ideation clearly need aggressive treatment, but may or may not need inpatient treatment, depending on numerous other factors.

Appendix A

Patient Assistance Programs

This is a list of addresses and telephone numbers of patient assistance programs offered by drug manufacturers. The list is limited to fairly expensive and commonly used psychotropic medications.

Drug Name	Address	Phone #
Anafranil	Patient Assistance Program Ciba-Geigy Corporation Building D 2058 556 Morris Avenue Summit, NJ 07901	1-800-257-3273
Clozaril (clozapine)	Novartis Patient Assistance Program P.O. Box 9764 McLean, VA 22102-9764	1-800-455-6655
Effexor (venlafaxine)	Wyeth-Ayerst Professional Services P.O. Box 8299 Philadelphia, PA 19101-8299	1-800-568-9938
Luvox (fluvoxamine)	Solvay Pharmaceuticals Marietta, GA 30062	1-800-788-9277
Paxil (paroxetine)	Paxil Access to Care Program Smithkline Beecham One Franklin Plaza FP 1510 P.O. Box 7404 Philadelphia, PA 19101-7404	1-800-729-4544

Prozac (fluoxetine)	Lily Cares P.O. Box 9105 McLane, VA 22102	1-800-545-6962
Revia (naltrexone)	Patient Assistance Program Dupont, Merck Plaza Hickory Run P.O. Box 80723 Wilmington, DE 19880-0723	1-800-474-2762
Risperdal (risperidone)	Janssen Cares Risperdal Patient Assistance Program 4828 Parkway Plaza Boulevard Suite 120 Charlotte, NC 28217-1969	1-800-652-6227
Serzone (nefazodone) (also Buspar)	Bristol-Myers-Squibb 2400 West Lloyd Expressway Mail Code R-22 Evansville, IN 47721	1-800-437-0994
Wellbutrin (bupropion)	Burroughs Wellcome Company Patient Assistance Program P.O. Box 52035 Phoenix, AZ 85072-9349	1-800-722-9294
Zoloft (sertraline)	Pfizer Indigent Program P.O. Box 25457 Alexandria, VA 22313-5457	1-800-646-4455
Zyprexa (olanzapine)	Zyprexa Patient Assistance Program P.O. Box 9105 McLean, VA 22102	1-800-488-2133

Appendix B

Alphabetical Listing of Drugs by Generic Names, with U.S. Brand Names

Generic Name	Brand Name
alprazolam	Xanax
amantadine	Symmetrel
amitriptyline	Elavil, Endep
amitriptyline + perphenazine	Triavil, Etrafon
amitriptyline + chlordiazepoxide	Limbitrol
amoxapine	Asendin
atenolol	Tenormin
benztropine	Cogentin
bethanechol	Urecholine
biperiden	Akineton
bromocriptine	Parlodel
bupropion	Wellbutrin
buspirone	Buspar
carbamazepine	Tegretol
chloral hydrate	Noctec
chlordiazepoxide	Librium
chlordiazepoxide + amitriptyline	Limbitrol
chlorpromazine	Thorazine

Generic Name	Brand Name
chlorprothixene	Taractan
clomipramine	Anafranil
clonazepam	Klonopin
clonidine	Catapres
clorazepate	Tranxene
clozapine	Clozaril
cyproheptadine	Periactin
dantrolene	Dantrium
desipramine	Norpramin, Pertofrane
dextroamphetamine	Dexedrine
diazepam	Valium
diphenhydramine	Benadryl
disulfiram	Antabuse
divalproex sodium	Depakote, Depakote sprinkle
donepezil	Aricept
doxepin	Sinequan, Adapin
estazolam	Prosom
fenfluramine	Pondimin
filgrastim	Neupogen
fluoxetine	Prozac
fluphenazine	Prolixin, Permitil
flurazepam	Dalmane
fluvoxamine	Luvox
gabapentin	Neurontin
guanfancine	Tenex
haloperidol	Haldol
hydroxyzine	Vistaril, Atarax

Generic Name	Brand Name
imipramine	Tofranil, Janimine
isocarboxazid	Marplan (discontinued)
lamotrigine	Lamictal
levothyroxine (T4)	Synthroid, Levoxine
liothyronine (T3)	Cytomel
lithium	Eskalith, Lithobid, Lithonate, Cibalith
lorazepam	Ativan
loxapine	Loxitane
maprotiline	Ludiomil
mesoridazine	Serentil
methylphenidate	Ritalin
metoclopramide	Reglan
mirtazapine	Remeron
molindone	Moban
naltrexone	Revia, Trexan
nefazodone	Serzone
nifedipine	Procardia
nortriptyline	Pamelor, Aventyl
olanzapine	Zyprexa
oxazepam	Serax
paroxetine	Paxil
pemoline	Cylert
perphenazine	Trilafon
perphenazine + amitriptyline	Triavil, Etrafon
phenelzine	Nardil
phenobarbital	Luminal
pindolol	Visken

Generic Name	Brand Name
prazepam	Centrax
prochlorperazine	Compazine
procyclidine	Kemadrin
propranolol	Inderal
protriptyline	Vivactil
quazepam	Doral
risperidone	Risperdal
selegiline	Eldepryl, Deprenyl
sertindole	Serlect
sertraline	Zoloft
sodium divalproex	Depakote
sodium valproate	Depakene
temazepam	Restoril
thioridazine	Mellaril
thiothixene	Navane
tranylcypromine	Parnate
trazodone	Desyrel
triazolam	Halcion
trifluoperazine	Stelazine
trihexyphenidyl	Artane
trimipramine	Surmontil
valproate	Depakene
valproic acid	Depakene
venlafaxine	Effexor
verapamil	Calan, Isoptin
yohimbine	Yocon
zolpidem	Ambien

Appendix C

Alphabetical Listing of Drugs by U.S. Brand Names, with Generic Names

Brand Name	Generic Name
Adapin	doxepin
Akineton	biperiden
Ambien	zolpidem
Anafranil	clomipramine
Antabuse	disulfiram
Aricept	donepezil
Artane	trihexyphenidyl
Asendin	amoxapine
Atarax	hydroxyzine
Ativan	lorazepam
Aventyl	nortriptyline
Benadryl	diphenhydramine
Buspar	buspirone
Calan	verapamil
Catapres	clonidine
Centrax	prazepam
Cibalith	lithium citrate (syrup)

Brand Name	Generic Name
Clozaril	clozapine
Cogentin	benztropine
Compazine	prochlorperazine
Cylert	pemoline
Cytomel	liothyronine (T3)
Dalmane	flurazepam
Dantrium	dantrolene
Depakene	valproate, valproic acid, sodium valproate
Depakote	divalproex sodium, sodium divalproex
Depakote sprinkle	divalproex sodium, sodium divalproex
Deprenyl	selegiline
Desyrel	trazodone
Dexedrine	dextroamphetamine
Doral	quazepam
Effexor	venlafaxine
Elavil	amitriptyline
Eldepryl	selegiline
Endep	amitriptyline
Eskalith	lithium
Etrafon	amitriptyline + perphenazine
Halcion	triazolam
Haldol	haloperidol
Inderal	propranolol
Isoptin	verapamil
Janimine	imipramine
Kemadrin	procyclidine
Klonopin	clonazepam

Brand Name	Generic Name
Lamictal	lamotrigine
Levoxine	levothyroxine (T4)
Librium	chlordiazepoxide
Limbitrol	chlordiazepoxide + amitriptyline
Lithobid	lithium
Lithonate	lithium
Lithotab	lithium
Loxitane	loxapine
Ludiomil	maproptiline
Luminal	phenobarbital
Luvox	fluvoxamine
Marplan	isocarboxazid (discontinued)
Mellaril	thioridazine
Moban	molindone
Nardil	phenelzine
Navane	thiothixene
Neupogen	filgrastim
Neurontin	gabapentin
Noctec	chloral hydrate
Norpramin	desipramine
Pamelor	nortriptyline
Parlodel	bromocriptine
Parnate	tranylcypromine
Paxil	paroxetine
Periactin	cyproheptadine
Permitil	fluphenazine
Pertofrane	desipramine

Brand Name	Generic Name
Pondimin	fenfluramine
Procardia	nifedipine
Prolixin	fluphenazine
Prosom	estazolam
Prozac	fluoxetine
Reglan	metoclopramide
Remeron	mirtazapine
Restoril	temazepam
Revia	naltrexone
Risperdal	risperidone
Ritalin	methylphenidate
Serax	oxazepam
Serentil	mesoridazine
Serlect	sertindole
Serzone	nefazodone
Sinequan	doxepin
Stelazine	trifluoperazine
Surmontil	clomipramine
Symmetrel	amantadine
Synthroid	levothyroxine (T4)
Taractan	chlorprothixene
Tegretol	carbamazepine
Tenex	guanfancine
Tenormin	atenolol
Thorazine	chlorpromazine
Tofranil	imipramine
Tranxene	clorazepate
Trexan	naltrexone

Brand Name	Generic Name
Triavil	amitriptyline + perphenazine
Trilafon	perphenazine
Urecholine	bethanechol
Valium	diazepam
Visken	pindolol
Vistaril	hydroxyzine
Vivactil	protriptyline
Wellbutrin	bupropion
Xanax	alprazolam
Yocon	yohimbine
Zoloft	sertraline
Zyprexa	olanzapine

Appendix D

Alphabetical Listing of Abbreviations

AC	before meals
ACE inhibitor	angiotensin converting enzyme inhibitor
ADD	attention deficit disorder
ADHD	attention deficit hyperactivity disorder
AM	in the morning
AV	atrioventricular
BID	twice a day
BUN	blood urea nitrogen
CAD	coronary artery disease
CBC	complete blood count
CFS	chronic fatigue syndrome
CHF	congestive heart failure
CMHC	community mental health center
CPK	creatine phosphokinase
DSM	*Diagnostic and Statistical Manual of Mental Disorders*
ECT	electroconvulsive therapy
EEG	electroencephalogram
EKG	electrocardiogram
EPS	extrapyramidal symptoms

FDA	Food and Drug Administration
GAD	generalized anxiety disorder
GAF	global assessment of functioning
GI	gastrointestinal
HS	at night; at bedtime
IM	intramuscular(ly)
IV	intravenous(ly)
MAO	monoamine oxidase
MAOI	monoamine oxidase inhibitor
mcg	microgram
mcl	microliter
mciu	microinternational unit
mEq/L	milliequivalent per liter
mg	milligram
ml	milliliter
ng	nanogram
NMS	neuroleptic malignant syndrome
NSAID	nonsteroidal anti-inflammatory drug
OCD	obsessive-compulsive disorder
OTC	over the counter
PC	after meals
po	by mouth
PRN	as needed
PTSD	post-traumatic stress disorder
QD	daily, every day
QOD	every other day
Qhs	every night
QID	four times a day

REM	rapid eye movement
SDA	serotonin-dopamine antagonist
SSRI	selective serotonin reuptake inhibitor (aka, serotonin-specific reuptake inhibitor)
TCA	tricyclic antidepressant
TD	tardive dyskinesia
TID	three times a day
TSH	thyroid stimulating hormone
UA	urinalysis
WBC	white blood cell count

Bibliography

American Medical Association. (1994). *Drug evaluations annual.* Washington, DC: Author.

American Psychiatric Association. (1994). *Diagnostic and statistical manual of mental disorders*, fourth edition. Washington, DC: Author.

American Society of Hospital Pharmacists. (1994). *Drug information 1994.* Bethesda, MD: Author.

Appleton, W. S. (1988). *Practical clinical psychopharmacology*, third edition. Baltimore, MD: Williams & Wilkins.

Ayd, F. J. (1994). Clozapine 1994: Clinical considerations. *International Drug Therapy Newsletter, 29* (May/June): 21-28.

Balon, R., Yeragani, V. K., Pohl, R., and Ramesh, C. (1993). Sexual dysfunction during antidepressant treatment. *Journal of Clinical Psychiatry, 54*: 209-212.

Beasley, C. M., Tollefson, G., Tran, P., Satterlee, W., Sanger, T., Hamilton, S., and the Olanzapine Study Group. (1996). Olanzapine versus placebo and haloperidol. *Neuropsychopharmacology, 14*(2): 83-85.

Blier, P., and Bergeron, R. (1995). Effectiveness of pindolol with selected antidepressant drugs in the treatment of major depression. *Journal of Clinical Psychopharmacology, 15* (June): 217-222.

Bodkin, J. A., Cohen, B. M., Salomon, M. S., Cannon, S. E., Zornberg, G. L., and Cole, J. O. (1996). Treatment of negative symptoms in schizophrenia and schizoaffective disorder by Selegiline augmentation of antipsychotic medication. *Journal of Nervous and Mental Disease, 184*: 295-301.

Borison, R. L. (1995). Clinical efficacy of serotonin-dopamine antagonists relative to classic neuroleptics. *Journal of Clinical Psychopharmacology, 15*(1) (suppl. 1): 24S-29S.

Breier, A., Buchanan, R. W., Kirkpatrick, B., Davis, O., Irish, D., Summerfelt, A., and Carpenter, W. (1994). Effects of clozapine on positive and negative symptoms in outpatients with schizophrenia. *American Journal of Psychiatry, 151*: 20-26.

Brenner, J. (1995). Double-blind comparison of org 3770, amitriptyline, and placebo in Major Depression. *Journal of Clinical Psychiatry, 56*: 519-525.

Ciraulo, D. A., and Shader, R. I. (1991). *Clinical manual of chemical dependence.* Washington, DC: American Psychiatric Press, Inc.

Coffey, C. E. (1993). *The clinical science of electroconvulsive therapy.* Washington, DC: American Psychiatric Press, Inc.

Compendium Publications Group. (1994) *Physicians' compendium of drug therapy.* Secaucus, NJ: Author.

DeVane, C. L. (1994). Pharmacogenetics and drug metabolism of newer antidepressant agents. *Journal of Clinical Psychiatry, 55*: 38-45.

Glaxo Wellcome USA, Inc. (1996). Lamictal package insert. Research Triangle Park, North Carolina.

Guttmacher, L. B. (1988). *Somatic therapies in psychiatry.* Washington, DC: American Psychiatric Press, Inc.

Hyman, S. E., Arana, G. W., and Rosenbaum, J. F. (1995). *Handbook of psychiatric drug therapy,* third edition. Boston, MA: Little, Brown.

Janicak, P. G., Davis, J. M., Preskorn, S. H., and Ayd, F. J. Jr. (1993). *Principles and practice of psychopharmacotherapy.* Baltimore, MD: Williams and Wilkins.

Joseph, S. (1997). *Personality disorders: New symptom-focused drug therapy.* Binghamton, NY: The Haworth Press.

Kane, J. M., Honigfeld, G., Singer, J., Meltzer, H. (1988). Clozapine for the treatment-resistant schizophrenic: A double-blind comparison with chlorpromazine. *Archives of General Psychiatry, 45*: 789-796.

Kaplan, H. I., and Sadeck, B. J. (Editors). (1989). *Comprehensive textbook of psychiatry/V,* fifth edition. Baltimore, MD: Williams & Wilkins.

Kehoe, W. A., and Schorr, R. B. (1996). Focus on mirtazapine: A new antidepressant with noradrenergic and specific serotonergic activity. *Formulary, 31*: 455-469.

Lieberman, J. A., Kane, J. M., and Johns, P. A. (1989). Clozapine: guidelines for clinical management. *Journal of Clinical Psychiatry, 50*: 329-338.

Marder, S. R., and Meibach, R. C. (1994). Risperidone in the treatment of schizophrenia. *American Journal of Psychiatry, 151*: 825-835.

Maxmen, J. S. (1991). *Psychotropic drugs–Fast facts.* New York: W. W. Norton & Company.

Mc Elroy, S. L., Dessain, E. R., Pope, H. G., Cole, J., Keck, P., Frankenberg, F., Aizley, H., and O'Brien, S. (1991). Clozapine in the treatment of psychotic mood disorder, schizoaffective disorder, and schizophrenia. *Journal of Clinical Psychiatry, 52*: 411-414.

Meltzer, H. Y. (editor). (1992). *Novel Antipsychotic Drugs*, New York, Raven Press.

Meltzer, H. Y. (1994). An overview of the mechanism of action of clozapine. *Journal of Clinical Psychiatry, 55* (suppl. B): 46-52.

Meltzer, H. Y., and Fibiger, H. C. (1996). Olanzapine: a new antipsychotic drug. *Neuropsychopharmacology, 14*(2): 83-85.

Nemeroff, C. B., DeVane, C. L., and Pollock, B. G. (1996). Newer antidepressants and the cytochrome P450 system. *American Journal of Psychiatry, 153*(3): 311-320.

Physicians' desk reference. (1995). Montvale, NJ: Medical Economics Company.

Preskorn, S. H. (1994). Antidepressant drug selection: criteria and options. *Journal of Clinical Psychiatry, 55* (suppl. A): 6-22.

Richelson, E. (1994). Preclinical pharmacology of antipsychotic drugs: relationship to efficacy and side effects. *Journal of Clinical Psychiatry, Monograph, 12*(2): 17-20.

Rosse, R. B., Giese, A. A., Deutsch, S. I., and Morihisa, J. M. (1989). *Laboratory diagnostic testing in psychiatry.* Washington, DC: American Psychiatric Press, Inc.

Roth, A. S., Ostroff, R. B., and Hoffman, R. E. (1996). Naltrexone as a treatment for repetitive self-injurious behavior: An open-label trial. *Journal of Clinical Psychiatry, 57*: 233-237.

Sandoz Pharmaceutical Corporation. (1993). *Clozaril–Management of adverse events.* East Hanover, NJ: Author.

Sandoz Pharmaceutical Corporation. (1994). *Standards of care in schizophrenia.* East Hanover, NJ: Author.

Sandoz Pharmaceutical Corporation. (1995). *Clozaril treatment trends.* East Hanover, NJ: Author.

Schatzberg, A. F., and Cole, J. O. (1991). *Manual of clinical psychopharmacology.* Washington, DC: American Psychiatric Press, Inc.

Schatzberg, A. F., and Nemeroff, C. B. (Editors). (1995). *Textbook of psychopharmacology.* Washington, D.C.: American Psychiatric Press, Inc.

Tollefson, G. D. (1994). Olanzapine: a novel antipsychotic with a broad spectrum profile. *Neuropsychopharmacology, 10* (suppl. 3): 805.

Van Kammen, D. P., Mc Evoy, J. P., Targum, S. D., Kardatzke, D., Sebree, T., and the Sertindole Study Group. (1996). A randomized, controlled, dose-ranging trial of sertindole in patients with schizophrenia. *Psychopharmacology, 124*: 168-175.

Index

Page numbers followed by the letter "t" indicate tables.